KU-484-220

OXFORD ASSESS AND PROGRESS

Series Editors

Katharine Boursicot
Director, Health Professional Assessment Consultancy (HPAC)
Honorary Reader in Medical Education St George's,
University of London

David Sales
Consultant in Medical Assessment

OXFORD ASSESS AND PROGRESS

Clinical Medicine

Third Edition

Edited by

Dan Furmedge MBBS MSc MRCP(UK) DRCOG
MAcadMEd FHEA AKC

Consultant Physician in Geriatric & General Internal Medicine
Honorary Clinical Lecturer in Medical Education
Guy's and St Thomas' NHS Foundation Trust
London, UK

Rudy Sinharay MBChB MRCP(UK) MD(Res)

Consultant Physician in Respiratory & General Internal Medicine
Guy's and St Thomas' NHS Foundation Trust
London, UK

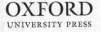

OXFORD
UNIVERSITY PRESS

OXFORD
UNIVERSITY PRESS

Great Clarendon Street, Oxford, OX2 6DP,
United Kingdom

Oxford University Press is a department of the University of Oxford.
It furthers the University's objective of excellence in research, scholarship,
and education by publishing worldwide. Oxford is a registered trade mark of
Oxford University Press in the UK and in certain other countries

© Oxford University Press 2019

The moral rights of the authors have been asserted

First Edition published in 2010
Second Edition published in 2014
Third Edition published in 2019
Impression: 2

Published in the United States of America by Oxford University Press
198 Madison Avenue, New York, NY 10016, United States of America

British Library Cataloguing in Publication Data
Data available

Library of Congress Control Number: 2018948241

ISBN 978-0-19-881296-8

Printed and bound in Great Britain by
Ashford Colour Press Ltd.

Series editor preface

The Oxford Assess and Progress series is a groundbreaking development in the extensive area of self-assessment texts available for medical students. The questions were specifically commissioned for the series, written by practising clinicians, extensively peer-reviewed by students and their teachers, and quality-assured to ensure that the material is up-to-date, accurate, and in line with modern testing formats.

The series has a number of unique features and is designed to be as much a formative learning resource as a self-assessment one. The questions are constructed to test the same clinical problem-solving skills that we use as practising clinicians, rather than only to test theoretical knowledge. These skills include:

- gathering and using data required for clinical judgement
- choosing the appropriate examination and investigations, and interpretation of the findings
- applying knowledge
- demonstrating diagnostic skills
- the ability to evaluate undifferentiated material
- the ability to prioritize
- making decisions and demonstrating a structured approach to decision-making.

Each question is bedded in reality and is typically presented as a clinical scenario, the content of which has been chosen to reflect the common and important conditions that most doctors are likely to encounter both during their training and in exams! The aim of the series is to build the reader's confidence in recognizing important symptoms and signs and suggesting the most appropriate investigations and management, and in so doing to aid the development of a clear approach to patient management which can be transferred to the wards.

The content of the series has deliberately been pinned to the relevant *Oxford Handbook* but, in addition, has been guided by a blueprint which reflects the themes identified in *Tomorrow's Doctors* and *Good Medical Practice* to include novel areas such as history taking, recognition of signs (including red flags), and professionalism.

Particular attention has been paid to giving learning points and constructive feedback on each question, using clear fact- or evidence-based explanations as to why the correct response is right and why the incorrect responses are less appropriate. The question editorials are clearly referenced to the relevant sections of the accompanying *Oxford Handbook* and/or more widely to medical literature or guidelines. They are designed to guide and motivate the reader, being multi-purpose in nature and covering, for example, exam technique, approaches to difficult subjects, and links between subjects.

Another unique aspect of the series is the element of competency progression, from being a relatively inexperienced student to being a more experienced junior doctor. We have suggested the following four degrees of difficulty to reflect the level of training, so that the reader can monitor their own progress over time:

- graduate should know ★
- graduate nice to know ★★
- foundation doctor should know ★★★
- foundation doctor nice to know ★★★★

We advise the reader to attempt the questions in blocks as a way of testing their knowledge in a clinical context. The series can be treated as a dress rehearsal for life on the ward by using the material to hone clinical acumen and build confidence by encouraging a clear, consistent, and rational approach, proficiency in recognizing and evaluating symptoms and signs, making a rational differential diagnosis, and suggesting appropriate investigations and management.

Adopting such an approach can aid not only success in examinations, which really are designed to confirm learning, but also—more importantly—being a good doctor. In this way, we can deliver high-quality and safe patient care by recognizing, understanding, and treating common problems, but at the same time remaining alert to the possibility of less likely, but potentially catastrophic, conditions.

David Sales and Katharine Boursicot
Series Editors

A note on single best answer questions

Single best answer questions are currently the format of choice being widely used by most undergraduate and postgraduate knowledge tests, and therefore all of the assessment questions in this book follow this format.

Single best answer questions have many advantages over other machine-markable formats, such as extended matching questions (EMQs), notably the breadth of sampling or content coverage that they afford.

Briefly, the single best answer or 'best of five' question presents a problem, usually a clinical scenario, before presenting the question itself and a list of five options. These consist of one correct answer and four incorrect options or 'distractors' from which the reader has to choose a response.

All of the questions in this book, which are typically based on an evaluation of symptoms, signs, or results of investigations, either as single entities or in combination, are designed to test *reasoning* skills, rather than straightforward recall of facts, and utilize cognitive processes similar to those used in clinical practice.

The peer-reviewed questions are written and edited in accordance with contemporary best assessment practice, and their content has been guided by a blueprint pinned to all areas of *Good Medical Practice*, which ensures comprehensive coverage.

The answers and their rationales are evidence-based and have been reviewed to ensure that they are absolutely correct. Incorrect options are selected as being plausible, and indeed they may appear correct to the less knowledgeable reader. When answering questions, the reader may wish to use the 'cover' test, in which they read the scenario and the question but cover the options.

Katharine Boursicot and David Sales
Series Editors

A note on single best
answer questions

Single-best answer questions

Katharine Boursicot and David Sales
Series Editors

Contents

Contents

Contributors

Thomas Coryndon, Consultant in Emergency Medicine, University College London Hospitals NHS Foundation Trust, London, UK

Doug Fink, Specialty Training Registrar in Infectious Diseases and General Internal Medicine, Hospital for Tropical Diseases, University College London Hospitals NHS Foundation Trust, London, UK

Dan Furmedge, Consultant Physician in Geriatric and General Internal Medicine and Honorary Clinical Lecturer in Medical Education, Guy's and St Thomas' NHS Foundation Trust, London, UK

Shelly Griffiths, Specialty Training Registrar in Colorectal and General Surgery, Gloucestershire Hospitals NHS Foundation Trust, London, UK

James Harnett, Senior Clinical Fellow in Emergency Medicine, University College London Hospitals NHS Foundation Trust, London, UK

Chris Parnell, Clinical Fellow in Emergency Medicine, University College London Hospitals NHS Foundation Trust, London, UK

Ross Paterson, Academic Clinical Lecturer in Neurology, National Hospital for Neurology and Neurosurgery, University College London Hospitals NHS Foundation Trust, London, UK

Maria Phylactou, Academic Clinical Fellow in Endocrinology and Diabetes, North West Thames, Imperial College London, London, UK

Ricky Sinharay, Specialty Training Registrar in Gastroenterology and Hepatology, Addenbrooke's Hospital, Cambridge University Hospitals NHS Foundation Trust, Cambridge, UK

Rudy Sinharay, Consultant Physician in Respiratory and General Internal Medicine, Guy's and St Thomas' NHS Foundation Trust, London, UK

Laszlo Sztriha, Consultant Neurologist and Stroke Physician, King's College Hospital NHS Foundation Trust, London, UK

Dominik Vogel, Senior Clinical Fellow in Critical Care, Echocardiography and ECMO, Guy's and St Thomas' NHS Foundation Trust, London, UK

William White, Specialty Training Registrar in Nephrology and General Internal Medicine, Royal Free London NHS Foundation Trust, London, UK

Normal and average values

	Normal value
Haematology	
White cell count (WCC)	$4–11 \times 10^9$/L
Haemoglobin (Hb)	M: 135–180 g/L F: 115–160 g/L
Packed cell volume (PCV)	M: 0.4–0.54 L/L F: 0.37–0.47 L/L
Mean corpuscular volume (MCV)	76–96 fL
Neutrophils	$2–7.5 \times 10^9$/L
Lymphocytes	$1.3–3.5 \times 10^9$/L
Eosinophils	$0.04–0.44 \times 10^9$/L
Basophils	$0–0.1 \times 10^9$/L
Monocytes	$0.2–0.8 \times 10^9$/L
Platelets	$150–400 \times 10^9$/L
Reticulocytes	$25–100 \times 10^9$/L
Erythrocyte sedimentation rate (ESR)	<20 mm/hour (but age-dependent; see OHCM, p. 356)
Prothrombin time (PT)	10–14 s
Activated partial thromboplastin time (aPTT)	35–45 s
International normalized ratio (INR)	0.9–1.2
Biochemistry	
Alanine aminotransferase (ALT)	5–35 IU/L
Albumin	35–50 g/L
Alkaline phosphatase (ALP)	30–150 IU/L
Amylase	0–180 U/dL
Aspartate aminotransferase (AST)	5–35 IU/L
Bilirubin	3–17 micromol/L
Calcium (total)	2.12–2.65 mmol/L
Chloride	95–105 mmol/L
Cortisol	450–750 nmol/L (a.m.) 80–280 nmol/L (midnight)
C-reactive protein (CRP)	<10 mg/L
Creatine kinase	M: 25–195 IU/L F: 25–170 IU/L

	Normal value
Creatinine	70–<150 micromol/L
Ferritin	12–200 micrograms/L
Folate	2.1 micrograms/L
Gamma-glutamyl transpeptidase (GGT)	M: 11–51 IU/L F: 7–33 IU/L
Lactate dehydrogenase (LDH)	70–250 IU/L
Magnesium	0.75–1.05 mmol/L
Osmolality	278–305 mOsmol/kg
Phosphate	0.8–1.4 mmol/L
Potassium	3.5–5 mmol/L
Protein (total)	60–80 g/L
Sodium	135–145 mmol/L
Thyroid-stimulating hormone (TSH)	0.5–5.7 mU/L
Thyroxine (T4)	70–140 nmol/L
Thyroxine (free)	9–22 pmol/L
Urate	M: 210–480 mmol/L F: 150–39 mmol/L
Urea	2.5–6.7 mmol/L
Vitamin B12	0.13–0.68 mmol/L
Arterial blood gases	
pH	7.35–7.45
Arterial oxygen partial pressure (PaO_2)	>10.6 kPa
Arterial carbon dioxide partial pressure ($PaCO_2$)	4.7–6.0 kPa
Base excess	± 2 mmol/L
Urine	
Cortisol (free)	<280 nmol/24 hours
Osmolality	350–1000 mOsmol/kg
Potassium	14–120 mmol/24 hours
Protein	<150 mg/24 hours
Sodium	100–250 mmol/24 hours

Abbreviations

A&E	Accident and Emergency
AAA	abdominal aortic aneurysm
ABCDE	airway, breathing, circulation, disability, exposure
ABG	arterial blood gas
ABPA	allergic bronchopulmonary aspergillosis
ABPI	ankle–brachial pressure index
ACE	angiotensin-converting enzyme
ACS	acute coronary syndrome
ACTH	adrenocorticotrophic hormone
ADH	antidiuretic hormone
ADP	adenosine diphosphate
ADPKD	autosomal dominant polycystic kidney disease
AF	atrial fibrillation
AFB	acid-fast bacilli
AIDS	acquired immune deficiency syndrome
AIHA	autoimmune haemolytic anaemia
AKI	acute kidney injury
ALL	acute lymphoblastic leukaemia
ALP	alkaline phosphatase
ALS	advanced life support
ALT	alanine aminotransferase
AML	acute myeloid leukaemia
AMR	anti-microbial resistance
AMTS	abbreviated mental test score
ANCA	antineutrophil cytoplasmic antibodies
aPTT	activated partial thromboplastin time
ARB	angiotensin receptor blocker
ARLD	alcohol-related liver disease
ART	anti-retroviral therapy
ASA	American Society of Anesthesiologists
AST	aspartate aminotransferase
ATP	adenosine triphosphate
AV	atrioventricular
AVNRT	atrioventricular nodal re-entry tachycardia

AVRT	atrioventricular re-entrant tachycardia
β-hCG	beta-human chorionic gonadotropin
BASHH	British Association for Sexual Health and HIV
bd	twice daily
BHIVA	British HIV Association
BHL	bilateral hilar lymphadenopathy
BiPAP	bi-level positive airway pressure
BMI	body mass index
BNP	B-type natriuretic peptide
BP	blood pressure
bpm	beat per minute
BPPV	benign paroxysmal positional vertigo
BTS	British Thoracic Society
CA125	cancer antigen 125
CAD	coronary artery disease
CADASIL	cerebral autosomal dominant arteriopathy with subcortical infarcts and leukoencephalopathy
CCP	cyclic citrullinated peptide
CCU	coronary care unit
CD4	cluster of differentiation 4
CDAD	*Clostridium difficile*-associated disease
CEA	carcinoembryonic antigen
CIN	contrast-induced nephropathy
CK	creatine kinase
CKD	chronic kidney disease
CLL	chronic lymphocytic leukaemia
CLO	*Campylobacter*-like organism
cm	centimetre
cmH_2O	centimetre of water
CML	chronic myeloid leukaemia
CMV	cytomegalovirus
CN	cranial nerve
CNS	central nervous system
COHb	carboxyhaemoglobin
COPD	chronic obstructive pulmonary disease
CPAP	continuous positive airway pressure
CPR	cardiopulmonary resuscitation
Cr	creatinine

CREST	calcinosis, Raynaud's syndrome, (o)esophageal dysmotility, sclerodactyly, telangiectasia
CRP	C-reactive protein
CRT	capillary refill time; cardiac resynchronization therapy
CSM	Committee on Safety of Medicines
CT	computed tomography
CTPA	computed tomography pulmonary angiogram
CVC	central venous catheter
CVP	central venous pressure
CXR	chest X-ray
DAPT	dual antiplatelet therapy
DC	direct current
DDP4	dipeptidyl peptidase 4
DEXA	dual-energy X-ray absorptiometry
DKA	diabetic ketoacidosis
dL	decilitre
DMARD	disease-modifying anti-rheumatic drug
DNA	deoxyribonucleic acid
DNACPR	Do Not Attempt Cardiopulmonary Resuscitation
DNAR	Do Not Attempt Resuscitation
DOAC	direct-acting oral anticoagulant
DOLS	Deprivation of Liberty Safeguard
DRE	digital rectal examination
dsDNA	double-stranded deoxyribonucleic acid
DVLA	Driver and Vehicle Licensing Agency
DVT	deep vein thrombosis
EBV	Epstein–Barr virus
EC	enteric-coated
ECG	electrocardiogram
ED	emergency department
EEG	electroencephalogram
eGFR	estimated glomerular filtration rate
EGPA	eosinophilic granulomatosis with polyangiitis
EPP	exposure-prone procedure
ERCP	endoscopic retrograde cholangiopancreatography
ESC	European Society of Cardiology
ESR	erythrocyte sedimentation rate
EVAR	endovascular aneurysm repair
FBC	full blood count

FFP	fresh frozen plasma
fL	femtolitre
FSGS	focal segmental glomerulosclerosis
ft	foot/feet
fT4	free thyroxine
FTD	frontotemporal dementia
g	gram
G	gauge
GALS	gait, arms, legs, and spine
GBM	glomerular basement membrane
GBS	Guillain–Barré syndrome
GCA	giant cell arteritis
GCS	Glasgow Coma Scale
GFR	glomerular filtration rate
GGT	gamma-glutamyl transpeptidase
GI	gastrointestinal
GMC	General Medical Council
GORD	gastro-oesophageal reflux disease
GP	general practitioner
GTN	glyceryl trinitrate
5-HIAA	5-hydroxyindoleacetic acid
HAART	highly active anti-retroviral treatment
HAV	hepatitis A virus
Hb	haemoglobin
HbA1c	glycosylated haemoglobin
HBc	hepatitis B core
HBs	hepatitis B surface
HBsAb	hepatitis B surface antibody
HBsAg	hepatitis B surface antigen
HBV	hepatitis B virus
hCG	human chorionic gonadotrophin
HCO_3	bicarbonate
HCV	hepatitis C virus
HCW	healthcare worker
HDV	hepatitis delta virus
HE	hepatic encephalopathy
HELLP	haemolysis, elevated liver enzymes, and low platelet count
HHS	hyperosmolar hyperglycaemic non-ketotic state
HHV-8	human herpesvirus 8

HiB	*Haemophilus influenzae* type B
HIDA	hepatobiliary iminodiacetic acid
HIT	heparin-induced thrombocytopenia
HIV	human immunodeficiency virus
HIVAN	human immunodeficiency virus-associated nephropathy
HNIG	human normal immunoglobulin
HOCM	hypertrophic obstructive cardiomyopathy
HR	heart rate
HS	heart sound
HSP	Henoch–Schönlein purpura
HSV	herpes simplex virus
HTLV	human T-lymphotropic virus
HUS	haemolytic uraemic syndrome
Hz	hertz
IBD	inflammatory bowel disease
IBS	irritable bowel syndrome
ICP	intracranial pressure
ICS	inhaled corticosteroid
IgA	immunoglobulin A
IgE	immunoglobulin E
IGF-1	insulin-like growth factor 1
IgG	immunoglobulin G
IgM	immunoglobulin M
IGRA	interferon gamma release assay
IIH	idiopathic intracranial hypertension
IM	intramuscular
IMCA	Independent Mental Capacity Advocate
in	inch
INH	inhaler
INR	international normalized ratio
ITP	idiopathic thrombocytopenic purpura
ITU	intensive therapy unit
IU	international unit
IV	intravenous
IVIG	intravenous immunoglobulin
IVU	intravenous urogram
JME	juvenile myoclonic epilepsy
JVP	jugular venous pressure
kg	kilogram

kPa	kilopascal
KS	Kaposi's sarcoma
KUB	kidneys, ureters, and bladder
L	litre
LABA	long-acting beta-agonist
LAD	left anterior descending artery
LCA	left main coronary artery
LCx	left circumflex coronary artery
LDH	lactate dehydrogenase
LFT	liver function test
LGI-1	leucine-rich glioma-inactivated 1
LGV	lymphogranuloma venereum
LMN	lower motor neurone
LMWH	low-molecular-weight heparin
LV	left ventricle/left ventricular
m	metre
MAC	*Mycobacterium avium* complex
MAHA	microangiopathic haemolytic anaemia
MC&S	microscopy, culture, and sensitivity
MCV	mean corpuscular volume
MDMA	3,4-methylenedioxy-methamphetamine
mg	milligram
MGUS	monoclonal gammopathy of uncertain significance
MHC	major histocompatibility complex
MI	myocardial infarction
min	minute
mIU	milli international unit
mL	millilitre
mmHg	millimetre of mercury
mmol	millimole
MMSE	mini-mental state examination
MoCA	Montreal Cognitive Assessment
mol	mole
mOsm	milliosmole
mph	mile per hour
MR	modified release
MRCP	magnetic resonance cholangiopancreatography
MRI	magnetic resonance imaging
ms	millisecond

MS	multiple sclerosis
MSM	men who have sex with men
MTX	methotrexate
mU	milliunit
mV	millivolt
NAC	N-acetylcysteine
NaHCO₃	sodium bicarbonate
NASH	non-alcoholic steatohepatitis
NCEPOD	National Confidential Enquiry into Patient Outcome and Death
NEB	nebulized
NEWS	National Early Warning Score
ng	nanogram
NG	nasogastric
NHS	National Health Service
NHSBT	NHS Blood and Transplant
NICE	National Institute for Health and Care Excellence
NIV	non-invasive ventilation
NMDA	N-methyl-D-aspartate
nmol	nanomole
NOAC	novel oral anticoagulant
NPSA	National Patient Safety Agency
NSAID	non-steroidal anti-inflammatory drug
NSTEMI	non-ST-elevation myocardial infarction
O₂	oxygen
od	once daily
OGD	oesophagogastroduodenoscopy
OGTT	oral glucose tolerance test
OHCM	*Oxford Handbook of Clinical Medicine*
OSA	obstructive sleep apnoea
OSCE	Objective Structured Clinical Examination
PaCO₂	partial pressure of carbon dioxide in arterial blood
p-ANCA	perinuclear antineutrophil cytoplasmic antibodies
PaO₂	partial pressure of oxygen in arterial blood
PCR	protein:creatinine ratio; polymerase chain reaction
PCV	packed cell volume
PDA	posterior descending artery
PE	pulmonary embolus
PEFR	peak expiratory flow rate

PEG	percutaneous endoscopic gastrostomy
PET	positron emission tomography
PHE	Public Health England
PID	pelvic inflammatory disease
pmol	picomole
PMR	polymyalgia rheumatica
PNH	paroxysmal nocturnal haemoglobinuria
PO	*per os* (by mouth)
PPI	proton pump inhibitor
PR	per rectum
PRN	*pro re nata* (when required)
PSA	prostate-specific antigen
PT	prothrombin time
PTH	parathyroid hormone
qds	four times daily
RA	rheumatoid arthritis
RCA	right coronary artery
RCP	Royal College of Physicians
RCT	randomized controlled trial
RDW	red cell distribution width
RhF	rheumatoid factor
RMSF	Rocky Mountain spotted fever
RNA	ribonucleic acid
RNP	ribonucleoprotein
RR	respiratory rate
RUQ	right upper quadrant
s	second
SA	sinoatrial
SAH	subarachnoid haemorrhage
SaO_2	arterial oxygen saturation
SC	subcutaneous
SCD	sickle-cell disease
SGLT2	sodium–glucose co-transporter 2
SIADH	syndrome of inappropriate antidiuretic hormone secretion
SIRS	systemic inflammatory response syndrome
SL	sublingual
SLE	systemic lupus erythematosus
SMV	superior mesenteric vein
SPC	Summary of Product Characteristics

SpO_2	oxygen saturation in blood
SpR	specialty registrar
STAT	immediately
STEMI	ST-elevation myocardial infarction
SVT	supraventricular tachycardia
T	temperature
T3	tri-iodothyronine
T4	thyroxine
TB	tuberculosis
Tc	technetium
TDD	total daily dose
tds	three times daily
TIA	transient ischaemic attack
TIBC	total iron-binding capacity
TRALI	transfusion-related acute lung injury
TSH	thyroid-stimulating hormone
TTE	transthoracic echocardiogram
TTP	thrombotic thrombocytopenic purpura
U	unit
U&E	urea and electrolytes
UKELD	United Kingdom Model for End-Stage Liver Disease
Ur	urea
US	ultrasound
USS	ultrasound scan
UTI	urinary tract infection
V/Q	ventilation/perfusion
VF	ventricular fibrillation
VKA	vitamin K antagonist
VT	ventricular tachycardia
VTE	venous thromboembolic disease
WCC	white cell count
WHO	World Health Organization
WPW	Wolff–Parkinson–White (syndrome)

How to use this book

Oxford Assess and Progress: Clinical Medicine has been carefully designed to ensure you get the most out of your revision and are prepared for your exams. Here is a brief guide to some of the features and learning tools.

Organization of content

Chapter editorials will help you unpick tricky subjects, and when it is late at night and you need something to remind you why you are doing this, you will find words of encouragement!

Answers can be found at the end of each chapter, in order.

How to read an answer

Unlike other revision guides on the market, this one is crammed full of feedback, so you should understand exactly why each answer is correct, and gain an insight into the common pitfalls. With every answer, there is an explanation of why that particular choice is the most appropriate. For some questions, there is additional explanation of why the distracters are less suitable. Where relevant, you will also be directed to sources of further information such as the *Oxford Handbook of Clinical Medicine*, websites, and journal articles.

→ www.nice.org.uk/guidance/cg43

Progression points

The questions in every chapter are ordered by level of difficulty and competence, indicated by the following symbols:

★   Graduate '*should know*'—you should be aiming to get most of these correct.
★★   Graduate '*nice to know*'—these are a bit tougher, but not above your capabilities.
★★★   Foundation Doctor '*should know*'—these will really test your understanding.
★★★★ Foundation Doctor '*nice to know*'—give these a go when you are ready to challenge yourself.

Oxford Handbook of Clinical Medicine

The OHCM page references are given with the answers to some questions (e.g. OHCM 10th edn → p. 402). Please note that this reference is to the **10th edition of the OHCM**, and that other editions are unlikely to have the same material in exactly the same place.

Chapter 1

Cardiovascular medicine

Dominik Vogel

The field of cardiovascular medicine is an inexhaustible source for clinical trials (→ OHCM 10th edition: p 93). The most feasible way of keeping up to date is referring to guidelines. In addition to those made available by the National Institute for Health and Care Excellence (NICE), the European Society of Cardiology (ESC) provides very useful Clinical Practice Guidelines that are accessible via: https://www.escardio.org/Guidelines/Clinical-Practice-Guidelines.

If you don't manage to read the full text of each of the provided guidelines, you might find the 'summary cards' useful that you can download for free using the same link.

QUESTIONS

1. A 62-year-old woman has had palpitations for 6 hours. Her electro-cardiogram (ECG) shows a narrow complex tachycardia at a rate of 160 bpm. The Valsalva manoeuvre is performed and she reverts to sinus rhythm. Which is the *single* most likely cause of her tachycardia? ★

A Atrial fibrillation

B Atrial flutter

C Atrial tachycardia

D Atrioventricular nodal re-entrant tachycardia

E Sinus tachycardia

2. A 30-year-old man is woken from sleep by central chest pain and breathlessness. The pain radiates through to his back, making him sit up in bed. He is otherwise fit and well, aside from having had a sore throat 2 weeks previously.

T 37.8°C, HR 110 bpm, BP 125/90 mmHg.

His chest X-ray is reported as 'normal', and an electrocardiogram (ECG) is performed (Figure 1.1).

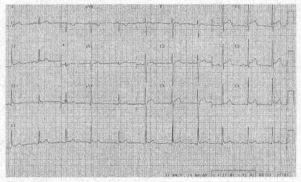

Figure 1.1

Which is the *single* most likely diagnosis? ★

A Acute pericarditis

B Hypertrophic obstructive cardiomyopathy (HOCM)

C Infective endocarditis

D Myocardial infarction (MI)

E Pulmonary embolus (PE)

3. A 71-year-old man has had central chest pain radiating to his left arm for 1 hour. His observations are:

T 37.1°C, HR 44 bpm, BP 110/65 mmHg, RR 22/minute.

Which is the *single* most likely occluded coronary artery? ★

A Left anterior descending artery (LAD)

B Left circumflex coronary artery (LCx)

C Left main coronary artery (LCA)

D Posterior descending artery (PDA)

E Right coronary artery (RCA)

4. A 65-year-old man has had central chest pain radiating to his left arm for 2 hours. He has had increasingly regular chest pain over the last 2 weeks. He has type 2 diabetes and takes metformin. An electrocardiogram (ECG) is performed (Figure 1.2).

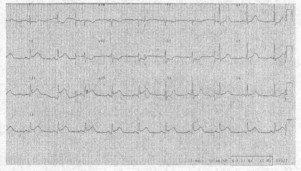

Figure 1.2

Which is the *single* most likely occluded coronary artery? ★

A Left anterior descending artery (LAD)

B Left circumflex coronary artery (LCx)

C Left main coronary artery (LCA)

D Posterior descending artery (PDA)

E Right coronary artery (RCA)

5. A 78-year-old man is recovering after an ST-elevation myocardial infarction (STEMI). In the past hour, his pulse rate has increased from 100 to 130 bpm, and his respiratory rate from 20 to 30/minute. The junior doctor is called. The patient has a productive cough and is sitting forward with his hands on his knees. Which *single* treatment is most likely to improve his condition? ★

A Bendroflumethiazide 2.5 mg oral (PO)

B Bumetanide 1 mg PO

C Furosemide 80 mg intravenous (IV)

D Heparin 5000 U IV

E Metoprolol 5 mg IV

6. A 72-year-old man has felt dizzy and short of breath for the past couple of hours. He is very conscious of his heart beating and is extremely anxious. He has hypertension and was discharged from hospital 3 months previously after a non-ST-elevation myocardial infarction (NSTEMI).

T 36.6°C, HR 200 bpm, BP 115/80 mmHg.

Chest: clear.

An electrocardiogram (ECG) is performed (Figure 1.3).

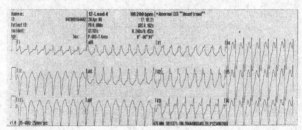

Figure 1.3

Which would be the *single* most appropriate immediate management? ★

A Adenosine

B Amiodarone

C Digoxin

D Lidocaine

E Synchronized cardioversion

7. A 44-year-old man has had sudden-onset chest pain radiating to his jaw, with sweating and nausea. An electrocardiogram (ECG) is performed and shows ST-elevation in V1–V6, I, and aVL leads. Which is the *single* most likely occluded coronary artery? ★

A Left anterior descending artery (LAD)

B Left circumflex coronary artery (LCx)

C Left main coronary artery (LCA)

D Posterior descending artery (PDA)

E Right coronary artery (RCA)

8. A 66-year-old woman has been feverish for the past 2 weeks, particularly at night. She was brought into the Emergency Department by her husband who found her shivering. She has type 2 diabetes mellitus and had a prosthetic mitral valve fitted 9 months previously.

T 38.4°C, HR 110 bpm, BP 95/50 mmHg.

Urine dipstick: blood 2+.

Which *single* additional fact from the woman's recent history would most support the likely diagnosis? ★

A She did a 10-km charity run

B She has had the 'flu' vaccine

C She recently started taking insulin

D She spent 2 weeks in southern Europe

E She underwent dental surgery

9. A 26-year-old woman has a routine medical assessment prior to travelling abroad for voluntary medical service.

T 36.6°C, HR 90 bpm, BP 115/80 mmHg.

Her heart sounds are normal, with no murmurs. An electrocardiogram (ECG) is performed (Figure 1.4).

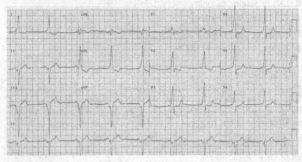

Figure 1.4
Reproduced with permission from Myerson S.G, Choudhury R.P, Mitchell A.R.J., *Emergencies in Cardiology*. Copyright (2006) with permission from Oxford University Press.

Which is the *single* most likely diagnosis? ★

A First-degree heart block

B Left bundle branch block

C Normal

D Sinus arrhythmia

E Wolff–Parkinson–White syndrome

10. A 45-year-old man suffers sudden central chest pain while at rest. It spreads across his chest and up to his neck. After 20 minutes, the pain has not eased and he feels sweaty and short of breath. This is the third such episode in the last 3 months. An electrocardiogram (ECG) is performed (Figure 1.5).

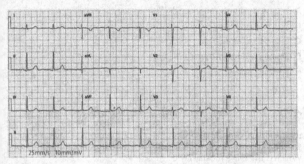

Figure 1.5

Reproduced with permission from Warrell D.A, Cox T.M., Firth J.D, *Oxford Textbook of Medicine*, fifth edition, figure 16.3.1.5. Copyright (2010) with permission from Oxford University Press.

12-hour troponin I <0.05 ng/mL.

Which would be the *single* most accurate classification of this event? ★

A Acute coronary syndrome

B Non-ST-elevation myocardial infarction

C ST-elevation myocardial infarction

D Stable angina

E Unstable angina

11. The on-call junior doctor receives a call from a nurse about a 55-year-old man who is experiencing palpitations on one of the medical wards. These started 5 minutes ago, and the nurse has taken an electrocardiogram (ECG) and asked for the patient to be reviewed. His heart rate is 140 bpm. It is a busy night shift, and there are five patients waiting to be seen in Accident and Emergency (A&E). Which *single* additional detail from the nurse should prompt an immediate review of the patient (i.e. within the next 5 minutes)? ★

A He is currently being loaded with digoxin

B Arterial oxygen saturation (SaO$_2$) 98% on 10 L oxygen (O$_2$)

C Systolic blood pressure 90 mmHg

D Temperature 38.1°C

E The patient is extremely anxious

12. A 59-year-old man has had several episodes of paroxysmal atrial fibrillation. His doctor is considering whether to start him on anticoagulation therapy. He calculates his stroke risk, using the CHA2DS2–VASc calculator, and finds that he scores 0. Which one further test would be most useful in planning his therapy? ★

A B-type natriuretic peptide (BNP)

B Echocardiogram

C Exercise tolerance test

D Seven-day Holter monitor

E 24-hour tape

13. A 73-year-old woman has been short of breath for the past 3 weeks. She now needs to sleep with four pillows, rather than two, and has swollen ankles by the end of the day. She uses a regular steroid inhaler for asthma but has never been in hospital for any reason. Which is the *single* most likely diagnosis? ★

A Acute exacerbation of asthma

B Angina

C Heart failure

D Pneumonia

E Pulmonary embolus

14. A 77-year-old woman has been referred to the Cardiology Department with paroxysmal atrial fibrillation. At her echocardiogram, she is found to have a left ventricular ejection fraction of 35%. She is advised to start anti-thrombotic therapy. Dabigatran is recommended. Which is the *single* most accurate description of its mechanism of action? ★

A Direct inhibitor of thrombin

B Indirect inhibitor of factor Xa

C Inhibitor of adenosine diphosphate (ADP) on platelet cell membranes

D Inhibitor of cyclo-oxygenase enzyme

E Inhibitor of the formation of vitamin K-dependent coagulation factors

15. A 72-year-old woman has noticed that her abdomen has swollen over the past 6 months. It has become uncomfortable and she has felt increasingly short of breath. She has been on home nebulizers for chronic obstructive pulmonary disease (COPD) for many years.

T 37.2°C, HR 90 bpm, BP 135/90 mmHg, RR 20/minute.

Her jugular venous pressure (JVP) is visible at 5 cm above the sternal angle, and she has bilateral ankle oedema pitting to the knee. Her abdomen is distended, but non-tender, with no organomegaly. Shifting dullness is demonstrated. Which is the *single* most likely cause of this woman's abdominal distension? ★

A Budd–Chiari syndrome

B Chronic persistent hepatitis

C Constrictive pericarditis

D Cor pulmonale

E Portal hypertension

16. A 20-year-old woman has had palpitations for 6 hours. She has had similar episodes before, but they have never lasted this long. An electrocardiogram (ECG) shows a regular rhythm of 160 bpm, with inverted P waves in leads II, III, and aVF, and narrow QRS complexes. Although vagal manoeuvres do not work, after adenosine 6 mg intravenous (IV), normal sinus rhythm at 90 bpm is restored.

Which is the *single* most likely origin of her tachycardia? ★ ★

A Atrium

B Atrioventricular (AV) node

C Bundle of His

D Sinoatrial (SA) node

E Ventricle

17. A 52-year-old man presents to the emergency department with epigastric pain and anorexia. He complains of nausea without vomiting and has not taken his regular medication for 3 days. His stool frequency and appearance are normal. On examination, you note a thoracotomy scar, which, according to the patient, is from a surgery he had 3 years ago. Auscultation reveals a clicking 1st heart sound. His abdomen is soft, with a tender epigastrium. Which *single* lab value is vital for the patient's management? ★ ★

A Bilirubin

B Haptoglobin

C International normalized ratio (INR)

D Lactate dehydrogenase (LDH)

E Reticulocytes

18. A 52-year-old man suffered sudden central chest pain whilst watching television. He described it as a 'suffocating' sensation that rose up to his neck and made it difficult to breathe. He arrived at the emergency department at 10 p.m. within 2 hours of the onset of pain. An electrocardiogram (ECG) was performed, showing normal sinus rhythm (85 bpm), with non-specific ST-segment changes, and troponin I was 0.09 ng/mL. The patient was admitted to the coronary care unit (CCU) where you see him 2 hours later.

Now, he looks pale, clammy, and anxious. The nurse at his bedside has just performed an ECG (Figure 1.6).

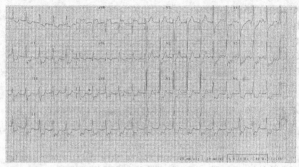

Figure 1.6

Which is the *single* most appropriate immediate course of action? ★★

A Measure blood pressure

B Measure creatinine kinase level

C Obtain an echocardiogram

D Proceed to coronary angiography

E Repeat troponin level

19. A 70-year-old man has had palpitations and been short of breath for the last 24 hours. He has hypertension and was recently discharged from hospital after a myocardial infarction. An electrocardiogram (ECG) is performed (Figure 1.7). The on-call registrar suggests giving the man adenosine 6 mg intravenous (IV).

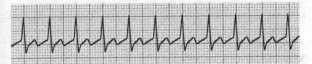

Figure 1.7

Which *single* description most accurately explains why adenosine works? ★★

A It blocks the atrioventricular (AV) node and thus may unmask flutter waves

B It increases vagal tone, thus slowing the atrial rate

C It reduces the force of contractions and thus corrects the arrhythmia

D It resets the sinoatrial (SA) node, thus correcting ventricular tachycardia (VT)

E It transiently stops the atria from fibrillating

20. A 42-year-old woman with highly symptomatic paroxysmal atrial fibrillation underwent pulmonary vein isolation. After recovering from her sedation, she was transferred to the coronary care unit. At 8 p.m., the nurse fast-bleeps you because the patient has become unwell.

Sinus tachycardia 160 bpm

Systolic blood pressure 85 mmHg

Which is the *single* next most important step in immediate management? ★★

A 12-lead electrocardiogram (ECG)

B Arterial line insertion for invasive blood pressure measurement

C Bedside transthoracic echocardiogram

D Central line insertion for central venous pressure (CVP) monitoring

E Supine chest X-ray

21. A 76-year-old woman has been short of breath on minimal exertion for 5 days. On walking upstairs, she has had several twinges of central chest tightness. She had been pain-free since being diagnosed with coronary artery disease 10 years previously.

Troponin (36 hours after onset of pain): 1.45 ng/mL

An electrocardiogram (ECG) shows T wave inversion in the inferolateral leads. Which is the *single* most appropriate immediate step in management? ★★

A Aspirin 75 mg oral (PO) + clopidogrel 75 mg PO

B Aspirin 300 mg PO + clopidogrel 300 mg PO

C Aspirin 300 mg PO + pantoprazole 40 mg PO

D Aspirin 300 mg PO + ticagrelor 180 mg PO

E Aspirin 75 mg PO + ticagrelor 90 mg PO

22. A 77-year-old man has had increasing breathlessness and leg oedema over the past few weeks. A recent transthoracic echocardiogram had shown a left ventricular ejection fraction of 35–40%. He takes lisinopril 20 mg oral (PO) once daily and bisoprolol 7.5 mg PO once daily. Choose the *single* medication that would be most appropriate to start from the following list of options. ★★

A Amlodipine 5 mg PO once daily

B Digoxin 62.5 micrograms PO once daily

C Furosemide 40 mg PO once daily

D Ivabradine 5 mg PO twice daily

E Losartan 50 mg PO once daily

23. A 68-year-old woman has been started on both ramipril and bisoprolol for chronic heart failure with reduced ejection fraction [New York Heart Association (NYHA) class II]. However, she develops an irritating tickly cough and wishes to change her prescription. Choose the *single* medication that would be most appropriate to start from the following list of options. ★★

A Amlodipine 5 mg oral (PO) once daily

B Digoxin 62.5 micrograms PO once daily

C Enalapril 5 mg PO once daily

D Losartan 50 mg PO once daily

E Spironolactone 25 mg PO once daily

24. A 54-year-old man is referred for an echocardiogram to assess a systolic murmur. On the parasternal long-axis view of a transthoracic echocardiogram, which part of the heart is the closest to the ultrasound-probe? ★ ★ ★

A Aortic valve

B Descending aorta

C Left atrium

D Left ventricle

E Right ventricle

25. A 52-year-old man has had pain in his upper chest for the last hour. It came on after he had climbed the stairs to his office. He felt breathless, as well as hot and uncomfortable. His symptoms subsided within a few minutes of sitting down. He recalls a similar episode a month ago after running for a bus. He is a non-smoker and takes no regular prescription medications.

12-hour troponin I <0.05 ng/mL.

An electrocardiogram (ECG) is performed (Figure 1.8).

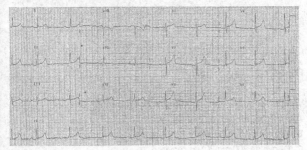

Figure 1.8

Which is the *single* most appropriate initial investigation of this man's symptoms? ★ ★ ★

A Computed tomography (CT) coronary angiography

B Echocardiogram at rest

C Exercise ECG

D Invasive coronary angiography

E Stress echocardiogram

26. A 55-year-old woman has noticed her heart beating fast. It happened three times within the last year and was not associated with any other symptoms. She is anxious about the cause of these attacks, as she has no other medical problems. The episodes lasted a couple of hours each time but were gone before she managed to see her general practitioner (GP). She had a 24-hour tape recently which did not show any arrhythmias, though she was asymptomatic throughout.

She is seen in the emergency department where she presents with palpitations that have been going on for 4 hours. Again there are no other symptoms such as dyspnoea or chest pain.

HR 80 bpm, BP 115/75 mmHg

12-lead electrocardiogram (ECG) (Figure 1.9):

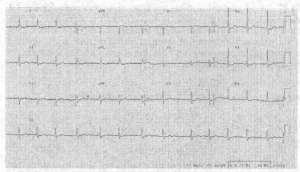

Figure 1.9

Which is the *single* most appropriate treatment? ★ ★ ★

A Amiodarone 100 mg oral (PO) once daily

B Digoxin 62.5 micrograms PO once daily

C Flecainide 200 mg PO, as required

D Metoprolol 25 mg PO twice daily

E Sotalol 40 mg PO twice daily

27. A 62-year-old woman is recovering on a medical ward after an exacerbation of her asthma. Her regular observations are checked.

BP 205/115 mmHg.

The nursing staff contact the junior doctor and discuss the patient over the telephone. Which *single* question would be most useful in the immediate assessment of this patient? ★★★

A Are her pupils equal and reactive to light?

B Does she have a headache?

C Has her medication been changed recently?

D Has this happened before?

E What is her heart rate?

28. A 62-year-old man has collapsed. He had felt fine beforehand, apart from a fluttering feeling in his chest. He turned very pale as he fell to the ground, but within seconds, his face flushed and full consciousness was regained. This has happened on two previous occasions. An electrocardiogram (ECG) is performed (Figure 1.10).

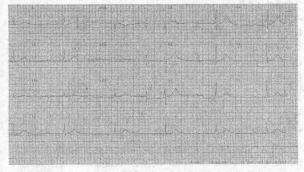

Figure 1.10

Reproduced with permission from Myerson S.G, Choudhury R.P, Mitchell A.R.J., *Emergencies in Cardiology*. Copyright (2006) with permission from Oxford University Press.

Which is the *single* most appropriate treatment for these episodes? ★★★

A Amiodarone 200 mg oral (PO) twice daily

B Flecainide 50 mg PO twice daily

C Implantable cardioverter–defibrillator

D Permanent pacemaker

E Radiofrequency ablation of the accessory pathway

29. A 54-year-old woman has collapsed. She cannot remember feeling unwell beforehand and has no residual symptoms afterwards. She has hypertension, type 2 diabetes, depression, and schizophrenia. She takes nifedipine, bendroflumethiazide, metformin, amitriptyline, and olanzapine. Her blood tests are within normal limits. An electrocardiogram (ECG) is performed (Figure 1.11).

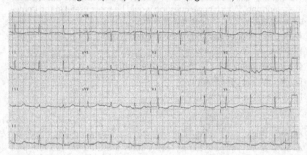

Figure 1.11

Which *single* medicine is most likely to have been responsible for her collapse? ★★★

A Amitriptyline

B Bendroflumethiazide

C Metformin

D Nifedipine

E Olanzapine

30. A 54-year-old man is recovering on a surgical ward after angioplasty to his right leg. Routine observations are carried out.

HR 100 bpm, BP 230/135 mmHg, SaO$_2$ 96% on air.

Over the next 4 hours, the man develops central chest pain radiating to his jaw. Serial electrocardiograms (ECGs) show dynamic T wave changes in the lateral chest leads. His blood pressure remains unchanged. Which is the *single* most appropriate approach to treating the blood pressure? ★★★

A Do not treat until the patient is pain-free

B Intermittent use of a sublingual spray

C Lower the BP with oral therapy over the next 24–48 hours

D Lower the BP urgently with intravenous (IV) therapy

E Use a one-off dose of a sublingual tablet

31. A 61-year-old man has been followed up a week after a syncopal episode where he lost consciousness for a few seconds whilst standing in a queue but was able to get back to his feet a few seconds later. He was fully investigated by cardiology, and although no other cause could be found, the risk of recurrence was deemed to be very low.

He is keen to continue driving his car and asks for advice from his doctor. Which is the *single* most appropriate advice? ★★★

A He can continue driving because no cause was found

B He can start driving 4 weeks after the episode

C He must discuss the episode with the Driver and Vehicle Licensing Agency (DVLA)

D He must stop driving for 6 months

E He should stop driving indefinitely

32. A 69-year-old woman has been increasingly breathless since suffering a non-ST-elevation myocardial infarction (NSTEMI) 4 weeks ago. She currently takes losartan 100 mg oral (PO) once daily, bisoprolol 5 mg PO once daily, aspirin 75 mg PO once daily, and ticagrelor 90 mg PO twice daily. Cardiac magnetic resonance imaging (MRI) had shown a left ventricular ejection fraction (LVEF) of 32% at a heart rate of 60 bpm. Choose the *single* medication that would be most appropriate to start from the following list of options. ★★★

A Furosemide 40 mg PO once daily

B Ivabradine 5 mg PO twice daily

C Ramipril 2.5 mg PO once daily

D Spironolactone 25 mg PO once daily

E Verapamil 120 mg PO once daily

33. A 75-year-old woman has been told that she has heart failure with reduced ejection fraction. She is already on bisoprolol 5 mg oral (PO) once daily and rivaroxaban 20 mg PO once daily for atrial fibrillation. Choose the *single* most appropriate medication to initiate from the following options. ★★★

A Amlodipine 5 mg PO once daily

B Ivabradine 5 mg PO twice daily

C Ramipril 2.5 mg PO once daily

D Spironolactone 25 mg PO once daily

E Valsartan/sacubitril 49 mg/51 mg PO twice daily

34. A 66-year-old Caucasian man has his quarterly appointment with his family doctor. He has been taking an angiotensin-converting enzyme (ACE) inhibitor for just over a year and uses allopurinol for gout.

BP 165/95 mmHg

Choose the *single* most appropriate medication to initiate from the following options. ★ ★ ★

A Alfuzosin 5 mg oral (PO) once daily

B Amlodipine 5 mg PO once daily

C Atenolol 25 mg PO once daily

D Bendroflumethiazide 2.5 mg PO once daily

E Spironolactone 25 mg PO once daily

35. A 38-year-old Afro-Caribbean woman has had repeatedly high blood pressure readings over the last 6 months. She also has type 1 diabetes.

BP 155/95 mmHg.

Choose the *single* most appropriate medication to initiate from the following options. ★ ★ ★

A Amlodipine 5 mg oral (PO) once daily

B Atenolol 25 mg PO once daily

C Bendroflumethiazide 2.5 mg PO once daily

D Losartan 25 mg PO once daily

E Ramipril 2.5 mg PO twice daily

36. A 62-year-old Caucasian man is struggling to control his blood pressure. He is asymptomatic, but his doctor is concerned as he is already on ramipril 10 mg oral (PO) once daily and amlodipine 10 mg PO once daily.

BP 190/100 mmHg.

Choose the *single* most appropriate medication to initiate from the following options. ★ ★ ★

A Alfuzosin 5 mg PO once daily

B Diltiazem 60 mg PO three times a day

C Furosemide 40 mg PO once daily

D Indapamide 2.5 mg PO once daily

E Losartan 25 mg PO once daily

37. A 59-year-old Caucasian woman has had increasing episodes of angina. She is already on perindopril 4 mg oral (PO) once daily, amlodipine 10 mg PO once daily, and indapamide 2.5 mg PO once daily.

BP 185/95 mmHg.

Choose the *single* most appropriate medication to initiate from the following options. ★★★

A Bendroflumethiazide 2.5 mg PO once daily

B Bisoprolol 2.5 mg PO once daily

C Losartan 25 mg PO once daily

D Ramipril 2.5 mg PO twice daily

E Spironolactone 25 mg PO once daily

38. A 66-year-old woman with metastatic bowel cancer is undergoing palliative chemotherapy. She had an inferior myocardial infarction 3 years ago but currently has no chest pain. An electrocardiogram (ECG) is performed (Figure 1.12).

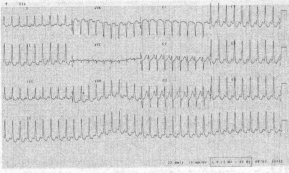

Figure 1.12
Reproduced with permission from Myerson S.G, Choudhury R.P, Mitchell A.R.J., *Emergencies in Cardiology*. Copyright (2006) with permission from Oxford University Press.

HR 160 bpm, BP 110/50 mmHg, SaO$_2$ 98% on 2 L O$_2$.

Chest: good air entry bilaterally. ★★★

Choose the *single* most appropriate immediate treatment from the following list of options.

A Amiodarone 300 mg intravenous (IV)

B Digoxin 500 micrograms IV

C Flecainide 150 mg oral (PO)

D Modified Valsalva manoeuvre

E Synchronized direct current (DC) cardioversion

39. A 48-year-old woman has had palpitations for the last 4 hours and now feels light-headed. She has no previous cardiac history. She has increased her alcohol consumption over the last few months and was at a party last night but cannot remember how much she drank. An electrocardiogram (ECG) is performed (Figure 1.13).

HR 135 bpm, BP 70/40 mmHg, SaO$_2$ 96% on 15 L O$_2$.

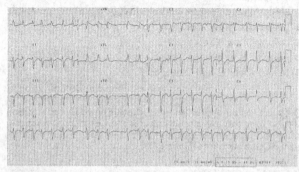

Figure 1.13

Choose the *single* most appropriate immediate treatment from the following list of options. ★★★

A Adenosine 6 mg intravenous (IV)

B Amiodarone 300 mg IV

C Flecainide 150 mg oral (PO)

D Modified Valsalva manoeuvre

E Synchronized direct current (DC) cardioversion

40. A 67-year-old man has felt his heart 'racing' for the last 6 hours. He suffered from this a few months ago but did not come to hospital. He has no chest pain and otherwise feels well.

HR 180 bpm, BP 110/70 mmHg, SaO$_2$ 97% on 15 L O$_2$.

A rhythm strip shows a regular narrow complex tachycardia. Blowing into the end of a 10-mL syringe and lying down with the legs up afterwards do not affect the rhythm.

Choose the *single* most appropriate immediate treatment from the following list of options. ★★★

A Adenosine 6 mg intravenous (IV)

B Amiodarone 300 mg IV

C Digoxin 500 micrograms IV

D Flecainide 150 mg oral (PO)

E Synchronized direct current (DC) cardioversion

41. A 72-year-old man has had palpitations over the last 8 hours and now has chest pain and feels more short of breath. He has never had any cardiac problems.

HR 180 bpm, BP 100/60 mmHg, SaO$_2$ 96% on 15 L O$_2$.

He has bibasal crepitations and a raised jugular venous pressure (JVP). An electrocardiogram (ECG) is performed (Figure 1.14).

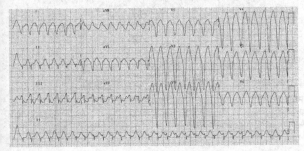

Figure 1.14

Choose the *single* most appropriate immediate treatment from the following list of options. ★★★

A Adenosine 6 mg intravenous (IV)

B Amiodarone 300 mg IV

C Digoxin 500 micrograms IV

D Furosemide 40 mg IV

E Synchronized direct current (DC) cardioversion

42. A 55-year-old man has had primary percutaneous coronary angioplasty for an inferior myocardial infarction. He is recovering well until he starts to experience palpitations. An electrocardiogram (ECG) is performed (Figure 1.15).

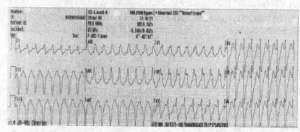

Figure 1.15

Reproduced with permission from Myerson S.G, Choudhury R.P, Mitchell A.R.J., *Emergencies in Cardiology.* Copyright (2006) with permission from Oxford University Press.

HR 175 bpm, BP 125/70 mmHg, SaO$_2$ 98% on air.

Choose the *single* most appropriate immediate treatment from the following list of options. ★★★

A Adenosine 6 mg intravenous (IV)

B Amiodarone 300 mg IV

C Digoxin 500 micrograms IV

D Furosemide 40 mg IV

E Synchronized direct current (DC) cardioversion

43. A 72-year-old man is given a new antihypertensive medication. His renal function is normal. Three weeks later, he feels unwell and a blood test shows the following results:

Sodium 139 mmol/L, potassium 4.9 mmol/L, creatinine 281 micromol/L, urea 15.2 mmol/L.

Choose the *single* most likely drug to be responsible for the symptoms described. ★★★

A Amlodipine

B Bendroflumethiazide

C Bisoprolol

D Doxazosin

E Lisinopril

44. A 42-year-old woman has type 2 diabetes mellitus and hypertension. She has recently been started on a new antihypertensive medication and has noticed that her blood glucose control is not as good as it was before.

Choose the *single* most likely drug to be responsible for the symptoms described. ★★★

A Alfuzosin

B Bendroflumethiazide

C Furosemide

D Spironolactone

E Valsartan

45. A 64-year-old woman has always had cold hands and feet, even in summer. She has recently started an additional antihypertensive medication and has found that her cold peripheries are even worse than usual.

Choose the *single* most likely drug to be responsible for the symptoms described. ★★★

A Atenolol

B Bendroflumethiazide

C Nifedipine

D Ramipril

E Verapamil

46. A 55-year-old man has noticed that his ankles are more swollen than is usual for him. Two weeks ago, he was started on an antihypertensive medication.

Choose the *single* most likely drug to be responsible for the symptoms described. ★★★

A Amlodipine

B Atenolol

C Indapamide

D Ramipril

E Verapamil

47. An 80-year-old woman has been feeling dizzy and lethargic for the past week. She has recently been started on a second antihypertensive medication, having been on a beta-blocker for many years.

HR 45 bpm, BP 75/40 mmHg.

Choose the *single* most likely drug to be responsible for the symptoms described. ★ ★ ★

A Amlodipine

B Bendroflumethiazide

C Enalapril

D Metoprolol

E Verapamil

48. A 40-year-old woman has become increasingly short of breath over a 24-hour period. She also has central chest pain that is made slightly easier if she sits forward. She has had no previous cardio-respiratory problems but does take prednisolone 20 mg oral (PO) once daily for a rheumatological condition.

T 37.2°C, HR 100 bpm, BP 115/75 mmHg.

She has several mouth ulcers and tender, swollen wrist joints. Which *single* examination finding is most likely to support the diagnosis? ★ ★ ★ ★

A Displaced apex beat

B Flushed cheeks

C Pericardial rub

D Red rash on trunk

E Splinter haemorrhages in fingernails

49. A 63-year-old man is taking digoxin 125 micrograms PO once daily for atrial fibrillation (AF). He returns to sinus rhythm for a few days before going back into AF. The decision is taken to start amiodarone. He is intravenously loaded with 300 mg over 1 hour, with a further 900 mg over 23 hours. Following this, he is commenced on an oral dose of 200 mg oral (PO) once daily. Which is the *single* most appropriate next step in management? ★ ★ ★ ★

A Continue both drugs at their current doses

B Decrease the amiodarone dose to 100 mg PO once daily

C Decrease the digoxin dose to 62.5 micrograms PO once daily

D Increase the amiodarone dose to 400 mg PO once daily

E Increase the digoxin dose to 250 micrograms PO once daily

50. A 74-year-old man is suffering with a progressive reduction in his exercise tolerance. He can now only manage a few steps before becoming breathless and light-headed. He takes bisoprolol 5 mg oral (PO) once daily, ramipril 10 mg PO once daily, furosemide 80 mg PO once daily, and spironolactone 50 mg PO once daily.

Heart rate at rest: sinus rhythm, 65 bpm (no bundle branch block, QRS 110 ms). Left ventricular ejection fraction (LVEF): 20–25%.

Choose the *single* most appropriate medication to initiate from the following options. ★★★★

A Bendroflumethiazide 2.5 mg PO once daily

B Cardiac resynchronization therapy (CRT)

C Digoxin 62.5 micrograms PO once daily

D Ivabradine 5 mg PO twice daily

E Valsartan/sacubitril 49 mg/51 mg PO twice daily

ANSWERS

1. D ★   OHCM 10th ed. → p. 126

Narrow complex tachycardias originate from within the atria or the atrioventricular (AV) node. They encompass atrial fibrillation, sinus tachycardia, and supraventricular tachycardias (atrial tachycardia, atrioventricular nodal re-entrant tachycardia, and atrioventricular re-entry tachycardia). If the tachycardia is 'junctional', i.e. it is dependent on the AV node (D), then interventions such as carotid sinus massage, the Valsalva manoeuvre, or adenosine—that transiently block the node— have a high chance of restoring sinus rhythm. If it is independent of the AV node (A, B, C, E), then these measures are more likely to reveal important information about the nature of the tachycardia.

Sohinki D and Obel O. Current trends in supraventricular tachycardia management. *Ochsner J.* 2014 Winter;**14**:586–95.

Whinnett ZI, Sohaib SMA, and Davies DW. Diagnosis and management of supraventricular tachycardia. *BMJ.* 2012;**345**:e7769.

2. A ★   OHCM 10th ed. → p. 154

In a young, previously healthy individual who has just had a minor infection, symptoms like this are strongly suggestive of pericardial inflammation. In about 60% of cases, the electrocardiogram (ECG) will be supportive of the diagnosis. An echocardiogram and a chest X-ray (CXR) are usually part of the workup. Therapy consists of restriction of physical activity and anti-inflammatory drugs [usually a non-steroidal anti-inflammatory drug (NSAID) plus colchicine].

Patients with one of the following risk factors should be admitted, as these are associated with poor prognosis: high fever (>38°C), subacute course, large pericardial effusion or cardiac tamponade, failure to respond to a 1-week course of NSAIDs, pericarditis associated with myocarditis (myopericarditis), immunodepression, trauma, and oral anticoagulant therapy.

B. Hypertrophic obstructive cardiomyopathy (HOCM) usually announces itself with a collapse, or even sudden death, and has a strong family history.

C. Endocarditis is unlikely to affect a previously healthy individual without risk factors (e.g. intravenous drug use, replacement valves); those who present with it are usually rather unwell, with a new heart murmur but a normal ECG.

D. Myocardial infarction (MI) in a young man is unlikely; however, young age does not exclude MI.

E. The sudden nature and distribution of the pain make pulmonary embolism possible, but the surrounding story is not supportive.

Adler Y, Charron P, Imazio M, *et al.* 2015 ESC Guidelines for the diagnosis and management of pericardial diseases: The Task Force for the Diagnosis and Management of Pericardial Diseases of the European Society of Cardiology (ESC). *Eur Heart J.* 2015;**36**:2921–64.

3. E ★   OHCM 10th ed. → p. 122

This man has had a myocardial infarction (MI) and is bradycardic. The most likely cause of bradycardia is an inferior MI as, in 60% of cases, the right coronary artery supplies the sinoatrial (SA) node (the left coronary artery supplying the other 40%).

4. E ★   OHCM 10th ed. → p. 99

This is an inferior myocardial infarction caused by an occlusion in the right coronary artery (RCA).

In the left coronary artery (LCA), the left main stem divides into the left anterior descending (LAD) and left circumflex arteries. The LAD supplies two-thirds of the interventricular septum, the anterior portion of the left ventricle (LV), and the apex of the heart. The LCA can branch again into the left marginal artery supplying the left atrium, the obtuse margin of the heart, and the posterior LV wall.

The RCA supplies blood to the right ventricle and 25–35% of the blood to the LV. In 90% of people, it supplies the atrioventricular node, in 60% the sinoatrial node, and in 85% of people, it gives off the posterior descending artery (PDA), which supplies the inferior wall, ventricular septum, and posteromedial papillary muscle.

5. C ★   OHCM 10th ed. → p. 800

This man is displaying the signs of severe acute left ventricular heart failure, common after a myocardial infarction, and requires intravenous diuresis. Sudden changes in physiology after a cardiac event should raise suspicion of failure and can be confirmed by eliciting the signs of fluid overload (jugular venous pressure, gallop rhythm, fine lung crackles). This deterioration should prompt immediate treatment and further investigations, making it likely that you need some help. Important tasks may include: monitoring SpO_2, blood pressure, ECG, and urine output, invasive monitoring of blood pressure, obtaining a bedside echocardiogram, starting non-invasive ventilation, and administering nitrates, morphine or—at the other end of the spectrum—inotropic agents.

6. B ★   OHCM 10th ed. → p. 804

The ECG shows a regular broad complex tachycardia. Adult advanced life support guidelines state that if the patient is not cardiovascularly compromised—as in this case where he is maintaining a good blood pressure—the first-line treatment is amiodarone 300 mg as a loading dose, followed by 900 mg over the course of the next 24 hours. In those who are compromised (chest pain, signs of heart failure, systolic BP <90 mmHg, syncope), the first-line treatment is with urgent synchronized cardioversion.

→ www.resus.org.uk/_resources/assets/attachment/full/0/6477.pdf

7. A ★   OHCM 10th ed. → pp. 108, 740

This is an anterior myocardial infarction caused by an occlusion in the left anterior descending artery (LAD).

In the left coronary artery (LCA), the left main stem divides into the left anterior descending and left circumflex arteries. The LAD supplies two-thirds of the interventricular septum, the anterior portion of the left ventricle (LV), and the apex of the heart. The LCA can branch again into the left marginal artery supplying the left atrium, the obtuse margin of the heart, and the posterior LV wall.

The right coronary artery (RCA) supplies blood to the right ventricle and 25–35% of the blood to the LV. In 90% of people, it supplies the atrioventricular (AV) node, in 60% the sinoatrial (SA) node, and in 85% of people, it gives off the posterior descending artery (PDA), which supplies the inferior wall, ventricular septum, and posteromedial papillary muscle.

8. E ★   OHCM 10th ed. → p. 150

Signs of sepsis/infection with a previous history of heart valve replacement raise suspicion of infective endocarditis. Recent evidence suggests that there is no clear association between interventional procedures and infective endocarditis, and therefore antibiotic prophylaxis is no longer recommended in these patients. However, with this history, together with the presentation, this is the most likely source of bacteraemia.

→ www.nice.org.uk/Guidance/CG64

9. E ★   OHCM 10th ed. → p.133

In Wolff–Parkinson–White syndrome, an accessory pathway—the bundle of Kent—is situated between the atria and ventricles. In comparison with the atrioventricular (AV) node, this pathway is able to conduct electrical impulses rapidly, leading to extremely fast rates and a risk of sudden death. Rapid conduction between the atria and ventricles causes a slurred upstroke (delta wave) and a short PR interval.

10. E ★   OHCM 10th ed. → p. 118

The term acute coronary syndrome includes cardiac events across the spectrum, from unstable angina (in which pain occurs at rest without causing myocardial damage) and non-ST-elevation myocardial infarction (NSTEMI) to ST-elevation myocardial infarction (STEMI). It does not include stable angina, which develops during exertion but settles with rest. Purely on the basis of a cardiac-sounding history and a convincing examination, scenarios can be labelled as acute coronary syndrome, while ECGs and cardiac markers are awaited. These can then be used to classify the event more specifically. In this man's case, there was cardiac-sounding pain at rest with no ST-elevation on the ECG and negative cardiac markers (Figure 1.16). Whilst technically this is an acute coronary syndrome, unstable angina would be a more accurate way to describe this with the information provided.

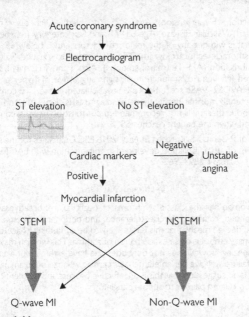

Figure 1.16
Reproduced with permission from Myerson S.G, Choudhury R.P, Mitchell A.R.J., *Emergencies in Cardiology*. Copyright (2006) with permission from Oxford University Press.

Thygesen K, Alpert JS, Jaffe AS, *et al.*; the Writing Group on behalf of the Joint ESC/ACCF/AHA/WHF Task Force for the Universal Definition of Myocardial Infarction. Third universal definition of myocardial infarction. *Eur Heart J.* 2012;**33**:2551–67.

11. C ★　　　OHCM 10th ed. → p. 779

In the context of a tachyarrhythmia, his blood pressure is unstable (systolic BP <90 mmHg = 'haemodynamically unstable'), and this should prompt an immediate review of the patient. Concurrent fever would obviously need investigating and treatment soon during the course of the night shift. The need for high-flow oxygen would also need to be reviewed soon, whilst the patient's anxiety could be monitored for a while prior to a review.

12. B ★　　　OHCM 10th ed. → p. 131

A risk factor-based approach is now favoured when considering the decision of whether or not to anticoagulate. The scoring system recommended is CHA2DS2–VASc [Congestive heart failure/left ventricular dysfunction, Hypertension, Age ≥75 (doubled), Diabetes, Stroke (doubled)–Vascular disease, Age 65–74, and Sex category (female)]. If a patient is without any of the major risk factors and is below 65, then a transthoracic echocardiogram (TTE) is needed to exclude 'valvular' atrial fibrillation (AF) (i.e. mitral stenosis). Also if the TTE might show impaired left ventricular function or signs suggestive of hypertension, the CHA2DS2–VASc score has to be recalculated. If the TTE confirms a structurally normal heart, then the diagnosis is 'lone AF' and anti-thrombotic therapy is not recommended but must be reassessed regularly and when the patient reaches 65.

Kirchhof P, Benussi S, Kotecha D, et al. 2016 ESC Guidelines for the management of atrial fibrillation developed in collaboration with EACTS. *Eur Heart J*. 2016;**37**:2893–962.

13. C ★   OHCM 10th ed. → p. 136

This woman has the classic symptoms of heart failure: breathlessness, orthopnoea, reduced exercise tolerance, and peripheral oedema. The gradual decline means that this is less likely to be something as acute as a pulmonary embolus or an exacerbation of asthma. This woman may well be wheezing, however, as not only does she have asthma, but also her heart failure will give her an element of cardiac wheeze on examination. There is no suggestion that this is an infective process and no mention of exertion-related pain or to support angina.

14. A ★   OHCM 10th ed. → p. 350

Whilst vitamin K antagonists (VKA) (E) used to be the first-line choice for anticoagulation in atrial fibrillation (AF) for decades, newer guidelines recommend discussing the options for anticoagulation [i.e. VKA vs direct-acting oral anticoagulants (DOACs)] with the patient and basing the choice on their clinical features and preferences. Dabigatran (A) is a twice-daily tablet that does not require monitoring. Its mechanism of action is direct thrombin inhibition. It is licensed for use in people with AF and one more risk factor, in a bid to reduce the risk of stroke and systemic embolism. The other DOACs are not listed here but are direct factor Xa inhibitors—rivaroxaban, edoxaban, and apixaban. Unfractionated heparin (B) may be used as a temporary anticoagulant but is usually not a sustainable choice. Clopidogrel (C) and aspirin (D) have not been shown to be effective as monotherapy in AF.

→ www.nice.org.uk/guidance/cg180

Faria R, Spackman A, Burch J, et al. Dabigatran for the prevention of stroke and systemic embolism in atrial fibrillation: a NICE single technology appraisal. *Pharmacoeconomics*. 2013;**31**:551–62.

15. D ★   OHCM 10th ed. → p. 194

This lady has cor pulmonale or right ventricular failure due to chronic hypoxic pulmonary vasoconstriction. Right ventricular hypertrophy, raised right atrial pressures [(raised jugular venous pressure (JVP)], and raised systemic venous pressure can cause ascites and peripheral oedema. Peripheral oedema in someone with chronic obstructive pulmonary disease (COPD) should always prompt assessment of right heart function.

A. This can present with ascites and ,abdominal pain, but symptoms and signs of liver failure, including hepatomegaly, would be expected.

B. There is no mention of jaundice.

C. This is a good differential for someone with features of right heart failure, but in someone with COPD, it is less likely to be the cause than cor pulmonale.

E. This can present with ascites but usually presents with organomegaly on a background of liver cirrhosis, most likely due to chronic alcohol use.

16. B ★ ★   OHCM 10th ed. → pp. 126, 806

The clues here are in the ECG and the fact that the tachycardia resolves with adenosine. Inverted P waves in the inferior leads are suggestive of retrograde atrial conduction. This phenomenon is common to junctional tachycardias, which would also fit with the patient—the fact that she has had them before—and the fact that it resolves once the atrioventricular (AV) node is blocked by adenosine.

Junctional tachycardias originate from the region of the AV node. They are either atrioventricular re-entrant tachycardias (AVRTs) or atrioventricular nodal re-entry tachycardias (AVNRTs). AVNRTs are the most common, usually affecting young, healthy individuals with no organic heart disease. They are caused by having two distinct pathways in the region of the AV node—a fast and a slow one.

In AVRT, there is an accessory pathway that actually bypasses the AV node and activates the ventricles prematurely. The most common type is Wolff–Parkinson–White syndrome.

Catheter ablation of the slow pathway in AVNRT and the accessory pathway in AVRT is well established and potentially curative.

Jackman M, Beckman KJ, McClelland JH, et al. Treatment of supraventricular tachycardia due to atrioventricular nodal reentry by radiofrequency catheter ablation of slow-pathway conduction. N Engl J Med. 1992;**327**:313–18.

17. C ★ ★

The patient has had a prosthetic mitral valve replacement and did not take his anticoagulant treatment for 3 days. If his international normalized ratio (INR) is <2.5, he is at higher risk for valve thrombosis, resulting in potentially fatal valve obstruction and/or stroke.

High reticulocyte count (B), lactate dehydrogenase (C), unconjugated bilirubin (D), and low haptoglobin (E) point towards haemolytic anaemia, which would be a good alternative differential to upper gastrointestinal bleeding if this patient had low haemoglobin.

18. A ★★   OHCM 10th ed. → p. 802

This question is a reminder to always ensure an ABCDE approach, especially in a complex clinical situation—it is vital to focus on the basics first. Measuring blood pressure will provide you with the answer to the essential question: can this be cardiogenic shock?

The patient has developed a heart rate of 100 bpm and the ECG is consistent with myocardial ischaemia. With the above history, the presence of hypotension would make 'cardiogenic shock' your working diagnosis, requiring senior help, alerting the cath lab for urgent reperfusion, and excluding cardiac tamponade with a bedside echocardiogram. You would not wait for lab results in this situation.

Note ST-elevation in aVR in this ECG. ST-elevations in aVR have to be distinguished from elevations in other leads (refer to determining the ECG axis—OHCM 10th ed. → p. 97) and need some special considerations. The presence of ST-depression of >0.1 mV in six or more surface leads, together with ST-elevation in aVR, is suggestive for ischaemia due to left main coronary artery (LCA) or multi-vessel obstruction, particularly if the patient presents with haemodynamic compromise.

The Task Force for the management of acute myocardial infarction in patients presenting with ST-segment elevation of the European Society of Cardiology (ESC). 2017 ESC Guidelines for the management of acute myocardial infarction in patients presenting with ST-segment elevation. *Eur Heart J.* 2017;**00**:1–66.

19. A ★★   OHCM 10th ed. → pp. 126, 806

Adenosine is used in narrow complex tachycardia after unsuccessful vagal manoeuvres, as it causes transient heart block at the atrioventricular (AV) node. This may interrupt the re-entry, hence terminate the episode of tachycardia in atrioventricular nodal re-entry tachycardia (AVNRT).

However, the depicted case looks rather like atrial flutter (note the heart rate of 150 bpm which suggests atrial flutter with a 2:1 ventricular response and hints of a saw-tooth pattern). After administration of adenosine, there will not be a ventricular response to the ongoing atrial activity for a few seconds—that can seem like forever! If you record this on a continuous ECG, you get proof of the underlying arrhythmia, thus 'unmasking' it. However, after the drug's effect on the AV node has ended, the atrial flutter will continue to cause a rapid ventricular response. Then it is time to think about anticoagulation (to prevent strokes), rhythm control (electrical cardioversion with lower energy than for atrial fibrillation/antiarrhythmic drugs), rate control (does not work very well in flutter), and electrophysiology.

20. C ★★   OHCM 10th ed. → pp. 154, 773

Ablation for atrial fibrillation requires advancement of catheters into the left atrium via puncture of the interatrial septum and delivery of thermal energy (i.e. heating or cooling) to electrically isolate the pulmonary vein ostia. Both puncture and heating/cooling can cause lesions that may subsequently result in pericardial effusion, leading to tamponade in approximately 1% of patients undergoing this procedure. This necessitates urgent bedside echocardiography.

Cardiac tamponade results in life-threatening shock. Clinical signs include hypotension with narrowed pulse pressure, muffled heart sounds, and jugular venous distension (Beck's triad). Central venous pressure (CVP) measurement (will be high) (D), and continuous blood pressure monitoring (showing pulsus paradoxus) (B) can be helpful if already established, while CXR (enlarged heart shadow) (E) and ECG (low-voltage) (A) might give you rather unspecific clues. A focused transthoracic echocardiogram (C) can establish the diagnosis within a few seconds, even in the hands of a relatively inexperienced operator. Furthermore, it can guide the lifesaving intervention—pericardiocentesis.

21. D ★★   OHCM 10th ed. → p. 798

With an ischaemic ECG (but without ST-segment elevations) and raised cardiac enzymes, this woman—known to have coronary artery disease—needs to be treated as per the protocol for an acute non-ST-elevation myocardial infarction (NSTEMI) which includes dual antiplatelet therapy (DAPT). DAPT with aspirin plus ticagrelor has been shown to reduce mortality, when compared to aspirin plus clopidogrel, in ST-elevation myocardial infarction (STEMI) and NSTEMI, as well as in high-risk patients with unstable angina. Ticagrelor has a faster onset of loading-dose effect than clopidogrel.

D. A proton pump inhibitor, in combination with DAPT, is recommended in patients at higher-than-average risk of gastrointestinal bleeds (e.g. history of gastrointestinal ulcer, corticosteroid use), but that does not mean the second antiplatelet agent should be withheld.

A and E. These are the dosages for maintenance therapy. Aspirin and clopidogrel are given once daily, whilst ticagrelor is given twice daily.

Task Force for the Management of Acute Coronary Syndromes in Patients Presenting without Persistent ST-Segment Elevation of the European Society of Cardiology (ESC). 2015 ESC Guidelines for the management of acute coronary syndromes in patients presenting without persistent ST-segment elevation. *Eur Heart J*. 2016;**37**:267–315.

Wallentin L, Becker RC, Budaj A, *et al*. Ticagrelor versus clopidogrel in patients with acute coronary syndromes. *N Engl J Med*. 2009;**361**:1045–57.

22. C ★★   OHCM 10th ed. → p. 136

At any stage in the treatment of confirmed heart failure, diuretics should be used to alleviate congestive symptoms and fluid retention. Therefore, furosemide is the only option here; after initiation, response to treatment and renal function need to be closely monitored and doses titrated.

→ www.nice.org.uk/guidance/cg108

Ponikowski P, Voors AA, Anker SD, *et al*.; ESC Scientific Document Group. 2016 ESC Guidelines for the diagnosis and treatment of acute and chronic heart failure. *Eur Heart J*. 2016;**37**:2129–200.

23. D ★★   OHCM 10th ed. → p. 136

This is a common side effect with angiotensin-converting enzyme (ACE) inhibitors such as ramipril or enalapril. Angiotensin receptor blockers (ARBs), such as losartan, are indicated at the same stage in the treatment of heart failure for those intolerant of ACE inhibitors.

24. E ★★★   OHCM 10th ed. → p. 111

The right ventricle is more anterior to the left; hence, when you 'look' at the heart from beside the sternum (i.e. parasternal), it is the first thing you 'see'. Therefore, you do not need to know a lot about echocardiography to be able to answer it, but if the question made you look at the image of an echocardiogram, its goal is achieved.

25. A ★★★   OHCM 10th ed. → pp. 108, 740

This is typical angina in a patient without clear ECG evidence of coronary artery disease (CAD). According to the National Institute for Health and Care Excellence (NICE) guidelines, the first-line test should be a 64-slice (or above) computed tomography (CT) coronary angiography. If this is non-diagnostic or shows CAD of uncertain significance, he should proceed to functional testing, looking for inducible ischaemia (e.g. stress echocardiogram, scintigraphy, or magnetic resonance imaging). NICE recommends not using exercise ECG to diagnose or exclude stable angina for people without known CAD.

→ www.nice.org.uk/guidance/cg95

26. C ★★★   OHCM 10th ed. → p. 130

In patients who have paroxysmal atrial fibrillation (AF), guidance is that a 'pill-in-the-pocket' strategy (i.e. a medicine to be taken as required) should be considered if the following criteria are met:

• There is no history of left ventricular dysfunction, or valvular or ischaemic heart disease.
• There are infrequent symptomatic episodes of paroxysmal AF.
• Systolic BP >100 mmHg and resting HR >70 bpm.
• Patients can understand how and when to take the medication.

Flecainide is a class IC antiarrhythmic agent and can be used in this way due to its rapidity of action. Studies have shown that it is effective in 80% of arrhythmic episodes in those with paroxysmal AF and so reduces the need for hospitalization.

A. Amiodarone can be used if beta-blockers have been unable to suppress paroxysms in those with poor left ventricular function.

B. Digoxin is not used in paroxysmal AF, but as a rate control in permanent AF for 'sedentary' patients.

D. Metoprolol (or another 'standard' beta-blocker) would be the first choice in paroxysmal AF where a pill-in-the-pocket strategy is not thought appropriate.

E. Sotalol would be the next choice after a standard beta-blocker if suppression of symptoms has not been achieved.

→ www.nice.org.uk/guidance/cg180

Alboni P, Botto GL, Baldi N, *et al*. Outpatient treatment of recent onset atrial fibrillation with the 'pill-in-the-pocket' approach. *N Engl J Med*. 2004;**351**:2384–91.

27. B ★★★   OHCM 10th ed. → p. 140

In severe hypertension, it is vital to establish whether the raised blood pressure is causing end-organ dysfunction, as it may need emergency treatment. This is obvious in cases of myocardial infarction, pulmonary oedema, and aortic dissection, but it can be present in rather more covert ways. One of these is hypertensive encephalopathy, which classically presents with a headache, change in consciousness, and some minor neurological dysfunction. In this case, the junior doctor should establish over the phone whether the patient has a headache: if she does, then he should head directly to the ward to perform an urgent assessment of her Glasgow Coma Scale (GCS) score, neurology, and fundi.

A. This is a reasonable examination to perform but is not as crucial as fundoscopy, as it will not help to assess end-organ damage.

C. This is useful in finding the cause of the problem but should take a back seat, whilst the problem is being dealt with.

D. This would provide valuable information and help stratify the risk of this being an emergency but is not a rate-limiting step.

E. This should clearly be asked but is not the key to the case.

Varounis C, Katsi V, Nihoyannopoulos P, *et al*. Cardiovascular hypertensive crisis: recent evidence and review of the literature. *Front Cardiovasc Med*. 2017;**3**:51.

28. D ★★★   OHCM 10th ed. → pp. 98, 132, 460

The history recounts a series of transient bradycardias due to lack of conduction through the atrioventricular (AV) node, causing decreased cardiac output and loss of consciousness. The ECG shows a lack of correlation between the P waves and the QRS complexes, and a ventricular rate of 25–30 bpm. This is complete heart block (also known as third-degree AV block). Emergency treatment involves continuous cardiac monitoring and may require urgent pacing if symptomatic, with a view to the placement of a definitive pacemaker, even if the patient is asymptomatic.

A. This is the treatment of choice for stable ventricular tachycardia (VT), shock, refractory ventricular fibrillation (VF), and various forms of atrial fibrillation (AF), but it is contraindicated in AV block.

B. This causes frequency-dependent inhibition of cardiac sodium channels and is used in the treatment of many tachyarrhythmias.

C. This is used for ventricular tachyarrhythmias causing syncope.

E. This is the definitive treatment for atrioventricular re-entrant tachycardia (AVRT) in Wolff–Parkinson–White syndrome (WPW syndrome).

→ www.escardio.org/static_file/Escardio/Guidelines/publications/CPWeb_Summary_Card_Cardiac_Pacing_2013.pdf

29. A ★★★   OHCM 10th ed. → p. 96

The ECG shows a long QT interval (i.e. QTc >420 ms), which has led to the collapse and is most likely due to the tricyclic antidepressant amitriptyline. A long QT interval is associated with polymorphic ventricular arrhythmias (torsades de pointes) and can cause syncope, seizures, and sudden death.

B. Bendroflumethiazide can precipitate electrolyte imbalances. Electrolyte imbalances (hypokalaemia, hypocalcaemia, and hypomagnesaemia) can, in turn, precipitate prolongation of the QT interval, but in this case, blood tests are normal.

C. There are no reports of this in the Summary of Product Characteristics (SPC) for metformin.

D. There are no reports of this in the SPC for nifedipine.

E. Some antipsychotics are associated with a prolonged QT interval, but from clinical trials, olanzapine is no more likely to cause this than a placebo.

Schwartz PJ and Woosley RL. Predicting the unpredictable drug-induced QT prolongation and torsades de pointes. *J Am Coll Cardiol.* 2016;**67**:1639–5.

30. D ★★★   OHCM 10th ed. → p. 140

Treating severe hypertension is a common, but difficult, clinical problem. The key to management is to appreciate the actual effect that the raised blood pressure is having. If the blood pressure is causing end-organ dysfunction, then it can be said to represent a hypertensive emergency; if it is not, then it is termed a hypertensive urgency. There are certain situations that are indicative of end-organ damage, and therefore an emergency:

- Acute myocardial infarction/unstable angina (as in this case);
- Acute pulmonary oedema;
- Acute renal failure;
- Acute aortic dissection;
- Hypertensive encephalopathy;
- Eclampsia.

The aim in emergencies is to stop ongoing end-organ damage. The most effective way of doing this (without dropping the blood pressure too quickly and adversely affecting cerebral perfusion) is via controlled IV therapy (labetalol is recommended), with the aim of reducing the diastolic blood pressure by 10–15%.

B. Sublingual nitrate sprays may be useful for pain relief but will not treat the blood pressure effectively.

C. A slower approach can be taken if the patient is asymptomatic, with the aim of reducing the blood pressure gradually over a couple of days.

E. The use of sublingual therapies, such as nifedipine, has been condemned due to the seriousness of adverse events reported because of the uncontrolled way in which it drops blood pressure.

Varounis C, Katsi V, Nihoyannopoulos P, et al. Cardiovascular hypertensive crisis: recent evidence and review of the literature. *Front Cardiovasc Med*. 2017;**3**:51.

31. A ★★★   OHCM 10th ed. → p. 158

This sounds like a classic vasovagal syncope on standing, with no real sinister features. Although he was investigated by cardiology, he probably did not need further formal investigation, as long as the episodes were not recurrent or atypical for vasovagal syncope. With a single one-off episode classic of vasovagal syncope, he can continue driving and does not need to inform the Driver and Vehicle Licensing Agency (DVLA), according to current guidance (January 2018).

32. D ★★★   OHCM 10th ed. → p. 136

Aldosterone antagonists are licensed for use in moderate to severe heart failure with reduced ejection fraction [i.e. New York Heart Association (NYHA) classes III–IV] or in those who have suffered a myocardial infarction within the last month.

Pitt B, Zannad F, Remme WJ, et al. The effect of spironolactone on morbidity and mortality in patients with severe heart failure. *N Engl J Med*. 1999;**341**:709–17.

33. C ★★★   OHCM 10th ed. → p. 136

Angiotensin-converting enzyme (ACE) inhibitors and beta-blockers should be offered in combination as first-line treatment for confirmed heart failure due to left ventricular systolic dysfunction (reduced ejection fraction), as there is evidence for a survival benefit.

34. B ★★★   OHCM 10th ed. → p. 136

If a patient is on an angiotensin-converting enzyme (ACE) inhibitor but remains hypertensive, add a calcium channel blocker; the next-line therapy would be a thiazide-like diuretic, but this would be contraindicated due to gout.

→ www.nice.org.uk/guidance/cg127

35. A ★★★   OHCM 10th ed. → p. 136

In any black or Afro-Caribbean patient, the first-line treatment is a calcium channel blocker or a thiazide-like diuretic. In this case, she has diabetes; therefore, a calcium channel blocker is advised.

36. D ★★★   OHCM 10th ed. → p. 136

Step 3 in the management of hypertension is to add a thiazide-like diuretic to an angiotensin-converting enzyme (ACE) inhibitor and a calcium channel blocker if there are no contraindications like gout or diabetes. Thiazide-like diuretics, such as indapamide, have replaced the more conventional thiazides, such as bendroflumethiazide, but can still cause similar side effects such as hyponatraemia.

37. B ★★★   OHCM 10th ed. → p. 136

Spironolactone is the preferred fourth-line antihypertensive, and it owes this status to the PATHWAY-2 trial. However, in this example, the patient has angina and a beta-blocker is first line for the treatment of angina. Therefore, in this situation, a beta-blocker is used as a dual agent before considering the addition of spironolactone.

Williams B, MacDonald TM, Morant S, et al. Spironolactone versus placebo, bisoprolol, and doxazosin to determine the optimal treatment for drug-resistant hypertension (PATHWAY-2): a randomised, double-blind, crossover trial. *Lancet*. 2015;**386**: 2059–68.

38. D ★★★   OHCM 10th ed. → p. 806

A regular narrow complex tachycardia should initially be treated with a vagal manoeuvre. This increases vagal tone at the atrioventricular (AV) node, in order to prevent conduction of impulses from the atria. This can be achieved by the strain of blowing into a 10-mL syringe to just move the plunger ('Valsalva manoeuvre').

The 'modified Valsalva manoeuvre' refers to this strain in a semi-recumbent position and immediately at the end of the strain, laying patients flat with their legs elevated for 15 s. This resulted in an increased frequency of conversion out of supraventricular tachycardia (SVT) to a sinus rhythm, compared to the standard Valsalva manoeuvre, in a randomized trial (43% vs 17% success rate).

Appelboam A, Reuben A, Mann C, et al. Postural modification to the standard Valsalva manoeuvre for emergency treatment of supraventricular tachycardias (REVERT): a randomised controlled trial. *Lancet*. 2015;**386**:1747–53.

39. E ★★★   OHCM 10th ed. → p. 806

Regardless of the cause of the tachyarrhythmia, signs that the patient is unstable include: (i) chest pain; (ii) signs of heart failure; (iii) reduced consciousness level or syncope; and (iv) systolic BP <90 mmHg. This should prompt urgent electrical cardioversion under sedation or general anaesthesia. The shock delivered is 'synchronized' with the pulse (i.e. the R-wave on the ECG), in contrast to the asynchronous shock used in cardiac arrest when there is no pulse present. 'Stable' atrial fibrillation is treated with either a beta-blocker or digoxin, although if it is <48 hours since the onset, amiodarone can be used.

40. A ★★★   OHCM 10th ed. → p. 806

The patient has a supraventricular tachycardia, but the modified Valsalva manoeuvre has not terminated the attack. The next step in a stable patient is to try adenosine 6 mg IV, followed by up to two doses of 12 mg. If this does not terminate the attack, expert help should be sought.

41. E ★★★   OHCM 10th ed. → p. 804

Chest pain and signs of heart failure indicate that this patient is unstable. The regular broad complex tachycardia is probably ventricular tachycardia (VT), and he will require up to three shocks with synchronized direct current (DC) cardioversion. If this fails, chemical cardioversion with amiodarone can be tried.

42. B ★★★   OHCM 10th ed. → p. 804

This man has a regular broad complex tachycardia (presumed to be ventricular tachycardia) but is haemodynamically stable, and therefore, chemical cardioversion can be attempted with amiodarone, as per the adult advanced life support algorithms.

43. E ★★★   OHCM 10th ed. → p. 668

Renal impairment may occur after starting an angiotensin-converting enzyme (ACE) inhibitor in patients with bilateral renal artery stenosis. These patients rely on angiotensin II to maintain the glomerular capillary pressure by vasoconstriction on the efferent more than the afferent arteriole, and if this is removed (by ACE inhibition), there is an abrupt fall in the glomerular filtration rate. This is why renal function must be monitored after commending an ACE inhibitor.

44. B ★★★   OHCM 10th ed. → p. 317

Thiazide diuretics can affect blood glucose control by decreasing both insulin secretion and peripheral insulin sensitivity. They can also lead to electrolyte imbalance, especially hypokalaemia, particularly in patients who have hepatic and renal impairment.

45. A ★★★   OHCM 10th ed. → p. 708

Beta-blockers are contraindicated in Raynaud's phenomenon due to peripheral vasoconstriction, which is mediated via peripheral β-receptor antagonism. They can exacerbate such symptoms and are also associated with low mood.

46. A ★★★   OHCM 10th ed. → p. 114

Dihydropyridine calcium channel blockers reduce systemic vascular resistance via peripheral vasodilatation and, as a result, can cause swollen ankles, headaches, and flushing. Verapamil is relatively more selective for the myocardium and has minimal vasodilatatory effects.

47. E ★★★   OHCM 10th ed. → pp. 114, 757

When co-administered, beta-blockers and non-dihydropyridine calcium channel blockers such as verapamil (both of which have negative inotropic effects on the heart) can lead to profound bradycardia, or even complete depression of ventricular contraction leading to asystole. Therefore, verapamil should never be used in conjunction with a beta-blocker, unless with specialist cardiology input.

48. C ★★★★   OHCM 10th ed. → p. 154

This scenario describes chest pain and breathlessness that has developed against the background of a rheumatological condition. The combination of mouth ulcers and arthritis in a woman of 40 years on maintenance steroids should be suspicious for systemic lupus erythematosus (SLE). One of the other diagnostic criteria for this condition is serositis (i.e. pleuritis or pericarditis). Given this woman's history, that her pain is relieved by sitting forward, and her low-grade temperature and tachycardia, it is likely that she is suffering from pericarditis or a pericardial effusion, which can be detected clinically by impaired venous return [raised jugular venous pressure (JVP)] and a superficial scratching sound on auscultation (pericardial rub).

A. This is most commonly a sign of left ventricular hypertrophy.

B. This is the malar flush of mitral stenosis and should not be confused with the fixed erythema that occurs over the malar eminences in SLE.

D. This is the rash of erythema marginatum that may be found in rheumatic fever.

E. This is a vasculitic effect of infective endocarditis.

49. C ★★★★   OHCM 10th ed. → p. 115

Digoxin is cleared both renally and metabolically. Chronic cardiac failure and hypothyroidism reduce the efficacy of clearance, leading to elevated levels. Drugs such as amiodarone, verapamil, and quinidine have the same effect and should prompt a reduction in digoxin dose once started, to avoid precipitating toxic levels. Watch out for bradycardia, nausea, loss of appetite, yellow vision, and confusion.

Nademanee K, Kannan R, Hendrickson J, et al. Amiodarone-digoxin interaction: clinical significance, time course of development, potential pharmacokinetic mechanisms and therapeutic implications. J Am Coll Cardiol. 1984;4:111–16.

50. E ★★★★ OHCM 10th ed. → pp. 115, 132, 136

If in heart failure with reduced ejection fraction, symptoms persist or even worsen, despite optimal therapy with angiotensin-converting enzyme (ACE) inhibitors, angiotensin receptor blockers, beta-blockers, and spironolactone; one of the following is then required: ivabradine, cardiac resynchronization therapy (CRT), or valsartan/sacubitril.

CRT (B) is essentially a biventricular pacemaker that co-ordinates the action of the right and left ventricles. There are various inclusion criteria, including left ventricular ejection fraction and width of the QRS complex. They are more effective with wider QRS complexes and left bundle branch block morphology. In this case, as the QRS is normal, CRT would not be indicated.

Ivabradine (D) reduces the heart rate at the sinus node via the funny channel and can be given to patients who are unable to tolerate a beta-blocker or with a heart rate >70 bpm on maximum tolerated beta-blocker dose.

This patient should be switched from ramipril to sacubitril/valsartan (E), the first substance of a novel drug class known as angiotensin II receptor–neprilysin inhibitor, as this was shown to reduce mortality. Switching will require a thorough assessment, a short period off ACE inhibitors, and vigilant monitoring.

A thiazide (A) can break through loop diuretic resistance, which might stop weight gain on high-dose furosemide by sequential nephron blockage. This may help if oedema is the main symptom, but the combination should be used with care.

Digoxin (C) is useful for rate control in atrial fibrillation. Using its inotropic effect for the treatment of heart failure in patients with sinus rhythm may reduce hospitalization rates, but there is no evidence of survival benefit.

McMurray JJ, Packer M, Desai AS, et al.; PARADIGM-HF Investigators and Committees. Angiotensin-neprilysin inhibition versus enalapril in heart failure. N Engl J Med. 2014;**371**:993–1004.

Swedberg K, Komajda M, Böhm M, et al. Ivabradine and outcomes in chronic heart failure (SHIFT): a randomised placebo-controlled study. Lancet. 2010;**376**:875–85.

Chest medicine

Rudy Sinharay

Respiratory conditions are common, and the burden of morbidity on the general population is high. You only have to take part in a few general medical takes as a junior doctor to realize this. As the on-call bleep goes off again, you are referred another exacerbation of chronic obstructive pulmonary disease (COPD) or asthma, a breathless patient (is it a pulmonary embolism, pneumothorax, or something less common?), or a patient with haemoptysis and weight loss [is it lung cancer or tuberculosis (TB)?] or productive cough (pneumonia or bronchiectasis?). The number of different respiratory conditions can be bewildering, and it is essential for the developing physician to be able to manage 'common presentations', as well as potentially life-threatening situations such as an asthma attack or an acute pulmonary embolism.

The nuances of history taking is often key to successfully clinching a diagnosis:

- What chronic conditions, respiratory or otherwise, do your patients have?
- What is the onset of symptoms? Sudden breathlessness may indicate a pneumothorax or pulmonary embolus. A chronic productive cough may indicate COPD or bronchiectasis.
- Social history—do they smoke, what are their living conditions, what is their occupation?

Luckily, we have other tools to help us. The age-old art of inspection, palpation, percussion, and auscultation during an examination is essential when assessing the patient. Combined with imaging techniques, including chest radiography, CT scanning, and bedside thoracic ultrasound, the answer is often easily obtained. Keeping an open mind to the less common causes of breathlessness, cough, and haemoptysis is important. Combined with lung function testing, autoimmune blood tests, and bronchoscopy, subtler diagnoses such as interstitial lung disease, fungal lung disease, and autoantibody-induced haemoptysis may be revealed. And a word to the wise—not all breathlessness originates from the lungs! For instance, an increased body mass index will cause a physical restriction on the mechanics of breathing and a compensated metabolic acidosis may cause tachypnoea.

As with all chronic diseases, the management of chronic respiratory disease is becoming increasingly complicated with the advent of biologics, immunotherapy, antifibrotic therapy, and a genuinely confusing array of inhalers. But with practice and using the skills described previously, we can be guided towards initiating the correct first-line treatment whilst planning longer-term management.

QUESTIONS

1. A 60-year-old man has right-sided chest pain. He is short of breath and is bringing up increasing volumes of foul-smelling, rusty sputum. These symptoms have persisted despite having been on intravenous antibiotics for the past 4 days. He says he was given oral tablets the previous week by his doctor but did not complete the course. His observation chart is shown in Figure 2.1. The medical team are concerned about the man's poor progress and request a chest X-ray.

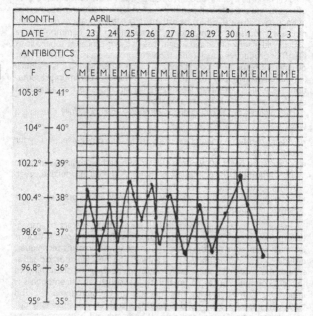

Figure 2.1

Which single X-ray finding would be most supportive of the likely diagnosis? ★

A Air within the right pleural space

B Obscured right heart border

C *Single* circular opacity in peripheral right hemithorax

D Tramlines and ring shadows in right hemithorax

E Walled-off cavity in right hemithorax with a fluid level

2. A 30-year-old woman has had an acute severe episode of asthma. This is her first acute episode for over 10 years and she is recovering in hospital. She has a salbutamol 100 micrograms inhaler that she uses occasionally and a beclometasone 200 micrograms inhaler that is prescribed for use twice daily. Which *single* measure is most likely to improve this woman's long-term asthma control? ★

A Add montelukast 10 mg oral (PO) once daily

B Add salmeterol 50 micrograms inhaler (INH) twice daily

C Ensure up-to-date spirometry and lung function tests

D Organize a review by an asthma specialist in 3 months' time

E Write a plan of how and when to take the inhalers

3. A 52-year-old woman is severely short of breath. She is confused and cannot respond to questions. There is no one accompanying her to shed light on her medical history.

T 37.1°C, HR 120 bpm, BP 105/65 mmHg, RR 26/min.

Her lips appear blue, her neck muscles are being used to assist breathing, and there is generalized wheeze on her chest. She is put on high-flow oxygen. Which is the *single* most appropriate course of immediate management? ★

A Aminophylline 300 mg intravenous (IV)

B Adrenaline 0.5 mg intramuscular (IM)

C Hydrocortisone 100 mg IV

D Magnesium sulfate 1.2 g IV

E Salbutamol 5 mg nebulized (NEB)

4. A 28-year-old woman has felt unwell for the last 4 days with coryzal symptoms and worsening breathlessness. She is asthmatic and has used her inhalers, without any relief for the last hour. On arrival in the Emergency Department, she is talking in broken sentences and her peak expiratory flow rate (PEFR) is 45% of predicted.

HR 115 bpm, RR 28/min.

She is assessed and given oxygen via a non-rebreather mask, whilst a salbutamol and ipratropium nebulizer is being prepared. An hour after admission, her PEFR is 80% of predicted. Which is the *single* most appropriate management? ★

A Contact the on-call anaesthetist for admission to the high-dependency unit

B Discharge home with medication and follow-up in 2 weeks

C Observe on the medical admissions ward for 24 hours

D Start bi-level positive airway pressure

E Start continuous positive airway pressure

5. A 69-year-old man has had a cough and myalgia, and felt feverish for the last 7 days. He is wheezy and is finding it particularly difficult to breathe. He has asthma and is using his usual inhalers every half an hour but feels that they are not having any effect on his symptoms. When assessing the severity of this asthma attack, which *single* finding is most consistent with a *severe* attack? ★

A Blood pressure (BP) 80/60 mmHg

B Inability to complete sentences

C Inaudible air entry bilaterally

D Peak expiratory flow rate (PEFR) <33% of predicted

E Arterial oxygen saturation (SaO_2) <75% on air

6. A 36-year-old man with asthma is seen as part of his annual asthma review. He has a salbutamol 100 micrograms inhaler prescribed, which he usually uses approximately twice a week. Which *single* feature from the following options would *not* concern you that his asthma is poorly controlled? ★

A Asthma attack in the last 2 years

B Increased use of the salbutamol inhaler to daily use

C An episode of pins and needles in his peripheries 1 month ago

D Waking at night with coughing

E Wheezing brought on by exercise

7. A 30-year-old woman is recovering in hospital after an episode of acute asthma. Overnight, she required hourly salbutamol 5 mg nebulizers, and after the morning ward round, she is now receiving them every 2 hours. She is intermittently using oxygen 3 L via a Hudson mask. She has regular admissions to hospital but has a young family and is keen for an early discharge home. Her normal regimen is a salbutamol 100 micrograms inhaler as required (PRN) and beclometasone 200 micrograms inhaler twice daily. She wants to be discharged by the end of the day. Which is the *single* most appropriate time for this woman to be discharged? ★

A When her nebulizers are stopped

B When she feels ready

C When she has been stable on inhalers for 24 hours

D When she has been stable on nebulizers for 24 hours

E When she is no longer requiring oxygen therapy

8. A 32-year-old woman has asthma and is increasingly short of breath in the mornings. She describes her chest feeling tight and says it is hard for her to catch her breath. As a result, she is taking two puffs of her salbutamol 100 micrograms inhaler at least three times before midday.

Peak expiratory flow rate: 310 L/min.

Which is the *single* most appropriate next step in her management? ★

A Beclometasone 200 micrograms inhaler (INH) twice daily

B Prednisolone 40 mg oral (PO) once daily for 5 days

C Salbutamol 200 micrograms INH four times daily

D Salmeterol 50 micrograms INH twice daily

E Seretide® 100/50 micrograms INH twice daily

9. A 17-year-old woman is leaving home to start further education. She has asthma and uses a salbutamol 100 micrograms inhaler three or four times a month. She has never had an acute episode before and is worried that she may not be able to recognize one if it were happening, and she asks for guidance as to what to look out for. Which is the *single* most important feature for the doctor to stress? ★

A Dizziness and tingling of peripheries

B Her inhaler does not improve symptoms

C Her inhaler gives her a tremor

D She is breathless after running for a bus

E She is breathless after running up a flight of stairs

10. A 20-year-old man has been diagnosed with asthma and is worried about the prospect of having an 'attack' and its treatment.

He is advised firstly to take one puff of his regular inhaler. Which is the *single* most appropriate additional instruction for the man to follow? ★

A Call for the emergency services

B Go into the open air and wait for the attack to pass

C Lie down, loosen clothing, and wait for the attack to pass

D Take one puff every 30–60 s up to a maximum of ten puffs

E Use the inhaler continuously until symptoms resolve

11. An 18-year-old man has had a cough for the last 6 weeks. It has got worse over the past week, such that he is now bringing up large volumes of green- and red-coloured sputum. He has had such exacerbations regularly. He uses insulin 12 U subcutaneous (SC) twice daily. Which is the *single* most accurate explanation for his sputum production? ★

A Chronic inflammation of lung parenchyma

B Chronic swelling of airway mucosa

C Permanent dilatation of the bronchioles

D Progressive fibrosis and remodelling of interstitium

E Prolonged bronchial muscle contraction

12. A 41-year-old man has felt unwell for 5 days. He has a cough productive of green sputum with an occasional reddish tinge. He has been feeling hot and cold, particularly at night, and has pain in the right side of his chest. He has smoked ten cigarettes a day for 25 years.

T 37.8°C, HR 100 bpm, BP 115/80 mmHg, RR 22/min, SaO₂ 93% on air.

There are basal crackles on the right side of the chest. Which is the *single* most likely diagnosis? ★

A Bronchial carcinoma

B Community-acquired pneumonia

C Granulomatosis with polyangiitis (Wegener's granulomatosis)

D Sarcoidosis

E Tuberculosis

13. An 83-year-old man is prescribed modified-release morphine tablets twice daily. He is seen in the outpatient lung cancer clinic, having run out. A new prescription must be written. Which is the *single* most important detail required on the prescription to satisfy legal requirements? ★

A Date of birth

B Dose in words and figures

C General Medical Council (GMC) number

D Handwritten prescription

E Patient's address

14. A 19-year-old woman has been coughing up copious amounts of sputum over the past week. It has been green with some rusty specks. For the third time this year, she is admitted for a course of intravenous (IV) antibiotics. Which *single* set of examination findings would be most supportive of the likely diagnosis? ★

A Enlarged supraclavicular lymph nodes + focal bronchial breathing

B Finger clubbing + coarse inspiratory crackles

C Mouth ulcers + unilateral dullness to percussion

D Pitting unilateral calf oedema + pleural rub

E Unilateral ptosis + unilateral reduced air entry

15. A 56-year-old man who has chronic obstructive pulmonary disease (COPD) and uses long-term oxygen therapy at home has not left his house for the last 2 weeks. He has started sleeping for large parts of the day, and his wife says that he has also occasionally been confused.

T 36.4°C, BP 146/90 mmHg, HR 90 bpm, SaO_2 89% on 2 L O_2.

Arterial blood gases (on 2 L O_2): pH 7.1, $PaCO_2$ 9.8 kPa, PaO_2 6.5 kPa, bicarbonate 36 mmol/L.

Which is the *single* most appropriate next step? ★

A Increase oxygen to 4 L/min

B Nebulized salbutamol 5 mg

C Non-rebreather mask at 15 L/min

D Trial of non-invasive ventilation (NIV)

E Trial of continuous positive airway pressure (CPAP)

16. A 68-year-old man becomes suddenly short of breath, with left-sided chest discomfort. He has chronic obstructive pulmonary disease (COPD) and is on home oxygen, regular nebulizers, and maintenance oral steroids.

T 37.1°C, HR 100 bpm, RR 24/min, SaO_2 86% on 2 L O_2.

A computed tomography (CT) pulmonary angiogram rules out a pulmonary embolus. Which *single* examination finding is most likely to support the diagnosis? ★

A Left-sided bronchial breath sounds

B Left-sided hyperresonant percussion note

C Left-sided hyporesonant percussion note

D Left-sided increased vocal resonance

E Left-sided stony dull percussion note

17. A 21-year-old woman has had left-sided chest pain for 1 week. It came on gradually and is sharp in nature and worse on deep inspiration.

T 36.6°C, HR 85 bpm, RR 18/min, SaO$_2$ 99% on air.

The left medial border of the sternum is tender to palpation, but her chest is otherwise clear. Which is the *single* most likely diagnosis? ★

A Acute pericarditis

B Community-acquired pneumonia

C Costochondritis

D Myocardial infarction

E Pulmonary embolus

18. A 70-year-old woman has had griping abdominal pain and constipation for the past month. As well as feeling generally 'achy', she admits to feeling mentally low. She has had a cough for the past 9 months, during which time she has lost more than 5 kg. She is an ex-smoker. She has been told that there is a 'shadow' on her chest X-ray and that her new symptoms may be related to this. Which is the *single* most likely mechanism that links her new symptoms to the X-ray findings? ★

A A carcinoid tumour is secreting serotonin

B A lung tumour has metastasized to the liver and brain

C A lung tumour is secreting parathyroid hormone

D A urogenital tumour has metastasized to the lung and bone

E An abdominal tumour has metastasized to the lung

19. A 60-year-old man has had a persistent cough for the past year. He has lost 5 kg during this time and has had increasing episodes of breathlessness. He has smoked heavily for many years. There are no specific chest signs, but he is cachectic and has a drooping eyelid on the right-hand side. A chest X-ray shows a *single* nodule in the right apical hemithorax, which it is suggested may be the cause of all of his symptoms. Which is the *single* structure that the nodule is most likely to be compressing? ★

A Accessory nerve

B Cervical sympathetic plexus

C Oculomotor nerve

D Superior vena cava

E Trigeminal nerve (ophthalmic division)

20. A 72-year-old woman is found confused and drowsy in her own home. She has recently been diagnosed with a bronchial carcinoma.

Sodium 124 mmol/L, potassium 4.4 mmol/L, urinary sodium 35 mmol/L.

Which is the *single* most likely type of carcinoma? ★

A Adenocarcinoma

B Alveolar cell

C Large cell

D Small cell

E Squamous cell

21. A 66-year-old man has been admitted with an episode of acute confusion. He does not respond, as he is having his 4-hourly observations. The attending nurse asks the junior doctor, who is on the ward, for urgent help. As the doctor approaches the man, he can hear gurgling. Which is the *single* most appropriate immediate management? ★

A Ask the nurse to put out a crash call

B Begin chest compressions at 30:2

C Give oxygen (O_2) 15 L/min via a non-rebreather mask

D Insert an oropharyngeal airway

E Suction the airway

22. A 70-year-old woman has a swollen left calf. She is admitted to a medical ward. Within 24 hours of admission, she dies. The junior doctor who attended to her on the ward is subsequently contacted by the hospital's legal department. They are concerned about one of the entries he made in the medical notes.

16/6/10 Junior Dr review, Watson #111

Asked to see patient: c/o chest pain

Pain in rt chest for last 2 hours

Came on suddenly—not had this pain before

Worse on inspiration

Rated 7/10, no shortness of breath

No radiation, nothing makes it better

T 36.8°C, HR 110 bpm, BP 110/70 mmHg, SaO$_2$ 95% on air, RR 24/min

Chest clear, no focal tenderness, HS I + II + 0

Plan: ECG, chest X-ray, regular paracetamol

Watson #111

Which is the *single* reason that is most likely to cause the legal team concern about this entry? ★

A Discussions with seniors either not sought or not documented

B Full examination either not performed or not documented

C Impression of clinical picture not documented

D No mention made of admitting complaint

E Time of review not documented

23. A 79-year-old woman has become acutely short of breath in hospital. The junior doctor notes that she has had a previous aspiration pneumonia and a pulmonary embolus and she is not for resuscitation. As the junior doctor is examining the woman, her respiratory effort dwindles and then ceases, and no pulses are palpable. Which is the *single* most appropriate next step? ★

A Ask a nurse to put out a cardiac arrest call

B Continue to examine for signs of life before confirming death

C Insert a Guedel airway and attempt ventilation

D Insert two large-bore cannulae into the antecubital fossae

E Start cardiac chest compressions immediately

24. The junior doctor on-call receives a bleep from a nurse during a busy night shift. A 63-year-old man has felt increasingly short of breath over the last 10 minutes. He has been admitted with an infective exacerbation of chronic obstructive pulmonary disease (COPD) and has been started on non-invasive ventilation (NIV). Suddenly he found it very difficult to breathe. He is on co-amoxiclav 1.2 g intravenous (IV). Which *single* additional detail from the nurse should prompt an immediate review of the patient, i.e. within the next 5 minutes? ★

A Heart rate (HR) 92 bpm

B Left-sided chest pain

C Respiratory rate 25/min

D Arterial oxygen saturation (SaO$_2$) 92% on 28% oxygen (O$_2$)

E Temperature 37.9°C

25. A 76-year-old woman has been reported as 'out of breath' for the past 12 hours. She has been sleepy and very quiet, refusing all meals in her care home. She has chronic obstructive pulmonary disease (COPD) and metastatic breast cancer.

T 37.5°C, HR 110 bpm, BP 100/70 mmHg, SaO$_2$ 65% on air, RR 7/min.

Which is the *single* most appropriate additional examination or bedside test to aid her treatment? ★

A Abbreviated mental test

B Lower limbs

C Peak flow

D Pupillary

E Respiratory

26. A 72-year-old man has been breathless for 2 days, with a cough productive of white sputum. It came on suddenly while he was running for a bus. He now has right-sided chest pain, which is worse on deep breaths in. He has been a smoker for 60 years but is not on any regular medication.

T 37.2°C, HR 110 bpm, SaO$_2$ 92% on air.

He has a generalized wheeze. Which is the *single* most likely diagnosis? ★

A Acute asthma

B Heart failure

C Infective exacerbation of chronic obstructive pulmonary disease (COPD)

D Myocardial infarction

E Pulmonary embolus

27. A 46-year-old woman has felt breathless for the last 48 hours and had an episode of haemoptysis this morning. She has recently undergone surgery to remove an ovarian carcinoma.

T 37.2°C, BP 110/58 mmHg, HR 90 bpm, SaO_2 95% on 2 L O_2.

Which *single* feature from the following history is consistent with the most likely diagnosis? ★

A 5 kg weight loss over the last month

B Breathlessness is maximal on exertion

C Cough productive of green sputum

D Pain worse on taking a deep breath in

E Swinging fevers and sweats, particularly at night

28. A 26-year-old man has sudden pain over his lower sternum. He feels breathless and nauseated but does not vomit. He has no other medical problems. There is decreased air entry at the right apex. Which is the *single* most likely diagnosis? ★

A Acute pericarditis

B Community-acquired pneumonia

C Costochondritis

D Pneumothorax

E Pulmonary embolus

29. A 19-year-old man becomes suddenly short of breath while playing football. He feels nauseated, with left-sided chest discomfort. He smokes ten cigarettes a day and admits to an occasional cough in the morning. He uses bronchodilators for his asthma but has never been admitted to hospital. Which *single* pair of examination findings is most likely to support the diagnosis? ★

A Bronchial breathing + dull to percussion on the left

B Decreased expansion + crackles on the left

C Decreased expansion + increased vocal resonance on the left

D Hyperresonant to percussion + diminished breath sounds on the left

E Stony dull to percussion + decreased vocal resonance on the left

30. A 23-year-old woman has suffered an infective exacerbation of her asthma. She has taken a 5-day course of prednisolone 40 mg oral (PO) once daily and is now ready to be discharged from hospital. This is her first hospital admission because of her asthma since childhood. Her discharge summary and prescription are being prepared. Which is the *single* most appropriate instruction for taking the prednisolone? ★

A Continue the same dose and see her general practitioner in 2 weeks

B No further prednisolone is needed

C Reduce by 5 mg every day for the next 8 days

D Reduce by 10 mg every day for the next 4 days

E Reduce by 10 mg every week for the next month

31. A 66-year-old man is breathless and being treated for an exacerbation of chronic obstructive pulmonary disease (COPD). It has not been possible to obtain a blood gas sample from the radial artery, and repeated attempts have left the patient in a great deal of distress. The registrar has asked the on-call junior doctor to take the blood from the femoral artery. The junior doctor has never performed this skill before.

RR 22/min, SaO_2 96% on O_2 5 L/min.

Which is the *single* most appropriate next step? ★

A Abandon the procedure as the man's oxygen saturation is within acceptable limits

B Analyse a venous sample obtained from the antecubital fossa instead

C Ask another doctor to explain the procedure before trying to take blood from the femoral artery

D Talk the patient into allowing another attempt at taking blood from the radial artery

E Tell the registrar that they have no experience of this procedure

32. A 66-year-old man has had abdominal pain with nausea for the past week. He has felt dizzy and fainted on two occasions. He has a chronic cough and was recently diagnosed with a bronchial carcinoma.

Lying BP 135/90 mmHg, standing BP 90/75 mmHg.

Which *single* category of complication is most likely to explain this man's new symptoms? ★

A Endocrine

B Local

C Metastasis

D Neurological

E Other

33. A 72-year-old man is said to be in a 'deep sleep' by the nursing staff. He is unrousable and does not even wake when he has his blood sugar checked. He is being treated with intravenous (IV) antibiotics for a lower respiratory tract infection and morphine liquid 5 mg oral (PO), as required, for associated chest pain. He is receiving 30% oxygen 10 L/min via a Venturi™ mask. The junior doctor who is on the ward is asked to see the man urgently. As the doctor reaches the man's bedside, he hears loud snoring.

Which is the *single* most appropriate immediate management? ★

A Head tilt and chin lift manoeuvres

B Insert a nasopharyngeal airway

C Naloxone 400 micrograms IV immediately (STAT)

D Reduce the oxygen flow rate

E Urgent cricothyroidotomy

34. A 28-year-old woman has had right-sided chest pain for the past week. It is worse when she breathes in and is accompanied by an intermittent dry cough. She has no other medical problems and has not suffered any recent periods of prolonged immobility. She takes the oral contraceptive pill.

BP 122/85 mmHg, HR 80 bpm, RR 18/min, SaO₂ 98% on air.

Which is the *single* most appropriate initial investigation to establish the diagnosis? ★

A Arterial blood gas

B Computed tomography pulmonary angiogram (CTPA)

C D-dimer

D Peak expiratory flow rate (PEFR)

E Ventilation/perfusion (V/Q) scan

35. A 59-year-old man is brought into the emergency department by ambulance. The crew present their findings: 'This is John, he's 59 with COPD. He's had difficulty breathing, especially for the past day or so. On arrival, his sats were 77% on air, pulse 125 bpm, BP 110/75 mmHg. We gave him a neb, and on 5 L of oxygen, his sats improved to 97%. He's more comfortable, but a bit confused.'

Which is the *single* most appropriate immediate management? ★

A Check his peak flow

B Give him another salbutamol 5 mg nebulized (NEB)

C Perform arterial blood gases

D Reduce the oxygen flow rate from 5 L to 2 L

E Start co-amoxiclav 1.2 g intravenous (IV)

36. A 32-year-old man who works as an IT consultant has been suffering from a productive cough and weight loss for the last 3 months. He is originally from India and has been living in the United Kingdom for 5 years. On closer questioning, he tells you he has felt inter-mittently feverish for the last 3 weeks. On examination, his temperature is 37.1°C, respiratory rate 16/min, and oxygen saturations 96%. A chest X-ray shows infiltrates in the right upper zone.

Which is the *single* most appropriate next investigation? ★

A Computed tomography (CT) scan of the chest

B Bronchoscopy

C Interferon gamma release assay (IGRA)

D Human immunodeficiency virus (HIV) test

E Send sputum samples for acid-fast staining and culture

37. A 68-year-old man has had several episodes of central abdom-inal pain, loose stools, and vomiting over the past 5 days. He has severe chronic obstructive pulmonary disease (COPD) and was recently treated with 2 weeks of antibiotics for a chest infection. He also takes aminophylline 450 mg oral (PO) twice daily and prednisolone 10 mg PO once daily. The patient suspects he may have suffered a reaction to the antibiotics. Which is the *single* most likely cause? ★

A Amoxicillin

B Cefalexin

C Co-amoxiclav

D Doxycycline

E Erythromycin

38. A 24-year-old woman has been diagnosed with smear-posi-tive pulmonary tuberculosis. She is started on rifampicin, iso-niazid, pyrazinamide, and ethambutol (standard quadruple therapy). Two weeks into treatment, she starts feeling nauseated and starts vomiting 2–3 times a day.

Which is the *single* most appropriate next step? ★

A Check her liver function tests (LFTs)

B Prescribe an antiemetic

C Stagger the administration of her medication

D Request an abdominal X-ray

E Check the sensitivities of the sputum culture

39. A 67-year-old woman has been admitted with increased tiredness over 2 weeks. On closer questioning, she has also lost 10 kg in weight in the last 6 weeks. Her medications include a tiotropium inhaler and furosemide 40 mg once daily (od). On examination, she is found to be cachectic, has nicotine stains on her hands, and is clubbed bilaterally. She is euvolaemic. Her serum sodium levels are 122 mmol/L. ★

What is the *single* most likely mechanism of the hyponatraemia?

A Dehydration

B Ectopic antidiuretic (ADH) production

C Effect of loop diuretic

D Heart failure

E Hypothyroidism driving increased ADH production

40. 22-year-old man is found to have a pneumothorax after presenting to the emergency department with sudden-onset chest pain. It completely resolves following on from a successful aspiration. He is due to go on holiday to Spain in a month and is concerned about flying.

What is the *single* most appropriate instruction you should give this man? ★★

A He should not fly until he has surgical pleurodesis of the affected lung

B He should not fly for 1 week

C He should not fly for 2 weeks

D He should not fly for 4 weeks

E He should not fly for 6 weeks

41. A 78-year-old woman has become suddenly breathless. She has left-sided chest pain that is worse on deep inspiration. One month ago, she had surgery to remove a pelvic tumour. She uses regular inhalers for chronic obstructive pulmonary disease (COPD).

BP 100/70 mmHg, HR 110 bpm, RR 24/min, SaO_2 94% on air.

Her chest is clear, but her left leg is noticeably swollen and tender posteriorly.

Which is the *single* most appropriate investigation to reach the diagnosis? ★★★

A Computed tomography (CT) chest/abdomen/pelvis

B Computed tomography pulmonary angiogram (CTPA)

C Ultrasound abdomen

D Ultrasound Doppler left leg

E Ventilation/perfusion (V/Q) scan

42. A 77-year-old man has had a cough with haemoptysis for over a year. During this time, he has lost 20 kg and developed pain in his upper abdomen. He is frail and has become increasingly dependent in his nursing home. The man's daughter tells the medical team that should they find anything worrying through the course of their investigations, they should not tell him as it would 'finish him off'. A subsequent computed tomography (CT) scan shows a primary bronchial malignancy with metastatic deposits in the liver. Which would be the *single* most appropriate course of action? ★ ★ ★

A Ask the man how much he would like to know about the ongoing investigations

B Refer the man to the palliative care team and allow them to deal with the information

C Tell the daughter and allow her to do what she likes with the information

D Tell the man that the scan was normal, as it would not be in his best interests to know the truth

E Wait until either the man or his daughter asks about the scan before venturing any information

43. A 38-year-old woman has had a productive cough with right-sided chest pain for 4 days. Prior to this episode, she had been fit and well.

T 38.4°C, HR 110 bpm, BP 110/75 mmHg, RR 26/min, SaO$_2$ 92% on 8 L O$_2$. There is bronchial breathing up to the mid zone on the right. After 48 hours of antibiotic therapy, this has progressed to include the upper zone. Her arterial oxygen saturation (SaO$_2$) has dropped to 86% on 8 L oxygen (O$_2$), and an arterial blood gas shows worsening type 1 respiratory failure. Which would be the *single* most appropriate course of action? ★ ★ ★

A Add a course of intravenous (IV) steroids

B Increase oxygen (O$_2$) delivery to 15 L/min

C Liaise with the Intensive Therapy Unit (ITU)

D Request an ultrasound scan of her chest

E Take blood cultures and switch antibiotics

44. A 45-year-old man has had a chest drain inserted for a large right-sided pneumothorax. The on-call junior doctor is asked to review a chest X-ray, checking the placement of the drain—the tip of the drain is pointing towards the apex, but a 3-cm pneumothorax remains and the underwater drain is not bubbling or swinging. Which is the *single* most appropriate next step? ★★★

A Advance the drain a few centimetres further and repeat the chest X-ray

B Clamp the drain for 12 hours

C Flush 20 mL of saline through the drain

D Remove the drain and leave air to be reabsorbed

E Remove the drain and replace with one further into the apex

45. An 88-year-old man is brought to the emergency department with a high fever, acute shortness of breath, and profuse diarrhoea. He is diagnosed with a chest infection and transferred to a ward but dies before any of the admitting team have seen him. The next morning, the hospital bereavement office asks the team's junior doctor to issue a medical certificate of the cause of death.

Which would be the *single* most appropriate course of action? ★★★

A Complete the certificate with 1a: Pneumonia

B Direct the office to the emergency department

C Gain permission from the family for a post-mortem

D Refer the case to the coroner

E Tell the office that the patient's general practitioner (GP) should complete the certificate

46. A 71-year-old man is transferred to the intensive therapy unit, following an aortic aneurysm repair. He has a long history of severe chronic obstructive pulmonary disease (COPD) and, as well as needing to use a number of inhalers, he takes prednisolone 20 mg oral (PO) once daily. He is nil by mouth following his surgery but still requires his daily steroid dose. Which is the *single* most appropriate equivalent intravenous (IV) hydrocortisone dose for this patient? ★★★

A Hydrocortisone 5 mg once daily

B Hydrocortisone 10 mg once daily

C Hydrocortisone 10 mg twice daily

D Hydrocortisone 20 mg three times daily

E Hydrocortisone 20 mg four times daily

47. A 32-year-old woman has been unwell for 3 weeks, initially with a headache and myalgia and latterly with a dry cough. She is a non-smoker and has no past medical history of note. She has reduced air entry bilaterally and symmetrical erythematous skin lesions that blister centrally on her arms and legs. Which is the *single* most likely causative organism? ★★★

A *Chlamydia pneumoniae*

B *Klebsiella pneumoniae*

C *Legionella pneumophila*

D *Mycoplasma pneumoniae*

E *Streptococcus pneumoniae*

48. A 21-year-old man experiences sudden right-sided chest pain while exercising. The pain persists in the emergency department, but he is not short of breath. He has no other medical problems.

T 36.6°C, HR 90 bpm, BP 115/80 mmHg, RR 18/min, SaO$_2$ 99% on air. An X-ray reveals a 1.5-cm sliver of air in the pleural space of the right lung.

Which would be the *single* most appropriate course of action? ★★★

A Admit for observation

B Aspirate the air with a needle and syringe

C Chest drain

D Discharge the man home

E Insert a 16G cannula into the second intercostal space

49. A 51-year-old man has become increasingly short of breath over a period of 3 years. He worked in ceramics and pottery until recently but has given up work early because he is unable to exert himself. He is a lifelong non-smoker. He has a chest X-ray performed. Which are the *single* most likely findings on the X-ray? ★★★

A Bilateral pleural effusions

B Large fibrotic masses in the upper zones

C Multiple bullae in the upper zones

D Nodular pattern in the upper and mid zones

E Reticulo-nodular shadowing in the lower zones

50. A 42-year-old man is being ventilated in the intensive therapy unit (ITU). He is quadriplegic, having contracted tuberculosis of the spine and has been told that he could not survive without respiratory support via his tracheostomy. His mental capacity has not been affected. He has told the doctors that he wants the ventilator to be switched off. Which is the *single* most appropriate course of action for the intensive care team? ★ ★ ★

A Continue ventilatory support as euthanasia is illegal

B Continue ventilatory support as his decision is irrational

C Stop ventilatory support only if the man has an advance directive

D Stop ventilatory support as his condition is terminal

E Stop ventilatory support if he is shown to have capacity

51. A 77-year-old man with metastatic prostate cancer dies on Sunday afternoon on a general medical ward. The junior doctor—part of the medical team looking after him—returns to work on Monday morning and is asked to fill out the required certificates. He completes the death certificate and the cremation form, thus confirming that he has seen the body after death—he plans to do this later on in the day. Unfortunately, he only remembers 3 days later. By the time he contacts the hospital mortuary, he is told the body has already been moved to the funeral directors. Which is the *single* most appropriate course of action? ★ ★ ★

A Attend the hospital mortuary and ask to see the documents relating to the man's death to confirm his identity

B Confirm the date and time of cremation with the crematorium, using that as proof of identity

C Confirm the identity of the patient with the doctor on-call at the weekend who certified the death on the ward

D Contact the patient's family and confirm that it was their relative that died at the weekend

E Go to the funeral directors and view the body before the cremation takes place

52. A 54-year-old man has felt increasingly irritable and tired over the last 6 months and on a number of occasions recently has briefly fallen asleep while driving. He has started to complain of regular headaches in the morning, and last week, quite out of character, he forgot his wife's birthday.

HR 80 bpm, BP 150/70 mmHg.

His body mass index (BMI) is 32 kg/m^2.

Which is the *single* most appropriate next step? ★★★

A Course of antidepressants

B Computed tomography (CT) scan of the head and neck

C Early morning arterial blood gases

D Sleep studies

E Thyroid function tests

53. A 72-year-old man has had a dry cough and increasing right-sided chest pain for 10 days. This is despite having just completed a 7-day course of amoxicillin 500 mg oral (PO) three times daily.

T 37.5°C, BP 85/55 mmHg, HR 100 bpm, SaO$_2$ 94% on air, RR 34/min.

Chest—decreased air entry in the right upper zone.

AMTS (abbreviated mental test score)—10/10.

Which is the *single* most appropriate next step in management? ★★★

A Amoxicillin 500 mg PO three times daily

B Amoxicillin 500 mg PO three times daily + clarithromycin 500 mg twice daily

C Ciprofloxacin 500 mg intravenous (IV) twice daily

D Co-amoxiclav 1.2 g IV three times daily + clarithromycin 500 mg twice daily

E Doxycycline 100 mg PO once daily

54. A 29-year-old lady complains of worsening intermittent wheeze and breathlessness that has been worsening despite several courses of antibiotics. She often coughs up thick brown sputum. She was given a diagnosis of asthma 3 years ago and is on a regular beclometasone 200 micrograms inhaler, two puffs twice daily (bd). She has positive immunoglobulin G (IgG) to *Aspergillus fumigatus*, a total serum immunoglobulin E (IgE) of 1024 ng/mL, and a blood eosinophil count of 1.1×10^3 cells/microlitre.

What is the *single* most appropriate next step in treatment? ★ ★ ★

A Change inhaler to inhaled corticosteroid (ICS)/long-acting beta-agonist (LABA)

B Refer for chest physiotherapy

C Start itraconazole 200 mg bd

D Start nebulized salbutamol

E Start prednisolone 40 mg once daily (od)

ANSWERS

1. E ★   OHCM 10th ed. → p. 170

If treatment for a pneumonia is not proving adequate, it is important to re-image the chest. This is especially true if the fever has not settled and continues to fluctuate, as in this example—a 'swinging pyrexia' is usually suggestive of a collection of pus somewhere. There may be an effusion amenable to drainage ('para-pneumonic'), pus in the pleural space (empyema), or, as here, an actual cavity of pus that will need a longer course of antibiotics (4–6 weeks) and may be postural drainage.

A. This indicates a pneumothorax.

B. This indicates focal consolidation.

C. This indicates a bronchial tumour.

D. This indicates bronchiectasis.

2. E ★   OHCM 10th ed. → p. 182

As per the British Thoracic Society (BTS) guidelines, any acute admission to hospital should be seen as a 'window of opportunity to review self-management skills'. Research has shown that the best way to do this is via personalized action plans. The BTS goes as far as saying that 'no patient should leave hospital without a written personalized action plan'. Certainly in cases such as this, where there has been a long gap since the last episode and where there is doubt as to what therapies have actually been taken, the best place to start is in formalizing a regimen and asking the patient to take ownership of it. The clearer the instructions, the more likely they are to be followed.

NB. As a note to option D, guidelines state that any admission should be followed up by an asthma specialist within 30 days.

3. E ★   OHCM 10th ed. → p. 810

This woman is short of breath, wheezy, and tachycardic. The most likely diagnosis is acute asthma, although anaphylaxis and a pneumothorax should be kept in mind. She is clearly compromised—unable to talk, confused, and cyanosed. This is at least a severe attack and would warrant an early call to the intensive therapy unit (ITU) while initial treatments are instigated. If her arrival had been telephoned through as a blue call by the paramedics, it would have been sensible to ensure that there was an anaesthetist on the scene to make a preliminary assessment.

However severe the case, the British Thoracic Society (BTS) guidelines are to use high-dose inhaled beta-2 agonists as first-line agents and to administer as early as possible.

A. Aminophylline infusions can be used if there has not been sufficient improvement with bronchodilators after 15–30 minutes. By this stage, however, it is likely that the ITU will have been called to make an assessment.

B. Adrenaline has a bigger role to play in anaphylaxis.

C. Give steroids in all cases of acute asthma.

D. Consider a one-off dose of magnesium sulfate in those who do not show a good initial response to bronchodilators or in life-threatening or near-fatal asthma.

British Thoracic Society, Scottish Intercollegiate Guidelines Network (2016). *British guideline on the management of asthma*. Revised 2016.

→ www.sign.ac.uk/sign-153-british-guideline-on-the-management-of-asthma.html

4. B ★   OHCM 10th ed. → p. 810

This is an acute severe asthma attack, but the woman's peak expiratory flow rate (PEFR) recovers to >75% of predicted within an hour after initial treatment, so she can be discharged, unless there are other reasons to prompt an admission. These would include: (1) she still has significant symptoms; (2) there are concerns about compliance; (3) she lives alone or is socially isolated; (4) she has psychological problems, a physical disability, or learning difficulties; (5) she has a previous history of near-fatal or brittle asthma; (6) exacerbation despite adequate-dose steroid tablets pre-presentation; (7) she presented at night; or (8) she is pregnant.

→ www.brit-thoracic.org.uk/document-library/clinical-information/asthma/btssign-asthma-guideline-2016/

5. B ★   OHCM 10th ed. → p. 810

Running out of breath before the end of a sentence, together with a peak expiratory flow rate (PEFR) of 33–50% of predicted and a heart rate (HR) >110 bpm, is consistent with a severe attack.

A and C. These indicate hypotension and a 'silent chest'.

D and E. All options suggest a life-threatening attack of asthma, largely due to poor respiratory effort as a result of exhaustion, leading to a hypercarbic state, which should prompt immediate referral to the high-dependency unit/intensive therapy unit.

6. C ★   OHCM 10th ed. → p. 182

Objective signs of losing control include:

- A history of waking at night with wheeze, cough, or chest pain (one night a week or more)
- Daytime symptoms (three times a week or more)
- Increased use of bronchodilator therapy (three times a week or more)
- Asthma attack within last 2 years
- Work days missed through asthma
- Any change in exercise tolerance.

C. This is a non-specific symptom that may suggest hyperventilation or dysfunctional breathing, but not asthma per se. It would not suggest poor asthma control, unlike the other listed options.

7. C ★   OHCM 10th ed. → p. 810

Patients should be 'stable' on their regular asthma therapy for 24 hours prior to discharge home. Their peak flow readings should be up to >75% of predicted or best. The prelude to discharge is also a good time to check the inhaler technique and that the patient has a firm management plan in place to prevent any further admissions.

→ www.sign.ac.uk/sign-153-british-guideline-on-the-management-of-asthma.html

8. A ★   OHCM 10th ed. → p. 182

The key in the management of asthma is to follow the step-up/step-down guidelines (as given in the *British Guideline on the Management of Asthma*). This woman is requiring more than one puff of her 'reliever' every day and so needs to move up to step 2 treatment, which is the addition of a regular 'preventer'. Note that Seretide® is an example of a combined preparation of a long-acting beta-agonist and an inhaled steroid (in this case, salmeterol and fluticasone), which would be a move up to step 3 treatment. The dose is always 50 micrograms of salmeterol but can be combined with 100, 250, or 500 micrograms of steroid. Inhaled corticosteroid doses may need to be titrated upward, depending on asthma control, up to a maximum dose equivalent of 1000 micrograms of beclometasone diproprionate. There are now a staggering number of new combined-preparation inhalers available on the market, so one should not be afraid to speak to your local respiratory clinical nurse specialist!

→ www.sign.ac.uk/sign-153-british-guideline-on-the-management-of-asthma.html

9. B ★   OHCM 10th ed. → p. 810

The definition of an asthma attack is: worsening cough, chest pain, breathlessness, or wheeze not relieved by a beta-agonist, resulting in breathlessness impairing speech, eating, or sleep.

→ www.asthma.org.uk/advice-asthma-attacks

10. D ★   OHCM 10th ed. → p. 810

The guidance from Asthma UK (which should form part of an asthma action plan) is as follows:

1. Sit up straight—do not lie down. Try to keep calm.
2. Take one puff of your reliever inhaler (usually blue) every 30–60 s, up to a maximum of ten puffs.

3. If you feel worse at any point while you are using your inhaler or you do not feel better after ten puffs or you are worried at any time, call 999 for an ambulance.
4. If the ambulance is taking longer than 15 minutes, you can repeat step 2.

→ www.asthma.org.uk/advice-asthma-attacks

11. C ★   OHCM 10th ed. → p. 173

The repeated lung infections that cystic fibrosis sufferers contract lead to the terminal airways remaining permanently open; the result is copious sputum production and the vicious circle of increasingly recurrent infections. Pancreatic insufficiency has led to the development of diabetes.

A. This indicates interstitial lung disease.

B and E. These indicate asthma.

D. This indicates idiopathic pulmonary fibrosis.

12. B ★   OHCM 10th ed. → p. 166

This man has the symptoms of an acute infection, with focal signs on his chest. As a smoker, he is at risk of community-acquired bacterial infections, the most common being *Streptococcus pneumoniae*. Although he is systemically unwell (rigors and tachycardia), he has no core adverse prognostic features, based on the simple and validated 'CURB-65' severity scoring system: new mental Confusion, RR >30/min, systolic BP <90 mmHg or diastolic BP <60 mmHg, and he is aged under 50. As he has no coexisting chronic illness, the British Thoracic Society guidelines are that he can be managed safely at home.

A. Although this man has a significant smoking history, early 40s would be young to develop lung cancer. This is an acute illness, with no suggestion of the kind of gradual decline that might be expected in a malignant process.

C. Granulomatosis with polyangiitis (formerly known as Wegener's granulomatosis) is a vasculitis that can present with cough and haemoptysis, but usually against a background of chronic symptoms (sinusitis, nasal ulceration, or other upper respiratory tract symptoms), rather than with an acute infection.

D. Sarcoidosis rarely presents with acute breathlessness.

E. The combination of haemoptysis and sweats means that tuberculosis is a reasonable differential diagnosis. A comprehensive travel and contact history should be taken from this man, and sputum should be sent for acid-fast bacilli, as well as microscopy, culture, and sensitivity. However, with such a short history, and with basal chest sounds and no history of weight loss, a pneumonia is more likely.

Lin WS, Baudouin SV, George RC, et al. BTS Guidelines for the management of community acquired pneumonia in adults: update 2009. 2009;*Thorax* **64**(suppl 3):iii1–55.

→ www.nice.org.uk/guidance/cg191

13. E ★

Prescriptions for controlled drugs cause confusion among doctors at all levels. They can now be computer-generated (including the date) but require the signature to be handwritten and the patient's address to be included, as well as the name and form of the medication to be supplied. The total quantity to be supplied must be written in words and figures, not the dose. The date of birth (unless for a child <12) and General Medical Council (GMC) number are not necessary.

14. B ★   OHCM 10th ed. → p. 173

This is suggestive of an infective exacerbation of cystic fibrosis, with a bronchiectatic picture. Chronic infection of the bronchi and bronchioles leads to permanent dilatation of these airways.

A. This indicates lung carcinoma.

C. This indicates systemic lupus erythematosus (SLE).

D. This indicates pulmonary embolism.

E. This indicates a Pancoast tumour.

15. D ★   OHCM 10th ed. → p. 188

This man is showing signs and symptoms of hypercapnia and type 2 respiratory failure. An increase in oxygen administration with non-rebreather masks or nasal oxygen will further increase his carbon dioxide. Although medical therapy, including nebulized bronchodilators, corticosteroids, and antibiotics, should be optimized, it is likely he will need ventilator support. Continuous positive airway pressure (CPAP) is delivered throughout the respiratory cycle but does not change during inspiration or expiration. Non-invasive ventilation (NIV) (also known as bi-level positive airway pressure or BiPAP) aids the inspiratory phase by delivering higher pressures during inspiration and dropping to CPAP during expiration. This allows retained carbon dioxide to be expired as a result of differences between the inspiratory and expiratory pressures, effecting sufficient tidal breathing. The positive end-expiratory pressure 'stents' the airways open, as well as recruits alveoli.

National Collaborating Centre for Chronic Conditions. Chronic obstructive pulmonary disease. National clinical guideline on management of chronic obstructive pulmonary disease in adults in primary and secondary care. *Thorax*. 2004;**59**(Suppl 1):1–232.

→ www.brit-thoracic.org.uk/standards-of-care/guidelines/btsics-guide-lines-for-the-ventilatory-management-of-acute-hypercapnic-respira-tory-failure-in-adults/

16. B ★   OHCM 10th ed. → p. 190

Pneumothoraces do not only afflict fit young men, but they also occur as secondary phenomena in those with established lung disease. If the volume of air in the pleural space is large enough, then classic signs elicited are: decreased air entry, reduced expansion, and a hyperresonant percussion note. These cases always require admission to hospital for either aspiration or insertion of a chest drain.

A, D, and C. These suggest consolidation, which would cause a more gradual decline in a chronic obstructive pulmonary disease (COPD) sufferer with an increasingly productive cough with or without fever.

E. This suggests fluid in the pleural space, which is unlikely to cause such sudden symptoms in someone with lung disease; indeed, there may be chronic effusions that fluctuate in volume and cause minimal symptoms.

MacDuff A, Arnold A, Harvey J; BTS Pleural Disease Guideline Group. Management of spontaneous pneumothorax: BTS pleural disease guideline 2010. *Thorax*. 2010;**65**(Suppl 2):ii8–31.

→ www.brit-thoracic.org.uk/Portals/0/Guidelines/PleuralDisease Guidelines/Pleural%20Guideline%202010/Pleural%20disease%20 2010%20pneumothorax.pdf

17. C ★   OHCM 10th ed. → p. 814

Inflammation of the costochondral joints presents insidiously until it causes severe, sharp pain originating from the anterior chest wall and often radiating around to the back. It should be on the differential diagnosis list for chest pain and—once more serious causes have been excluded—should be considered likely if there is point tenderness over the medial ribs (typically 2nd to 5th).

Although this woman has pleuritic chest pain, her observations are almost entirely normal—this would not be the case in **E** (tachycardia with or without hypoxia) or **B** (fever and tachycardia with hypoxia), whilst **D** would be very unlikely in a young woman without risk factors and would more likely present with sudden exertional pain and breathlessness, rather than gradually increasing pleuritic pain.

A may be the next most likely cause, as it can present with insidious pleuritic chest pain; however, there is also likely to be at least one additional finding: fever, tachycardia and/or tachypnoea, and not associated with tenderness on palpation.

18. C ★   OHCM 10th ed. → p. 174

The new symptoms are those of hypercalcaemia—either from skeletal metastasis or, as here, from secretion of parathyroid hormone by a squamous cell tumour. Hypercalcaemia as a result of primary hyperparathyroidism can be remembered, using:

- 'Stones'—renal stones
- 'Bones'—pain and sometimes pathological fractures (classically due to osteitis fibrosa cystica)
- 'Groans'—abdominal pain from ulcers, nausea, indigestion, or constipation
- 'Psychic moans'—lethargy, fatigue, and depression.

19. B ★   OHCM 10th ed. → p. 708

Based on the history, this nodule is likely to be a bronchial carcinoma. The right ptosis suggests that it is a Pancoast tumour, i.e. one that causes Horner's syndrome by compressing the sympathetic plexus. Features include anhidrosis, ptosis, miosis, and enophthalmos. As the tumour enlarges, it can involve the brachial plexus or recurrent laryngeal nerve.

A. This is cranial nerve (CN) XI, which innervates the trapezius and sternocleidomastoid.

C. This is CN III; this would cause a 'down-and-out', dilated pupil.

D. This would be expected to produce facial and upper limb oedema and dilated neck veins.

E. This would result in sensory loss around the eye.

20. D ★   OHCM 10th ed. → p. 175

Hyponatraemia in someone with lung cancer is suggestive of the syndrome of inappropriate antidiuretic hormone secretion (SIADH), caused by ectopic hormone secretion by a small cell tumour. These make up about 20% of lung cancers. The remainder are non-small cell and include squamous cell carcinoma, adenocarcinoma, and large cell carcinoma.

21. E ★   OHCM 10th ed. → p. 779

Audible gurgling suggests the presence of liquid material in the upper airways, which needs to be removed by a suction device such as the wide-bore rigid Yankauer sucker. Although a crash/peri-arrest call should be put out, suctioning the airway may be enough to allow sufficient ventilation to restore this man's full consciousness.

22. E ★

Although writing in notes may not always be an explicit part of the medical undergraduate curriculum, a junior doctor has to do it every day. It is also one of the few things for which he can be clearly held accountable. Even if the junior is not confident in what s/he is writing and is nervous about making bold pronouncements of diagnosis or management plans, s/he can help himself by obeying a few very simple rules:

1. Write the name and designation, and sign with the bleep number.
2. Write the time and date of review.
3. Write the reason for the review and who was present.

In cases such as this, where clinical events probably happened very quickly, it is vital in the aftermath to be able to follow them in chronological order. Omitting the time makes this very difficult. It also lessens the credibility of the entry and calls into question the professionalism of the doctor. Whilst the legal team—and indeed other doctors—may feel that this entry was also lacking for some of the other options listed, the only feature that will actually impair their dissection of events is the lack of a time.

23. B ★   OHCM 10th ed. → p. 895

Not for resuscitation means not for resuscitation. Although it is hard as a junior doctor not to react instinctively in situations like this and call the arrest team, all that is needed is careful monitoring of breathing and circulation until it is clear that death can be confirmed.

24. B ★   OHCM 10th ed. → p. 190

Sudden shortness of breath in a patient with chronic obstructive pulmonary disease (COPD) on non-invasive ventilation (NIV) should make you think of a spontaneous pneumothorax. The other findings are to be expected in someone with COPD and would not, in isolation, prompt an immediate review.

25. D ★   OHCM 10th ed. → p. 842

The key to this case is the discrepancy between the oxygen saturations and the respiratory rate—in someone who has ventilation problems, why would they be breathing so slowly? Their respiratory muscles are either tiring or being prevented from working. This patient has a reason to be on high-dose analgesia, so it would be important to examine her pupils urgently—if they are contracted, it may be that naloxone 200 micrograms intravenously (IV) will go a long way to reversing her current problems (repeated, if necessary, as it has a very short half-life and can be better given as an infusion). If opioid overdose is responsible, her ventilation rate will improve, as will her oxygen saturations and her level of consciousness.

26. E ★   OHCM 10th ed. → p. 190

Sudden-onset pleuritic chest pain is highly suggestive of a thromboembolic event, as is residual hypoxia. This man will need a computed tomography (CT) pulmonary angiogram. His wheeze is probably a sign of existing chronic obstructive pulmonary disease (COPD), but there is no evidence for an acute exacerbation such as increased sputum volume or purulence. There are no signs of cardiac ischaemia or failure.

27. D ★   OHCM 10th ed. → p. 190

The diagnosis is pulmonary embolism and, although not universal, it is most likely to cause pleuritic chest pain, which is classically worse on inspiration.

A. This would indicate a neoplastic diagnosis.

B and C. These indicate infection.

E. This indicates a lung abscess/empyema.

28. D ★ OHCM 10th ed. → p. 190

Sudden pain with breathlessness in a young man should make a primary spontaneous pneumothorax top of the list. The patient may be concerned that there is a cardiac cause and this can lead the junior doctor astray; it is therefore vital that, even with a satisfactory arterial oxygen saturation (SaO_2), if the story is convincing, a chest X-ray is performed. Often, in small pneumothoraces, there are no (or very subtle) clinical signs; indeed, tachycardia and tachypnoea may be the only findings.

A. This is a reasonable differential in a young man but is unlikely to announce itself so suddenly and does not fit with the clinical sign elicited.

B. Sudden pain is unlikely to be the presenting complaint of a chest infection. A young man is more likely to feel gradually short of breath, with an increasingly troublesome cough.

C. This is a differential not to forget but is more likely to present gradually. It should be considered once other diagnoses have been excluded and is suggested by tenderness on palpation of the costochondral joints.

E. This would also present this suddenly and possibly with the same symptoms. However, it is extremely unlikely in a young man with no risk factors, and typically there are no signs on examination of the chest.

Mackenzie SJ and Gray A. Primary spontaneous pneumothorax: why all the confusion over first-line treatment? *J R Coll Physicians Edinb.* 2007;**37**:335–8.

→ www.rcpe.ac.uk/sites/default/files/mackenziegrey.pdf

29. D ★ OHCM 10th ed. → p. 190

A hyperresonant percussion note with decreased air entry on the same side suggests that there is air in the pleural space—a pneumothorax should be top of the list when young men become suddenly breathless with chest pain, particularly when they have risk factors, as in this case (asthma and smoking), when it is classified as a secondary pneumothorax and managed differently from a primary spontaneous pneumothorax.

A, B, and C. These are all suggestive of consolidation, which would present gradually with fever and a cough.

E. This implies fluid in the pleural cavity, which again would be unlikely to cause sudden symptoms and is more likely to be the result of another process (such as pneumonia, tuberculosis, or malignancy), which would cause symptoms of its own first.

30. B ★ OHCM 10th ed. → p. 376

Patients who have had a course of steroids for shorter than 3 weeks and of doses <40 mg do not need gradual weaning, unless they have a history of repeated steroid use or previous adrenal suppression.

31. E ★

The doctor's duty is not to be protective of their own clinical reputation in front of their seniors, but to provide the safest level of patient care possible. Although it may be tempting to 'have a go', one of the most important skills for junior doctors is to recognize the limits of their abilities and not to be afraid of admitting if they are unable to carry out a particular task. To this end: 'In providing care you must recognize and work within the limits of your competence'. The arterial blood gases will give information on acid–base balance and carbon dioxide, as well as oxygen, levels and are a better indicator than peripheral saturations. The patient should not be coerced into another attempt, and the doctor would not be deemed competent just because another doctor has described the procedure to them.

General Medical Council (2013). *Good Medical Practice*, paragraph 14.

→ www.gmc-uk.org/guidance/good_medical_practice.asp

32. C ★   OHCM 10th ed. → pp. 174, 226

Abdominal pain with postural hypotension is suggestive of adrenocortical insufficiency. In a patient with lung cancer, this is most likely to be due to metastasis of the cancer to the adrenal glands, causing secondary Addison's disease.

33. A ★   OHCM 10th ed. → p. 895

Snoring occurs when the pharynx is partially occluded by the tongue or palate. It therefore heralds partial airway obstruction. In someone who is requiring assistance with his ventilation because of lower respiratory compromise, it should be reversed before too long. The aim of the manoeuvres is to stretch the anterior neck structures. If these measures succeed in stopping the snoring, but the man remains drowsy, then other issues, such as opioid or carbon dioxide toxicity, would need to be addressed. However, as in the first instance of any emergency situation, the airway needs to be managed to allow adequate ventilation.

34. C ★   OHCM 10th ed. → p. 190

As pulmonary embolism (PE) is a vital diagnosis not to miss, acute medical teams look for it everywhere. The result is a huge increase in the number of computed tomography (CT) scans performed and a decrease in the positive yield. The National Institute for Health and Care Excellence (NICE) guidance on assessing PE advocates the use of a two-level PE Wells score in order to work out the clinical probability of PE. This is a scoring system taking into account clinical evidence of deep vein thrombosis (DVT), heart rate (HR) >100 bpm, previous venous thromboembolism (VTE) episodes, haemoptysis, recent malignancy or immobility, and whether there is a more likely alternative diagnosis. If the score is >4, PE is likely, and if 4 or less PE is unlikely. In this case, the clinical probability is low. Therefore, the best first test would be a

D-dimer; if this is negative, then PE has been excluded and the diagnosis is elsewhere.

National Institute for Health and Care Excellence (2012). *Venous thromboembolic diseases: diagnosis, management and thrombophilia testing*. NICE Clinical guideline [CG144].

→ www.nice.org.uk/guidance/cg144

35. C ★   OHCM 10th ed. → pp. 184, 188

When being handed over the care of a patient by another professional, it is always important to review what has been done so far. In this case, the receiving doctor has been told that a chronic obstructive pulmonary disease (COPD) sufferer has shortness of breath that has improved with bronchodilators and low oxygen saturations that have reached 97% on 5 L.

His approach should begin with ABCDE (Airway, Breathing, Circulation, Disability, Exposure). Having assessed his airway, the next port of call is breathing—does a COPD sufferer need to have oxygen saturations in the high 90s? Could this be why he has become confused? Before considering antibiotics and imaging, it is important to ensure that oxygen delivery is sufficient and appropriate without causing compromise in other ways. The best way to do this in COPD sufferers is by titrating controlled oxygen therapy (via a Venturi mask) according to bedside oximetry, with target saturations of 88–92%. A baseline blood gas would be prudent once target saturations have been achieved, to ensure the patient is not in type 2 respiratory failure with acidosis, or indeed if there were any signs of hypercapnia such as drowsiness, confusion, or carbon dioxide (CO_2) flap. Whilst it is important to be vigilant for hypercapnia, it is also illogical to leave patients hypoxaemic. In cases where the balance is proving difficult, non-invasive ventilation (NIV) will need to be considered or, if appropriate, escalation to the Intensive Care Unit as invasive mechanical ventilation may be indicated.

→ www.brit-thoracic.org.uk/standards-of-care/guidelines/bts-guideline-for-emergency-oxygen-use-in-adult-patients/

36. E ★   OHCM 10th ed. → p. 393

This man has a history consistent with pulmonary tuberculosis. He has a productive cough that has persisted, along with weight loss and fevers, as well as classical X-ray findings. The next step would be to send sputum samples for Ziehl–Neelsen staining and culture, then to start drug treatment.

A. Computed tomography (CT) scanning may show characteristic changes such as 'tree in bud' or enlarged mediastinal lymph nodes, but is unlikely to change the treatment.

B. This man is producing sputum which can be sent for analysis and culture; therefore, bronchoscopy is not necessary.

C. Interferon gamma release assay (IGRA) testing is used for the diagnosis of latent tuberculosis.

D. Human immunodeficiency virus (HIV) would be routinely requested when investigating and treating patients with tuberculosis but would not be the *single most appropriate* next investigation.

37. E ★   OHCM 10th ed. → p. 689

The drug reaction referred to is aminophylline toxicity following the prescription of antibiotics. This is a common problem in patients with chronic obstructive pulmonary disease (COPD) who are using theophyllines, which have a narrow therapeutic range. The antibiotics most likely to cause toxicity are those that inhibit the cytochrome P450 enzyme system—erythromycin, as in this case, and ciprofloxacin.

38. A ★   OHCM 10th ed. → p. 394

This patient may have drug-induced hepatitis, which can be fatal. Symptoms include vomiting and abdominal pain, and there may be signs of jaundice. The patient should be advised to cease their medications immediately, and urgent liver function tests (LFTs) taken.

B and C. If there is no evidence of drug-induced hepatitis, using antiemetics or staggering the times of drug ingestion are strategies that may be employed to increase the tolerability of these medications.

E. Tuberculosis (TB) culture can take up to 6 weeks for a complete result but should be checked in due course to ensure the patient has fully sensitive TB.

39. B ★   OHCM 10th ed. → p. 175

Clinically, this lady has lung cancer, as evidenced by weight loss and clubbing in a smoker. She has hyponatraemia secondary to syndrome of inappropriate antidiuretic production (SIADH) that is usually caused by either ectopic antidiuretic hormone (ADH) production or stimulation of normal ADH production. This can occur in up to 10% of lung cancers (usually small cell lung cancer).

40. B ★ ★   OHCM 10th ed. → p. 814

An ascent to 5000 ft (1500 m) increases gas trapped in closed compartments by 20%, and an ascent to 8000 ft (2400 m) by 40%. A pneumothorax would therefore increase in volume by this much, and thus patients with a current pneumothorax should not fly. Previously, the British Thoracic Society's advice was to advise not to fly within 6 weeks of a pneumothorax; however, this has now changed to 1 week (slightly higher chance of recurrence) after full resolution of the pneumothorax. In the event of a traumatic pneumothorax, the advice is to wait until 2 weeks after resolution.

British Thoracic Society (2011). *Managing passengers with stable respiratory disease planning air travel: British Thoracic Society recommendations*.

→ thorax.bmj.com/content/66/Suppl_1/i1

41. D ★★★   OHCM 10th ed. → p. 190

This woman's history is suspicious for a pulmonary embolism (PE) and, as she has two major risk factors (recent surgery, malignancy), the clinical probability is high. She therefore warrants anticoagulation and imaging. It should be remembered that in 70% of cases of proven PE, there is a proximal deep vein thrombosis (DVT). Therefore, as she has clinical signs of a DVT, guidance is that leg ultrasound is the best initial test, as identification of a DVT would then preclude the need for further tests.

If there were no signs of a DVT, then a computed tomography pulmonary angiogram (CTPA) (**B**) would be preferable to a ventilation/ perfusion (V/Q) scan (**E**), as she has lung disease, which would affect the integrity of the nuclear imaging. As she has had recent pelvic surgery and now presents with a DVT, further imaging of the abdomen and pelvis (**A** and **C**) may be required at some point, but not before the DVT is clarified and the acute presentation is dealt with.

British Thoracic Society Standards of Care Committee Pulmonary Embolism Guideline Development Group. British Thoracic Society guidelines for the management of suspected acute pulmonary embolism. *Thorax*. 2003;**58**:470–84.

→ www.brit-thoracic.org.uk/document-library/clinical-information/ pulmonary-embolism/bts-guideline-for-the-management-of-suspected- acute-pulmonary-embolism/

42. A ★★★

The key to this scenario is the recognition that it is the man who is the patient, and not his daughter. Her opinion has been made clear—she may well be right about how the bad news would affect her father, but it is incumbent on every medical professional in such a situation to seek the patient's desires or 'information needs' before proceeding.

C. This singularly misses this point.

B. This would initiate the untenable situation of a man being palliated before he knows he has palliative disease.

D. This is plain deception.

E. This is cowardice that simply postpones a potentially difficult conversation. If bad news exists, then it needs to be broken. The process should begin by setting out initial goals for delivering it by listening—yes, to the patient's family, but crucially to the patient.

Rabow M and McPhee S. Beyond breaking bad news: helping patients who suffer. *Student BMJ*. 2000;**8**:45–88.

43. C ★★★

This woman's worsening clinical findings and blood gas show that her current treatment is not working. Although all options may add value at some stage, given her deterioration after 2 days of treatment, it is likely that she will need some assistance to improve her ventilation, probably in the form of continuous positive airway pressure (CPAP).

The key, however, is recognition of the downward trend. Following national guidelines, there should be appropriate local systems in place to ensure that this happens. The Royal College of Physicians (RCP) has set up a working party to standardize the National Early Warning Score (NEWS) across the National Health Service (NHS), with the aim of stratifying those patients at risk of clinical deterioration, based on their physiological observations. Those that fall into the low-risk group require continued monitoring; those in the medium-risk group need assessment by their medical team, and those in the high-risk group need urgent attention from a critical care team. The woman in this case would probably be in the high-risk group. The challenge for the junior doctor is that the information will not always be presented in this way. When confronted with a set of abnormal observations, it is vital that junior doctors perform their own risk stratification, based on local systems; they will then be more able to make the appropriate management decision, i.e. increase the frequency of observations, arrange assessment by the senior doctor from the medical team, or—as in this case—call for an urgent critical care review.

National Institute for Health and Care Excellence (2007). *Acutely ill patients in hospital: recognition of and response to acute illness in adults in hospital*. NICE Clinical guideline [CG50].

→ www.nice.org.uk/guidance/cg50

→ www.rcplondon.ac.uk/projects/outputs/national-early-warning-score-news

44. C ★★★   OHCM 10th ed. → p. 724

The drain may not be patent for a number of reasons. The holes may be occluded or in a lung fissure, or the drain may just not be in the right place to drain the remaining air. The first step is to try to unblock the tube with saline. Consultation with a respiratory physician with regard to putting the drain on a high-volume/low-pressure suction may also be worthwhile before it is removed and another re-sited, if needed.

A. For infection control reasons, drains should never be advanced.

B. This will not help the collection of air that remains and could cause a tension pneumothorax.

D. The collection of air is too large for this.

E. This is what will be required if efforts to unblock the drain are unsuccessful.

Laws D, Neville E, and Duffy J. BTS guidelines for the insertion of a chest drain. *Thorax*. 2003;**58**(Suppl 2):ii53–9.

45. B ★★★

The law requires that the certificate be completed by a doctor who attended to the patient during their last illness; 'attended to' means that they should have seen the patient at least twice. For this reason, both A and E are wrong. As this patient died within 24 hours of being in hospital, the case will need to be referred to the coroner's office. However, this should not be done by a doctor who has not seen the patient at all prior to death. Discussions about post-mortems should also be kept between the coroner and the 'attending' doctor. For these reasons, the most appropriate course of action for the junior doctor would be to direct the bereavement office back to the Emergency Department and to the attending doctor.

Dosani S. Dead cert: a guide to death certificates. *Student BMJ*. 2002;**10**:45–88.

Fertleman M. A doctor's life after a patient's death: guide to coroners and certificates. *Student BMJ*. 1997;**5**:12–13.

46. E ★★★

Prednisolone is four times the strength of hydrocortisone.

47. D ★★★   OHCM 10th ed. → p.168

The insidious presentation with 'flu-like' symptoms is classical. The skin rash is erythema multiforme.

B. *Klebsiella pneumoniae* infection is a rare cause of pneumonia. It produces cavitations, particularly in the upper lobes, in compromised populations such as the elderly and alcoholics.

48. D ★★★   OHCM 10th ed. → p. 814

As this is not secondary to other medical causes, this is a primary pneumothorax. Although the patient has some pain, he is not breathless and has a small defect; patients with small primary pneumothoraces and minimal symptoms do not require admission to hospital, but they should return should they become breathless. He will require early outpatient follow-up in a chest clinic within 2–4 weeks.

A. Admission in a primary pneumothorax may only be needed after repeated attempts to aspirate have been unsuccessful and a chest drain has been placed. Observation is more useful in secondary pneumothoraces, e.g. after a successful aspiration.

B. Aspiration can be attempted if the patient is breathless and/or there is a >2-cm rim of air on the chest X-ray. A maximum of two aspirations can be tried.

C. An intercostal chest drain should be inserted if the second attempt at aspiration of air is unsuccessful. Once air has stopped leaking, the drain should be left *in situ* for a further 24 hours prior to removal and discharge.

E. This is needle decompression and is used for tension pneumothoraces.

British Thoracic Society (2010). *Management of spontaneous pneumothorax: British Thoracic Society pleural disease guideline 2010.*

→ www.brit-thoracic.org.uk/Portals/0/Guidelines/PleuralDisease Guidelines/Pleural%20Guideline%202010/Pleural%20disease%20 2010%20pneumothorax.pdf

49. D ★★★ OHCM 10th ed. → p. 201

This man has progressive dyspnoea, following his exposure to silica during his work in ceramics. The chest X-ray appearance would show a 'miliary' or nodular pattern in the upper and mid zones and eggshell calcification of the hilar nodes.

A. This would indicate cardiac failure.

B. This would indicate progressive massive fibrosis due to progression of coal workers' pneumoconiosis.

C. This would indicate emphysematous changes.

E. This would indicate pulmonary fibrosis.

50. E ★★★ OHCM 10th ed. → p. 15

'A competent patient has the right to refuse treatment and their refusal must be respected, even if it will result in their death.'

General Medical Council (2008). Re B (Adult, refusal of medical treatment) [2002] 2 All ER 449. Right of a patient who has capacity to refuse life-prolonging treatment. In: *Consent: patients and doctors making decisions together.* General Medical Council: London.

→ www.gmc-uk.org/ethical-guidance/ethical-guidance-for-doctors/ consent

51. E ★★★

This is a strange scenario, but one in which many junior doctors find themselves. The most important point to remember is that the death certificate that is completed by the doctor is a legal document and that if he signs to say he has seen the body when he has not, he is breaking the law. The body must be seen after death by the doctor, unless he was present at the death or certified the death of the patient. If the body has left the hospital, it can be viewed at the funeral directors to satisfy this requirement.

52. D ★★★ OHCM 10th ed. → p. 194

This man has obstructive sleep apnoea (OSA) and probably snores very badly too if you asked his wife! It would be useful for this man and his wife to complete an Epworth Sleepiness Scale questionnaire. This will allow a subjective assessment of the degree of pre-treatment sleepiness. Pulse oximetry studies might be considered as a first-line approach, but in a man who has symptoms suggestive of OSA and has been sleepy while driving, he should be referred urgently to a sleep centre.

A. This man's problems will not be resolved by antidepressants.

B. He has had recurrent headaches and a change in personality, but his obesity and daytime somnolence should be investigated first to rule out OSA, as this is the overall clinical picture. If these investigations prove normal, a computed tomography (CT) head scan could be warranted.

C. This would be useful if obesity hypoventilation causing overnight hypercapnia were suspected. Early-morning blood gases reflect the overnight changes in ventilation and gas exchange.

E. This might be useful to check, considering his irritability and high body mass index (BMI), but it is not the first choice.

→ cks.nice.org.uk/obstructive-sleep-apnoea-syndrome#!topicsummary

53. D ★★★   OHCM 10th ed. → pp. 166–71

Both clinical and radiological findings are suggestive of a pneumonia affecting the right upper lobe. When planning treatment for a patient with pneumonia, it is useful to be able to stratify the severity of the infection. In the United Kingdom, this should be done using the CURB-65 scoring system.

In view of this man's age, hypotension, and tachypnoea, he scores 3; this grades his pneumonia as of high severity and therefore in need of hospital admission (this is without even taking the urea into account, as here—as is often the case in clinical practice—it is not available when the assessment has to be made). For those in this category, immediate treatment with parenteral antibiotics is advised. The antibiotics of choice are a broad-spectrum beta-lactamase stable antibiotic such as co-amoxiclav, together with a macrolide like clarithromycin.

→ www.brit-thoracic.org.uk/standards-of-care/guidelines/bts-guide-lines-for-the-management-of-community-acquired-pneumonia-in-adults-update-2009/

54. E ★★★   OHCM 10th ed. → p. 177

This lady has allergic bronchopulmonary aspergillosis (ABPA), which affects 1–5% of asthmatics. It results from type 1 and type 2 hypersensitivity reactions to *Aspergillus fumigatus*. In this case, the patient is losing control of her asthma, is producing purulent sputum, and has biochemical evidence of ABPA, with positive *Aspergillus* precipitins, total serum immunoglobulin E (IgE) >1000 ng/mL, and blood eosinophilia. The mainstay of treatment would be to start a course of prednisolone 30–40 mg per day, weaning down to a maintenance dose of 5–10 mg per day. The differential would include Churg–Strauss/eosinophilic granulomatosis with polyangiitis (EGPA), eosinophilic pneumonia, parasites, and drug-induced eosinophilic pneumonia.

A. This may help with the overall control of her asthma but is unlikely to treat ABPA.

B. This lady may need chest physiotherapy, as ABPA can cause thick mucus plugs that patients find difficult to expectorate.

C. Treatment with itraconazole has been shown by several randomized controlled trials (RCTs) to reduce steroid requirements and improve symptoms, but it is not the first-line treatment.

D. Nebulized bronchodilators are usually used in the context of an acute asthma attack.

Chapter 3

Endocrinology

Maria Phylactou

Since 1905, when Professor Ernest Starling first used the term 'hormone' in one of four Croonian lectures at the Royal College of Physicians, a lot has changed in the world of endocrinology. Endocrinology is the study of hormones and subsequent pathologies that arise from their imbalance. Endocrinology is also a specialty of common sense where application of basic physiological principles, such as negative feedback loops, can help any doctor appropriately interpret blood test results and form a management plan.

Diabetes forms a large part of the specialty and is becoming one of the most prevalent conditions of our time. A solid understanding of its diagnosis, management, and complications is a paramount skill that every doctor should possess in this day and age. New developments in the management of type 1 diabetes with insulin pumps and new drug-targeted treatments of obesity and the metabolic syndrome make this an exciting and ever changing field. But diabetes also offers the treating clinician the challenge of investing in their patient's education and identifying and addressing the lifestyle, social, and psychological impacts of the disease.

Whilst the main aim of this chapter is to arrive at a working practical knowledge of diabetes, it will also raise awareness of the other glands, so that their dysfunction can be recognized and investigated where appropriate.

QUESTIONS

1. A 32-year-old woman has lost 3 kg of weight over the past 3 months. She has no loss of appetite but has felt rather irritable and 'stressed'.

T 37.1°C, HR 120 bpm, BP 100/65 mmHg.

There is a fine tremor of both hands.

Her thyroid function tests are returned as follows:

Thyroid-stimulating hormone (TSH) 0.15 mU/L, free thyroxine (fT4) 36 pmol/L.

She is started on propranolol three times daily. Which is the *single* most appropriate next step in management? ★

A Amiodarone

B Carbimazole

C Levothyroxine

D Radioiodine therapy

E Tri-iodothyronine

2. A 68-year-old man undergoes annual retinal screening for his type 2 diabetes, for which he uses insulin twice daily. Following the scan, he asks his doctor what causes the presence of 'cotton-wool' spots in his report.

Which is the *single* most appropriate response? ★

A Areas of tissue starved of oxygen

B Deposits of fat

C Formation of new blood vessels

D Small bleeds

E Small swollen vessels

3. A 40-year-old man is acutely confused. He has an uncontrollable thirst, along with regular polyuria of >5L a day.

Serum osmolality 296 mOsmol/kg

Urine osmolality 280 mOsmol/kg; increases to 620 mOsmol/kg after desmopressin 20 micrograms nasally.

Which is the *single* most appropriate explanation for his symptoms? ★

A Decreased secretion of antidiuretic hormone (ADH) by the pituitary

B Impaired response of the kidney to ADH

C Inappropriately high secretion of ADH by the pituitary

D Primary polydipsia

E Renal hypersensitivity to ADH

4. An 18-year-old man has had abdominal pain for the past 24 hours. He has been unwell for the last few weeks. He has lost 10 kg in weight and has been taking a large bottle of water to bed every night.

T 37.5°C, HR 115 bpm, BP 110/70 mmHg, RR 30/min.

He is clammy, aggressive, and confused. Which is the *single* most likely diagnosis? ★

A Addisonian crisis

B Diabetes insipidus

C Diabetic ketoacidosis (DKA)

D Hyperaldosteronism

E Syndrome of inappropriate antidiuretic hormone secretion (SIADH)

5. A 78-year-old woman is admitted for elective repair of a femoral hernia. She is assessed the night before her surgery, at which time the examination reveals a previously undocumented finding (Figure 3.1). The patient has not noticed it before and seems untroubled by it. Which *single* further feature from the history is most likely to support the diagnosis? ★

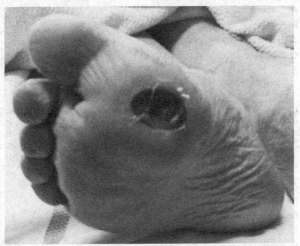

Figure 3.1

A Aching calves after long periods of standing

B Impaired sensation in feet

C Pain in feet when walking

D Persistent swelling resistant to treatment

E Recent history of trauma

6. A 28-year-old man has noticed that the tissue around his breasts has become increasingly swollen. They are non-tender. He has recently started chemotherapy for testicular cancer. Which is the *single* most likely biochemical cause for this change? ★

A Decreased androgen

B Decreased dopamine

C Increased growth hormone

D Increased oestrogen:androgen ratio

E Increased prolactin

7. A 70-year-old man has been feeling progressively more tired for 2 weeks. He has been drinking increasingly large volumes of fluid each day and passing more urine than normal.

Random capillary blood glucose: 42 mmol/L.

Arterial blood gases: pH 7.37, PaO₂ 10.9 kPa, PaCO₂ 4.8 kPa, HCO₃ 20 mmol/L.

Which is the *single* most likely precipitant for these symptoms? ★

A Diabetes insipidus

B First-presentation type 1 diabetes

C First-presentation type 2 diabetes

D Pancreatic cancer

E Poorly controlled type 1 diabetes

8. A 28-year-old woman has felt increasingly irritable over the last few months. She describes herself as 'hot and bothered'—she is always trying to cool herself down and is always sweating. She has lost 5 kg in weight during this time. She smokes 20 cigarettes a day and drinks 30 units of alcohol a week. Which *single* examination finding is most likely to support the diagnosis? ★

A Dry skin and hair

B Exophthalmos

C Hyperpigmented skinfolds

D Lymphadenopathy

E Malar rash

9. An 82-year-old man has become unresponsive. Earlier that morning, he had been talking with the nursing staff, although he declined breakfast. He has atrial fibrillation and type 2 diabetes, and uses high-dose analgesia for severe osteoarthritis.

T 35.2°C, HR 120 bpm, BP 175/100 mmHg, RR 22/min, SaO$_2$ 95% on air.

Glasgow Coma Scale (GCS) score: 10/15 (E2, V3, M5).

He is pale and shaking. There is weakness in all four limbs. Which is the *single* most likely cause of his sudden deterioration? ★

A Gastrointestinal haemorrhage

B Hypoglycaemia

C Hypothermia

D Opioid overdose

E Stroke

10. A 58-year-old man has been attempting to control his blood glucose using dietary measures and exercise for the past 9 months. At the start of this period, his fasting blood glucose was 6.8 mmol/L. Despite his efforts, his fasting glucose is now 8.4 mmol/L. His body mass index (BMI) is 32 kg/m^2. Which would be the *single* most appropriate course of action? ★

A Gliclazide

B Metformin

C No drug treatment indicated

D Pioglitazone

E Sitagliptin

11. A 78-year-old woman has a lump in her neck, which was first noticed by her daughter 3 months ago. There is an obvious midline swelling. It is hard, but non-tender and contains several discrete lumps. It moves on swallowing, but not on protrusion of the tongue. There are no associated lymph nodes and no dullness to percussion over the sternum. Which is the *single* most likely cause of the swelling? ★

A Graves' disease

B Hashimoto's thyroiditis

C Multinodular goitre

D Physiological goitre

E Subacute thyroiditis

12. A 60-year-old woman has felt generally weak and unwell with a headache for the past year or so. Apart from mild central obesity, the only point of note on examination is the loss of lateral gaze in the right eye. A magnetic resonance imaging (MRI) scan reveals a tumour originating from the pituitary fossa. Which *single* structure is the tumour most likely to have impinged? ★

A Cavernous sinus

B Internal carotid artery

C Optic chiasm

D Sphenoid sinus

E Suprasellar cistern

13. A 68-year-old man undergoes retinal screening. He has type 2 diabetes and uses insulin twice daily. He is told that there is evidence of new vessel formation and asks his doctor for the significance of this finding. Which is the *single* most appropriate response? ★

A Areas of the eye that had previously been damaged have regenerated

B He is likely to lose sight in this eye within 3 months

C His diabetic control is good and his vision is improving

D His disease is progressing and getting harder to control

E This is a normal finding in someone with type 2 diabetes

14. A 40-year-old woman is on a self-imposed fast. She has insulin-dependent diabetes, a transplanted kidney, and paranoid schizophrenia.

Urine dipstick: ketones 3+.

Random capillary blood glucose: 28 mmol/L.

She is refusing all medical help. Which is the *single* most appropriate course of action? ★

A Assess her capacity to make such a decision

B Gain consent for treatment from her next of kin

C Respect her wishes and withhold treatment

D Treat her under 'common law'

E Treat her under a section of the Mental Health Act 2007

15. A 17-year-old man has lost 6 kg over the past 2 months. He has also been excessively thirsty and not his usual self. His random lab glucose was 16 mmol/L.

Which is the *single* most appropriate next step in management? ★

A 24-hour capillary glucose diary

B Fasting venous blood glucose

C Oral glucose tolerance test (OGTT)

D Repeat random venous blood glucose

E Start treatment for diabetes

16. A 72-year-old man has had progressively severe pain, tingling, and tightness in both feet, especially at night, over the past year. He has type 2 diabetes and takes metformin 850 mg twice daily. Which *single* examination finding would be most likely to confirm the cause? ★

A Decreased distal vibration sense

B Excessive haemosiderin deposition

C Increased ankle reflexes

D Tenderness over the short saphenous veins

E Wasted quadriceps muscles

17. A 33-year-old woman stopped menstruating 3 months ago. She has also noticed milky discharge from her breasts.

She is currently being treated for type 1 diabetes, depression, benign positional vertigo, and back pain.

Serum beta-human chorionic gonadotropin (β-hCG) was negative.

Which *single* drug is most likely to have caused these new symptoms? ★

A Codeine phosphate

B Gabapentin

C Insulin

D Prochlorperazine

E Venlafaxine

18. A 49-year-old woman has felt tired over the last few months, and her thyroid function tests are returned as follows:

Thyroid-stimulating hormone (TSH) 6.8 mU/L, free thyroxine (fT4) 19 pmol/L.

She has no detectable goitre. Which is the *single* most likely explanation for the blood results? ★

A Hashimoto's thyroiditis

B Iodine deficiency

C Sick euthyroidism

D Subclinical hypothyroidism

E Unknown use of levothyroxine

19. A 50-year-old woman presents with a 3-day history of tingling in her fingers, followed by an intense 4-hour period where her jaw and right hand locked up. She recalls a similar episode 20 years ago that required hospital admission. She is housebound due to bad osteo-arthritis, has hypertension, and has been treated for depression in the past. Her body mass index (BMI) is 40 kg/m². Which *single* investigation would be most useful in the immediate management of symptoms? ★

A Calcium

B Cortisol

C Random blood glucose

D Thyroid-stimulating hormone (TSH)

E Urea and electrolytes

20. A 44-year-old man has had a hoarse voice for the past year. He has otherwise been well, but in passing he mentions that his shoe size has increased over the past 3 or 4 years. He has a protruding jaw and a large tongue. Which is the *single* most appropriate definitive test to support the likely diagnosis ★

A Insulin-like growth factor 1 (IGF-1)

B Insulin tolerance test, with growth hormone

C Oral glucose tolerance test (OGTT), with growth hormone

D Random capillary blood glucose

E Random growth hormone

21. A 64-year-old woman had a blood test for an insurance medical. Her results are all normal, except for her thyroid function tests, which are as follows:

Thyroid-stimulating hormone (TSH) 8.7 mU/L, free thyroxine (fT4) 11 pmol/L.

She has no symptoms or detectable goitre. Which is the *single* most appropriate initial management? ★

A Measure serum thyroid peroxidase antibodies

B Refer for radioiodine therapy

C Review thyroid function in 1 year

D Start a 'block and replace' regimen

E Start levothyroxine

22. A 36-year-old man has had intermittent abdominal pain associated with nausea for several years. He has recently started to feel faint, particularly on standing. He has areas of dark skin, most notably in the creases of his palms. Which is the *single* most appropriate option below that, in *high circulating levels*, could explain these skin changes? ★

A Adrenocorticotrophic hormone (ACTH)

B Aldosterone

C Caeruloplasmin

D Growth hormone

E Iron

23. A 77-year-old woman is delirious, drowsy and intermittently agitated. Her daughter reports that she stopped eating and drinking a few days ago and was diagnosed with a urinary tract infection by her general practitioner (GP). Her venous gas shows a glucose level of 47 mmol/L.

T 37.8°C, HR 120 bpm, BP 100/75 mmHg.

She is dehydrated and struggling to stay awake. Which is the *single* most appropriate course of action? ★

A Glucagon 4 mg intravenous (IV) immediately (STAT)

B Glucose 10% 200 mL IV

C Insulin 4 U IV STAT

D Sodium bicarbonate (NaHCO₃) 500 mL IV

E Saline 0.9% 1 L IV

24. A 44-year-old woman has had intermittent palpitations over the past 6 months. They are associated with anxiety and make it difficult for her to breathe normally. She also feels hot during these episodes and sweats.

T 36.6°C, HR 120 bpm, BP 115/85 mmHg.

Thyroid-stimulating hormone (TSH) 0.33 mU/L, thyroxine (T4) 198 nmol/L.

Which is the *single* most appropriate initial treatment for this woman's symptomatic relief? ★

A Carbimazole 40 mg oral (PO) once daily

B Digoxin 125 micrograms PO once daily

C Levothyroxine 125 micrograms PO once daily

D Propranolol 40 mg PO four times daily

E Propylthiouracil 30 mg PO once daily

25. A 45-year-old man has felt unwell for a year. He reports low libido and an inability to sustain an erection. He has also noticed that he is shaving less frequently and has occasional milk production from the nipples. After extensive investigations, a magnetic resonance imaging (MRI) scan shows an 8-mm tumour originating from the pituitary fossa. He is started on a drug to increase a particular hormone/neurotransmitter. Which is the *single* most likely target of his drug therapy? ★

A Dopamine

B Growth hormone

C Oestrogen

D Prolactin

E Testosterone

26. A 52-year-old woman has felt more tired than usual over the last 6 months, and her thyroid function tests are returned as follows:

Thyroid-stimulating hormone (TSH) 11.1 mU/L, free thyroxine (fT4) 14 pmol/L.

She has no detectable goitre. Which is the *single* most appropriate initial management? ★

A Measure anti-TSH antibodies

B Measure total tri-iodothyronine (T3) levels

C Refer for radioiodine therapy

D Start a 'block and replace' regimen

E Start levothyroxine

27. A 24-year-old man has suffered a headache with blurred vision for the past year. He has felt continually tired and also reports having to pass urine much more regularly than before. A range of preliminary tests are run:

Random venous blood glucose 10.7 mmol/L, fasting venous blood glucose 8.9 mmol/L, glycosylated haemoglobin (HbA1c) 6.4%, random capillary glucose 14.4 mmol/L.

Urine dipstick: glucose 2+.

Which *single* result should be given the most consideration in making a diagnosis of diabetes? ★

A Fasting venous blood glucose

B HbA1c

C Random capillary blood glucose

D Random venous blood glucose

E Urine dipstick

28. A 57-year-old man is started on a drug to reduce his blood glucose. The general practitioner (GP) warns him that it can cause hypoglycaemia. Which is the *single* most likely medication he is taking? ★

A Dapagliflozin

B Gliclazide

C Metformin

D Pioglitazone

E Sitagliptin

29. A 27-year-old woman has recently become constipated despite using a good dose of macrogol (osmotic laxative) given by a previous doctor. She feels exhausted, has lost her appetite, and is getting recurrent episodes of abdominal pain.

She has multiple areas of paler skin on her face.

T 36.3°C, HR 82 bpm, BP 90/60 mmHg.

Abdomen—soft, general discomfort, not distended.

Which *single* pathological process is most likely to have caused these symptoms? ★

A Autoimmune

B Infarction

C Infection

D Malignancy

E Vasculitis

30. A 19-year-old woman with type 1 diabetes has been vomiting and had diarrhoea for the last 24 hours. She is thirsty but has not vomited for the last 4 hours. She is assessed in the emergency department.

Normally she uses:

Novorapid® during the day: 10–12 U at breakfast, 16–20 U at lunch and dinner

Insulin glargine 38 U at night.

T 37.7°C, HR 90 bpm, BP 100/60 mmHg, glucose 15.8 mmol/L.

Urine dipstick: ketones 1+.

What is the *single* most appropriate advice in this situation? ★

A Admission for intravenous (IV) fluids

B Give extra rapid-acting insulin

C Halve the rapid-acting insulin dose, in line with her reduced calorie intake

D Limit her to just sips each hour for the next 12 hours to prevent vomiting

E Omit long-acting insulin in the evening until vomiting has stopped

31. You are asked to review a 27-year-old patient on the post-natal ward who is complaining of a headache, abdominal pain, and drowsiness. She gave birth 48 hours ago and has not been able to breastfeed since. Before you see her, you review her delivery notes and realize she had a postpartum haemorrhage that required a blood transfusion. BP 90/50 mm/Hg, Glasgow Coma Scale (GCS) score 13/15 (E3, V4, M6). Biochemistry: sodium (Na) 119 mmol/L, potassium (K) 3.7 mmol/L, urea (Ur) 9.2 mmol/L, creatinine (Cr) 56 micromoles/L.

Which is the *single* best explanation for the pathological process behind her symptoms? ★

A Addisonian crisis

B Diabetes insipidus

C Hypoglycaemia

D Metabolic acidosis

E Pituitary necrosis

32. A 42-year-old woman is referred by her general practitioner (GP) with constipation, low mood and a history of renal stones. Her GP organized some blood tests after she was found to have a frac-ture of her lumbar spine.

Corrected calcium 2.82 mmol/L, parathyroid hormone (PTH) 12.7 pmol/L, vitamin D 73 nmol/L, creatinine (Cr) 43 micromoles/L.

Which is the *single* best explanation for the pathological process behind her symptoms? ★

A Primary hyperparathyroidism

B Sarcoidosis

C Malignancy

D Hyperthyroidism

E Tertiary hyperparathyroidism

33. A 33-year-old woman has had two 'funny turns' in the past month. She has recently finished a long course of steroids, having been diagnosed with ulcerative colitis 1 year ago.

Which *single* investigation is most likely to support the diagnosis? ★★

A Calculate the aldosterone:renin ratio

B Collect urine for 24-hour free catecholamines

C Collect urine for 24-hour free cortisol

D Give dexamethasone, checking cortisol before and after

E Give tetracosactide, checking cortisol before and after

34. A 52-year-old man has gained 10 kg in weight in the past year. He feels as though he has lost all his energy and is low in mood.

8 a.m. cortisol: 678 mg/L.

His abdomen is distended and is shown in Figure 3.2.

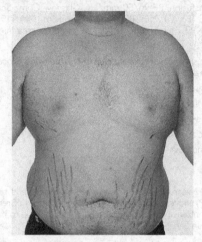

Figure 3.2

Reproduced with permission from Gardiner M.D, and Borley N.R., *Training in Surgery*, figure 3.18, p. 59. Copyright (2009) with permission from Oxford University Press.

Which is the *single* most appropriate subsequent investigation? ★★

A Computed tomography (CT) of the adrenal glands

B Dexamethasone suppression test

C Midnight cortisol levels

D Magnetic resonance imaging (MRI) of the pituitary gland

E Plasma adrenocorticotrophic hormone (ACTH) levels

35. A 40-year-old woman has had recurrent faints. Most recently, she had been sitting on a bus and as she stood, she felt instantly light-headed and could not stop herself from falling.

T 36.6°C, HR 90 bpm, BP (lying) 125/80 mmHg, BP (standing) 85/55 mmHg. Sodium 128 micromoles/L, potassium 5.8 mmol/L, urea 4.4 mmol/L, creatinine 88 micromoles/L.

Which is the *single* most appropriate medical management? ★★

A Doxazosin 4 mg oral (PO) once daily

B Enalapril 2.5 mg PO once daily

C Fludrocortisone 100 mg PO once daily

D Furosemide 40 mg PO once daily

E Midodrine 10 mg PO once daily

36. A 66-year-old woman is leaving hospital, having been treated for a broad complex tachycardia. She received two doses of amiodarone 300 mg intravenous (IV) and then an oral loading dose, before being discharged on 100 mg oral (PO) once daily. Which is the *single* most appropriate management of potential side effects? ★★★

A Check thyroid function in 6 months

B Only check thyroid function if symptoms develop

C Prophylactic carbimazole 20 mg PO once daily

D Prophylactic levothyroxine 50 micrograms PO once daily

E Ultrasound scan of thyroid gland in 3 months

37. A 72-year-old woman attends a routine diabetes outpatient clinic. At her previous check-up 1 year ago, she was told that her eyes were 'normal'. She takes metformin 500 mg oral (PO) twice daily. Fundoscopy is performed (Figure 3.3).

Which is the *single* most likely mechanism behind the appearance seen on fundoscopy? ★★★

A Capillary endothelial change

B Fibrosis of vessels

C Microvascular haemorrhage

D Neovascularization

E Retinal ischaemia

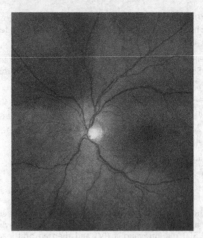

Figure 3.3

Reproduced with permission from Sundaram V., Barsam A., Alwitry A., Khaw P.T., *Training in Ophthalmology*, figure 4.13, p. 157. Copyright (2009) with permission from Oxford University Press.

38. A 55-year-old man has suffered intermittent bouts of extreme anxiety over the last 6 months. He has also experienced recurrent headaches and occasional palpitations and lost 5 kg. He has recently started taking lisinopril, bendroflumethiazide, and atenolol.

HR 60 bpm, BP 190/105 mmHg.

Which *single* hormone or hormone group is most likely to be the cause? ★★★

A Aldosterone

B Catecholamines

C Glucocorticoids

D Growth hormone

E Parathyroid hormone

39. A 33-year-old man has had diarrhoea and vomiting for the last 24 hours. He is starting to feel weak and very lethargic. He takes hydrocortisone 20 mg oral (PO) once daily for Addison's disease.

T 38.1°C, HR 100 bpm, BP 105/70 mmHg.

Which is the *single* most appropriate management? ★ ★ ★

A Double the daily dose to hydrocortisone 40 mg

B Give hydrocortisone 100 mg intramuscular (IM) immediately (STAT)

C Halve the daily dose to hydrocortisone 10 mg

D Increase the daily dose to hydrocortisone 25 mg

E Stop steroids immediately

40. A 75-year-old man has been increasingly irritable, lethargic, and low in mood for 6 months. He has hypertension, chronic kidney disease, and type 2 diabetes, and had an anterior circulation stroke last year. He takes metformin, phenytoin, and bendroflumethiazide. His 8 a.m. cortisol is marginally raised and remains so, even after suppression with dexamethasone 1 mg oral (PO). Which *single* factor from the history might explain a false positive result? ★ ★ ★

A Decreased glomerular filtration rate (GFR)

B Diuretic use

C Phenytoin use

D Presence of diabetes

E Presence of peripheral vascular disease

41. A 66-year-old man has been referred to an ophthalmologist. He was seen 9 months ago in a diabetes clinic with what the registrar described at the time as 'pre-proliferative' changes. He is currently on metformin 850 mg oral (PO) twice daily and gliclazide 160 mg PO twice daily. Fundoscopy is performed and reveals new vessel formation (Figure 3.4).

Which *single* mechanism is most likely to be responsible for the changes seen on fundoscopy? ★ ★ ★

A Excessive deposition of lipids

B Fibrosis of vessels

C Neovascularization

D Osmotic change in the lens

E Retinal ischaemia

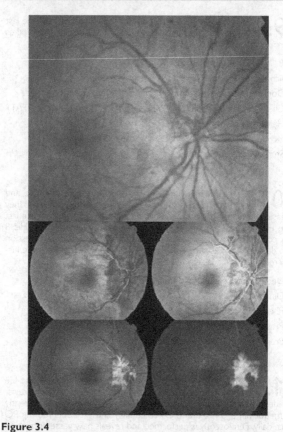

Figure 3.4

Reproduced with permission from Sundaram V, Barsam A, Barker L, Khaw PT, *Training in Ophthalmology*, Second edition, figure 6.17, p. 209. Copyright (2016) with permission from Oxford University Press.

42. A 66-year-old man is admitted with abdominal pain and distension and vomiting, and his bowels have not opened for 3 days. He is rehydrated with intravenous (IV) fluids, and his abdominal X-ray shows multiple distended loops of small bowel. He has recently been diagnosed with type 2 diabetes and takes metformin 500 mg oral (PO) three times daily. A computed tomography (CT) abdomen with IV contrast is booked for the following day. The nursing staff ask you whether metformin should be continued.

Sodium 137 mmol/L, potassium 4.3 mmol/L, creatinine 67 micromoles/L.

Which is the *single* most appropriate course of action? ★ ★ ★ ★

A Continue metformin and give IV fluids for 24 hours after the scan

B Continue metformin, but do not give IV contrast with the scan

C No additional precautions are required

D Stop metformin before the scan and restart 48 hours after

E Stop metformin before the scan and restart the morning after

ANSWERS

1. B ★   OHCM 10th ed. → p. 218

Having addressed symptom control with a beta-blocker, the next stage is to reduce circulating levels of thyroid hormones. This can be achieved with the use of antithyroid medication: carbimazole or propylthiouracil. Two strategies can be used: titration of the antithyroid drug according to thyroid function tests; or block and replace, with simultaneous administration of the antithyroid medication with levothyroxine.

A. Amiodarone is a cause of thyroid disease, rather than a cure.

C. More thyroid hormone without an appropriate blocking agent would clearly make things worse.

D. Radioiodine therapy is used in cases of relapse or after a period of medical therapy in resistant cases of hyperthyroidism.

E. Tri-iodothyronine (T3) is sometimes used in the treatment of hypo-thyroidism where there is difficulty achieving a euthyroid state with levothyroxine alone.

2. A ★   OHCM 10th ed. → p. 210

Cotton-wool spots are also known as 'soft exudates' and are yellowish-white discolorations of the retina. They are local infarcts of the surface of the retina that occur due to impaired blood supply. Along with haemorrhages (**D**) and venous beading, they are signs of retinal ischaemia, which constitutes pre-proliferative retinopathy. Good blood glucose and blood pressure control are vital to prevent progression to proliferative retinopathy. The patient should be referred to an ophthalmologist.

B. Lipid deposits are known as 'hard exudates' and are seen in background retinopathy.

C. Once new vessels start forming, proliferative retinopathy has begun, which requires urgent referral for laser treatment.

E. This refers to microaneurysms, or 'dots', that are also seen in background retinopathy.

3. A ★   OHCM 10th ed. → p. 241

This is diabetes insipidus, which can be cranial or nephrogenic. In this case, the fact that the urine becomes concentrated after administration of synthetic antidiuretic hormone (ADH) (desmopressin) shows that the problem lies in the pituitary (production of ADH), rather than the kidneys (site of action). The high serum osmolality points against primary polydipsia where you would expect a low serum and urine osmolality.

4. C ★   OHCM 10th ed. → p. 832

This is a typical first presentation of type 1 diabetes: weight loss, lethargy, polydipsia, and polyuria. The lack of insulin and subsequent hyperglycaemia are causing osmotic diuresis. Untreated, this will result in increasing confusion, coma, and death.

A. This is a reasonable differential for a young man presenting with increasing lethargy culminating in shock, but is much less likely than diabetic ketoacidosis (DKA). It is not associated with polyuria and polydipsia but rather causes hypoglycaemia instead.

B. This is a good thought in cases of polydipsia but is a much less common cause than DKA. It is less likely to result in profound dehydration and shock.

D. This is usually asymptomatic, although it can present with polydipsia (more as a result of hypokalaemia, rather than dehydration).

E. This causes hyponatraemia, and therefore confusion, but without the other features of this case—especially thirst. It is unlikely to develop without a precipitant such as a head injury, malignancy, or specific drug use.

5. B ★   OHCM 10th ed. → p. 212

This is the classical image of a diabetic foot ulcer induced by peripheral neuropathy—'punched out' and over an area of hard callus. Patients are usually pain-free and suffering from reduced sensation in a 'glove and stocking' distribution. These are at very high risk of deterioration and need urgent input from a specialist diabetic foot multidisciplinary team.

A. This is suggestive of venous disease.

C. This occurs in arterial disease.

D. This is lymphoedema.

E. Traumatic or thermal injuries sometimes precipitate these ulcers, but the hallmark of presentation is peripheral sensory neuropathy.

6. D ★   OHCM 10th ed. → p. 230

Increased breast tissue (gynaecomastia) should not be confused with galactorrhoea (spontaneous flow of milk from the nipples), which is caused by high levels of prolactin (E and, by association, B). A range of drugs and some oestrogen-secreting tumours—such as testicular—alter the oestrogen:androgen ratio. Low androgen levels (A) on their own do not cause breast tissue growth—it is how they relate to oestrogen levels that is crucial. High levels of growth hormone (C) do cause excessive soft tissue growth but do not commonly affect breast tissue and are not implicated in this scenario.

7. C ★   OHCM 10th ed. → p. 834

The very high blood glucose, coupled with a normal pH, points away from diabetic ketoacidosis, being more typical of a hyperosmolar hyperglycaemic non-ketotic state (HHS).

A. The history of polyuria and polydipsia would fit, but the very high blood sugar and the lethargy would not.

B. It would be unlikely for type 1 diabetes to present at this age. It does not usually present with glucose levels quite this high, as patients tend to present earlier due to acidosis.

D. Although diabetes can (rarely) be an early sign of pancreatic cancer (particularly in the elderly), such a short history, on a background of no other suspicious symptoms, makes this unlikely in this case.

E. This is possible in theory, but someone with type 1 diabetes is unlikely to allow sugars to creep this high without adjusting their insulin regimen. The protracted history is unlikely in someone with known disease, as they are more attuned to the fluctuation of their sugars and better equipped to take appropriate action more quickly.

8. B ★ OHCM 10th ed. → p. 218

The features described (overheating, sweating, weight loss, tachycardia) are those of a hypermetabolic state often associated with hyperthyroidism. Exophthalmos is suggestive of Graves' disease, which is the most common cause of thyrotoxicosis, especially in this age group.

A. This is a feature of hypothyroidism in which metabolism is slowed down, leading to cold intolerance, weight gain, and constipation.

C. These are found in Addison's disease (adrenocortical insufficiency), which is more likely to present with lethargy, dizziness, and aches and pains.

D. Lymphoproliferative disease could also present in a similar way, but thyroid dysfunction is more common. This patient should be examined for lymphadenopathy and organomegaly.

E. This is suggestive of systemic lupus erythematosus (SLE)—a reasonable differential in a young woman with vague systemic symptoms, but more likely to present alongside more concrete findings such as arthritis, serositis, or a rash.

9. B ★ OHCM 10th ed. → p. 214

All patients with a low Glasgow Coma Scale (GCS) score should have a capillary blood glucose check, as part of their initial ABCDEFG assessment (DEFG = Don't Ever Forget Glucose!). Furthermore all inpatients with diabetes should have close monitoring of their blood glucose. Their intercurrent illness and potential change in diet will affect their glycaemic control. This patient might have received his insulin in the morning, even though he did not have breakfast or may be on oral antiglycaemic agents which could have accumulated in acute renal impairment.

A. This is possible if he were on high-dose non-steroidal anti-inflammatory drugs (NSAIDs), but there are no suggestive symptoms. Furthermore, such an episode would cause hypotension.

C. Hypothermia is defined as a body temperature below 35° C but is unlikely to cause such severe symptoms, unless the temperature is <32°C.

D. This is another cause of a low GCS score but would cause a low respiratory rate and constricted pupils.

E. This would present with focal, rather than global, weakness due to the focal nature of blood vessel blockage from the thrombus.

10. B ★ OHCM 10th ed. → p. 207

This man has progressed from a diagnosis of impaired fasting glucose to type 2 diabetes and cannot continue on dietary control alone (**D**). Metformin is the first-line drug of choice, particularly given his raised body mass index (BMI).

A. Sulfonylureas should be considered as a first-line treatment if the patient does not tolerate metformin (or if metformin is contraindicated). They can be added as dual therapy to metformin if HbA1c is still >58 mmol/mol.

D. Thiazolidinediones can also be added as dual therapy with metformin or as third-line therapy with metformin and sulfonylureas.

E. Dipeptidyl peptidase 4 (DDP4) inhibitors can be added to metformin if HbA1c is >58 mmol/mol or as triple therapy to metformin and sulfonylureas.

National Institute for Health and Care Excellence (2015). *Type 2 diabetes in adults: management. NICE guideline* [NG28].

→ www.nice.org.uk/guidance/ng28

11. C ★ OHCM 10th ed. → p. 219

If there are discrete lumps in a thyroid swelling, then it is a nodular goitre. In this case, all options, apart from **C**, cause a diffuse 'smooth' goitre. *Single*-nodule goitres can represent cysts, adenomas, or—very rarely—cancers.

12. A ★ OHCM 10th ed. → p. 234

Lateral gaze is controlled by the abducens nerve (cranial nerve VI). It courses through the cavernous sinus, lateral and beneath the pituitary fossa where it has been affected by invasion or pressure from the tumour.

13. D ★ OHCM 10th ed. → p. 210

This patient has evidence of proliferative retinopathy. New vessel formation, or 'neovascularization', is the growth of new fragile blood vessels from the retina. As they tend to form on ischaemic areas, they represent worsening diabetic retinopathy and imply suboptimal blood glucose control. The vessels can bleed, cause scarring, and even cause retinal detachment. Despite this, it would be wrong to tell the patient that he will lose his sight in 3 months (**B**). The patient should be referred to a specialist on an urgent basis for consideration of laser treatment of the new vessels, whilst stressing the need to strive for optimal blood glucose control.

14. A ★　　　　　OHCM 10th ed. → p. 15

The fact that she has schizophrenia does not automatically mean she lacks capacity to make a decision about medical treatment. Patients who have capacity (i.e. who can understand, retain, and weigh up the necessary information and communicate their decision and can demonstrate this through a formal assessment of capacity) can make their own decisions. They can therefore refuse treatment, even if this is considered unwise or irrational to the doctor or may place the patient's health or their life at risk.

B. No other adult can consent on her behalf.

C. If she has capacity to make the decision, and this is entirely voluntary, then this is correct.

D. To treat under 'common law' without the patient's consent, the doctor would first have to prove that the patient lacked capacity to make the decision and then that it was in their best interests. The only other exception is in an emergency where the doctor feels the patient is at immediate harm or they are at risk of harming others, or to prevent a crime.

E. The Mental Health Act 2007 provides a statutory framework, which sets out when patients can be compulsorily treated for a mental disorder without consent, to protect them or others from harm. This can only be used when treating mental health disorders.

General Medical Council (2008). *Consent: patients and doctors making decisions together.*

→ www.gmc-uk.org/guidance/ethical_guidance/consent_guidance_contents.asp

15. E ★　　　　　OHCM 10th ed. → p. 207

The World Health Organization criteria for the diagnosis of diabetes state that one random glucose reading of >11.1 mmol/L, accompanied by symptoms of hyperglycaemia, is enough for diagnosis.

A. This is useful once treatment has started.

B. A fasting glucose reading of >7 mmol/L is also diagnostic if accompanied by symptoms or if it remains high once repeated.

C. An oral glucose tolerance test (OGTT) should be used for people with a fasting reading of 6.1–6.9 mmol/L. It is the only means of identifying people with impaired glucose tolerance.

D. This would be sensible if the patient were asymptomatic.

World Health Organization (2006). *Definition and diagnosis of diabetes mellitus and intermediate hyperglycaemia.*

→ www.who.int/diabetes/publications/diagnosis_diabetes2006/en/

16. A ★　　　　　OHCM 10th ed. → p. 212

The symptoms are typical of painful diabetic sensory neuropathy. Classical examination findings are decreased sensation (especially vibration sense) in a 'glove and stocking' distribution, with reduced ankle reflexes and foot deformities.

B. Haemosiderin is an iron storage complex that is released from erythrocytes, as they extravasate into the skin in venous ulcer disease. It stimulates melanin production, thus turning the skin brown.

C. These are seen in an upper motor neurone lesions.

D. Tenderness over the veins at the back of the calf (short saphenous system) is indicative of phlebitis and is common in venous disease.

E. This is not suggestive of sensory neuropathy, but rather of diabetic amyotrophy, which is painful wasting of muscles, chiefly of the pelvifemoral group.

17. D ★   OHCM 10th ed. → p. 236

This woman is suffering from galactorrhoea which is due to hyperprolactinaemia. Antiemetics act by reducing the levels of dopamine, which, in turn, stimulates prolactin release from the anterior pituitary. Thus, a common 'side effect' of some antiemetic treatment is hyperprolactinaemia. Other drugs, such as antipsychotics and oestrogens, can also raise prolactin levels.

18. D ★   OHCM 10th ed. → p. 217

The biochemistry shows subclinical hypothyroidism with raised thyroid-stimulating hormone (TSH) and normal free thyroxine (fT4). The likelihood of progression to overt hypothyroidism depends on the presence of antibodies.

A. This is an autoimmune destruction of the thyroid gland, resulting in hypothyroidism.

B. This would give rise to a goitre.

C. This is usual in acute illness, with low-to-normal TSH and low/high T4/tri-iodothyronine (T3).

E. This would result in high/normal fT4 with low/normal TSH.

19. A ★   OHCM 10th ed. → p. 222

The symptoms described are those of hypocalcaemia. Despite the distracting elements—overweight, hypertension, and depression—they are very typical, especially in someone whose social history suggests likely vitamin D deficiency. The fact that she suffered this many years previously raises the possibility of a genetic abnormality. A subsequent check of parathyroid hormone (PTH) level would help decide this, but in the acute setting, the focus should be on the calcium levels and correcting them appropriately. Failure to do so can induce cardiac arrhythmias (prolonged QT interval).

20. C ★   OHCM 10th ed. → p. 238

This man has features of acromegaly: feet enlargement, prognathism, macroglossia, and hoarseness due to laryngeal soft tissue swelling. The oral glucose tolerance test (OGTT) is the gold standard test for confirming the diagnosis. A rise in glucose fails to suppress the release of growth hormone. Insulin-like growth factor 1 (IGF-1) can also be measured (it will be high in acromegaly) but is not as conclusive as a dynamic test like the OGTT. The insulin tolerance test is used for the diagnosis of growth hormone deficiency.

21. A ★   OHCM 10th ed. → p. 221

This patient has subclinical hypothyroidism. Ten per cent of the general population aged >55 years have raised thyroid-stimulating hormone (TSH). It does not require thyroxine replacement. If thyroid peroxidase antibodies are present, the patient has an increased risk of progression to overt hypothyroidism. These patients should be monitored with annual TSH test (**C**) or earlier if symptoms are present.

B and D. These are indicated for hyperthyroidism.

22. A ★   OHCM 10th ed. → p. 226

The symptoms described suggest primary adrenal failure, which is characterized by low levels of cortisol and high levels of adrenocorticotrophic hormone (ACTH). The pigmentation is due to ACTH cross-reaction with melanocortin. Both arise from the same pre-hormone pro-opiomelanocortin.

B. This is tested in patients with resistant or early-onset hypertension or in those with hypertension associated with hypokalaemia.

C. Serum levels of caeruloplasmin and copper are actually decreased in Wilson's disease, which presents with hepatitis in children and with neuropsychiatric symptoms in young adults.

D. High levels of growth hormone occur in acromegaly, which affects soft tissues, rather than skin colour.

E. This will be raised in haemochromatosis due to increased intestinal iron absorption and deposition in organs, including the skin, causing generalized slate-grey skin pigmentation.

23. E ★   OHCM 10th ed. → p. 834

Confusion and drowsiness on a background of reduced oral intake in a 77-year-old patient should be treated as hyperosmolar hyperglycaemic state (HHS) until proven otherwise. These patients are severely dehydrated and need fluid resuscitation. The fluid normally used in the emergency situation is 0.9% sodium chloride (saline), and the aim is to reduce the osmolality and glucose levels slowly.

A. Glucagon is used in the emergency treatment of hypoglycaemia.

B. Glucose is avoided, as patients are hyperglycaemic

C. Insulin may be required if the glucose levels do not drop with rehydration.

D. There is no evidence for the use of sodium bicarbonate in the management of patients with HHS.

Joint British Diabetes Societies and Inpatient Care Group (2012). *The management of hyperosmolar hyperglycaemic state in adults with diabetes.*

→ diabetes-resources-production.s3-eu-west-1.amazonaws.com/ diabetes-storage/migration/pdf/JBDS-IP-HHS-Adults.pdf

24. D ★   OHCM 10th ed. → p. 218

Beta-blockers are used in the immediate management of the symptoms of hyperthyroidism. Propranolol is preferred over other beta-blockers, due to the added benefit of also partly blocking the peripheral conversion of thyroxine (T4) to tri-iodothyronine (T3). Patients who cannot tolerate beta-blockers may be treated with calcium channel blockers such as diltiazem. An antithyroid drug such as propylthiouracil or carbimazole is used to lower thyroid hormone levels, but the effect will not be immediate.

→ cks.nice.org.uk/hyperthyroidism

25. A ★   OHCM 10th ed. → p. 236

This man is displaying signs of hyperprolactinaemia. He was started on a dopamine agonist that would increase prolactin inhibition. The two commonly used drugs are cabergoline and bromocriptine.

26. E ★   OHCM 10th ed. → p. 221

This is subclinical hypothyroidism. The overall consensus is that patients can be offered treatment if thyroid-stimulating hormone (TSH) is >10 mU/L, as this could prevent cardiac deaths.

A. Thyroid peroxidase antibodies would be useful in predicting future hypothyroidism, not TSH receptor antibodies.

B. This is not an accurate measure of thyroid activity.

C and D. These are indicated for hyperthyroidism.

27. A ★   OHCM 10th ed. → p. 207

The symptoms of hyperglycaemia, along with one fasting glucose of >7.1 or one random glucose (D) of >11.1, are enough to diagnose diabetes. Glycosylated haemoglobin (HbA1c) levels (B) can be used to diagnose diabetes now (although the level here is in the impaired fasting range). Capillary glucose readings (C) should not be used for diagnosis purposes, and glycosuria (E) can be a normal finding. If the patient is asymptomatic, two samples are needed.

World Health Organization (2006). *Definition and diagnosis of diabetes mellitus and intermediate hyperglycaemia.*

→ www.who.int/diabetes/publications/diagnosis_diabetes2006/en/

28. B ★ OHCM 10th ed. → p. 208

Sulfonylureas work by activating adenosine triphosphate (ATP)-sensitive potassium channels on the pancreatic beta cells, thus causing insulin secretion. They therefore have the potential to cause a hypoglycaemic episode. Metformin (a biguanide), pioglitazone, dipeptidyl peptidase 4 (DDP4) inhibitors, and sodium–glucose co-transporter 2 (SGLT2) inhibitors do not cause hypoglycaemia, unless they are combined with sulfonylureas or insulin.

29. A ★ OHCM 10th ed. → p. 223

This lady was later diagnosed with Addison's disease. The areas of paler skin represent vitiligo.

Unexplained abdominal symptoms, particularly with associated existing autoimmune disease (pernicious anaemia/diabetes/hypothyroidism/ vitiligo), should certainly raise the question of adrenal insufficiency. This patient might be suffering from autoimmune polyendocrine syndrome type 1 or 2.

30. B ★ OHCM 10th ed. → p. 213

It is crucial that patients with type 1 diabetes know the 'sick day rules'. The additional insulin dose will depend on the degree of ketonuria. Trace or small amounts should prompt an additional 10% of the total daily insulin dose, whilst those with moderate to large amounts of ketonuria should take an additional 20%. However, in this situation, there would also be a low threshold for admission and observation with intravenous (IV) fluids.

A. This is the appropriate next step if the patient has ongoing vomiting, as she will need to be started on a variable-rate IV insulin infusion.

C and E. The patient should know to never stop taking insulin, to increase the frequency of blood tests (2- to 3-hourly), and to check the blood or urine for ketones.

D. Drinking adequate amounts (200 mL/hour) of sugar-free/diet drinks/water flushes out the ketones. If the patient cannot eat, they should replace their normal meals with 10 g of carbohydrate every 1–2 hours. Examples include 100 mL of Coke/fruit juice, one scoop of ice cream, half a pot (75 g) of fruit yoghurt, 200 mL of milk, and three glucose tablets.

→ www.nhslanarkshire.org.uk/Services/Diabetes/patient-info/ Documents/Sick%20Day%20Rules%20for%20Type%201%20 Diabetes%20Oct%2016.pdf

31. E ★ OHCM 10th ed. → p. 223

This lady has evidence of Sheehan's syndrome, which represents pituitary necrosis following postpartum haemorrhage. Note that the patient has evidence of acute adrenal insufficiency, due to the lack of adrenocorticotrophic hormone (ACTH), but has normal potassium, as mineralocorticoid production is intact.

An Addisonian crisis is not the case, as the pathology arises from the pituitary, and not from autoimmune destruction of the adrenal glands. Diabetes insipidus is associated with hypernatraemia. Hypoglycaemia can occur in the context of ACTH insufficiency; however, it is not the final diagnosis. Metabolic acidosis would not cause this clinical picture.

32. **A** ★   OHCM 10th ed. → p. 222

This lady has evidence of primary hyperparathyroidism, as evidenced by high calcium and inappropriately high parathyroid hormone (PTH). She is symptomatic from it and should have localization studies before being referred for a parathyroidectomy. Tertiary hyperparathyroidism would also present with high PTH and high calcium, but this is associated with chronic kidney disease when the glands act autonomously. The rest are causes of hypercalcaemia associated with low PTH.

33. **E** ★★   OHCM 10th ed. → p. 226

The concern is that this woman's adrenal glands have been suppressed by long-term steroid use, which has now come to an end. The initial investigation for this would be a short Synacthen® test, which uses exogenous synthetic adrenocorticotrophic hormone (ACTH) (tetracosactide, brand name: Synacthen®) to stimulate the adrenal gland into releasing cortisol.

A. The aldosterone:renin ratio is a good initial screening test for hyperaldosteronism.

B. Two 24-hour urinary collections are performed as a screening test to look for free catecholamines that would signify a phaeochromocytoma.

C and D. Both of these are used as screening tests to investigate suspected Cushing's syndrome (D is the dexamethasone suppression test).

34. **B** ★★   OHCM 10th ed. → p. 225

Interpretation of *single* cortisol readings, even if these are done early in the morning, is difficult. Therefore, a dynamic test, such as the dexamethasone suppression test, is the most appropriate way to diagnose Cushing's syndrome. In this condition, dexamethasone would fail to suppress cortisol. A high midnight cortisol (C) would also suggest Cushing's, but the most appropriate test is a dynamic test. Imaging is done after biochemical tests confirm the cortisol excess.

35. **C** ★★   OHCM 10th ed. → p. 226

Postural hypotension associated with hyponatraemia and hyperkalaemia is suggestive of adrenocortical insufficiency. It is the lack of mineralocorticoids that causes the postural drop—therefore, it is useful to check renin and aldosterone levels. If deficient and symptomatic, they need to be replaced by an exogenous steroid, i.e. fludrocortisone which is the most appropriate choice from the options provided. As a general point, measurement of the postural blood pressure is an easily performed bedside test that should not be forgotten in the assessment of a patient who has collapsed.

A. This is an alpha-blocker used in the treatment of hypertension and prostatic hypertrophy that is more likely to cause postural hypotension than prevent it.

B. This is an angiotensin-converting enzyme (ACE) inhibitor that is used as a first-line treatment for hypertension.

D. This is a loop diuretic used to relieve the symptoms of heart failure.

E. This is an alpha sympathomimetic that causes vasoconstriction and is therefore useful in the treatment of orthostatic hypotension. This is a second-line treatment that can be used if patients develop hypokalaemia or supine hypertension on fludrocortisone.

36. **A** ★★★ OHCM 10th ed. → p. 220

Despite the range of potential side effects of amiodarone (partly due to its very long half-life of 2 months), thyroid toxicity is the most common complication that requires intervention. Indeed, it has been described in up to 10% of patients on long-term amiodarone therapy. Both hyper- and hypothyroidism are possible, although hypothyroidism is more than twice as common. Whilst **C** and **D** may be indicated if toxicity develops, there is no place for **E** in the early stages of routine follow-up.

Siddoway L. Amiodarone: guidelines for use and monitoring. *Am Fam Physician.* 2003;**68**:2189–96.

→ www.aafp.org/afp/20031201/2189.html

37. **A** ★★★ OHCM 10th ed. → p. 210

The image shows background diabetic retinopathy with microaneurysms and hard exudates. At the root of this is hyperglycaemia-induced high retinal blood flow, which disturbs the endothelium of the capillaries—all subsequent changes stem from this. Retinal ischaemia (**E**) is responsible for neovascularization (**D**), which then opens up the possibility of these new vessels fibrosing (**B**). Microvascular haemorrhages (**C**) are the blots seen in background and pre-proliferative retinopathy; they are features, rather than the cause.

38. **B** ★★★ OHCM 10th ed. → p. 228

Hypertension in a young person demands that consideration be given to a possible endocrine cause. All of the hormones listed can cause hypertension, but it is catecholamines—phaeochromocytoma—that cause the symptoms seen in this man: the general features of anxiety, headaches, and the cardiovascular features of palpitations and hypertension.

A. Hyperaldosteronism should be suspected in young patients with hypertension or drug-refractory hypertension. The patients might suffer from hypokalaemia but are otherwise asymptomatic.

C. High circulating levels of cortisol occur in Cushing's syndrome and would be more likely to produce a range of physical and psychiatric findings.

D. Acromegaly does cause hypertension but presents with features of soft tissue enlargement.

E. Hyperparathyroidism can cause hypertension if left untreated for a long time. Patients will have symptoms of hypercalcaemia: lethargy, weakness, depression, and abdominal pain.

39. B ★★★   OHCM 10th ed. → p. 836

This patient is at risk of an adrenal crisis, as he might not be absorbing his steroid tablets due to vomiting. He should be educated to seek urgent medical attention in this instance and also be competent to inject an immediate (STAT) dose of hydrocortisone before arriving at the hospital. This is a lifesaving intervention that should not be delayed.

40. C ★★★   OHCM 10th ed. → p. 217

This is an example of pseudo-Cushing's syndrome, in which cortisol is falsely high due to increased metabolism of dexamethasone, in this case due to a liver enzyme inducer. In other words, this man's symptoms cannot be explained by adrenal gland dysfunction. Whilst this is not a common clinical problem, it serves as a reminder to be careful when interpreting results in patients who are on multiple medications.

41. E ★★★   OHCM 10th ed. → p. 210

The image indicates new vessels have been formed (thus, C describes what is happening, but not the mechanism behind it). This happens in the diabetic eye, as a result of occlusion of the microvasculature leading to local hypoxia and areas of the retina becoming ischaemic. This is a serious development, as these new vessels have the potential to bleed and fibrose and can detach the retina.

A. This refers to hard exudates that are seen in background retinopathy, i.e. a stage that this man has already been through.

B. This is not seen on the image but is the concern once neovascularization has taken place.

D. Acute hyperglycaemia can induce a cataract-like state that reverses once normal blood glucose levels are reached.

42. D ★★★★   OHCM 10th ed. → p. 748

This is a common situation. This man has small bowel obstruction and type 2 diabetes, but normal renal function, and will need contrast to visualize the bowel properly.

Worldwide, 110 cases of metformin-induced lactic acidosis were reported between 1968 and 1991, with seven developing it following iodinated intravenous (IV) contrast. Metformin is renally cleared, and the greatest concern is in those with known renal impairment. Hydration and limiting the dose of contrast can reduce the risk.

The American College of Radiologists Committee on Drugs and Contrast Media states that metformin can be continued in patients with normal renal function and no known co-morbidities associated with lactic acidosis until the time of the scan, but it should then be withheld for 48 hours. In those with normal renal function, but with co-morbidities, reassessment of renal function prior to restarting metformin is advised. In those with pre-existing renal dysfunction, much more cautious reinstitution of metformin is advised.

American College of Radiologists (2008). *Manual on contrast media*, Version 6.

→   www.scribd.com/doc/2952016/Contrast-Media-Administration-Guidelines-by-the-ACR-American-College-of-Radiology-Version-6-2008

Chapter 4

Gastroenterology

Ricky Sinharay

Gastroenterology and hepatology encompass a vast array of organs that have diverse structure and function and are affected by a multitude of disease processes. Diseases of the digestive tract are a major cause of morbidity and mortality in the United Kingdom (UK) and worldwide. There have been great advances in our understanding, diagnosis, and management of gastrointestinal (GI) disease, and knowledge continues to develop at a great pace. Understanding the physiology and cellular and molecular events that drive pathological processes, as well as the development of sophisticated endoscopic and radiological tests, have transformed diagnostic capability. Therapeutic endoscopy has progressed to replace surgical management of common GI emergencies such as upper GI tract bleeding and decompressing biliary tract obstruction. However, as ever, there is still much work to be done. For example, the advances in biologic immunotherapy in inflammatory bowel disease has greatly improved patients' quality of life and a reduction in the need for surgery, though the overall impact of these medications on the natural history of the disease is debatable at present.

Hepatology is a greatly misunderstood specialty. The physiological changes that occur as cirrhosis and portal hypertension develop are the key to understanding all manifestations of a decompensating liver. Recently, there has been a significant increase in the prevalence of chronic liver disease in the UK, and as a result, hospital admissions have increased.

Liver disease is the only major cause of death still increasing year on year, and twice as many people now die from liver disease than in 1991. The 2013 National Confidential Enquiry into Patient Outcome and Death (NCEPOD) of patients with alcohol-related liver disease (ARLD) found that less than half the number of patients who died from ARLD received 'good care', and avoidable deaths were identified.

Allied to this, the enquiry shed light on a cultural pessimism regarding outcomes and prognosis of chronic liver disease and, in particular, ARLD from both the public and the medical profession as a whole. There is now a concerted drive towards improving awareness of chronic liver disease, and initial simple supportive treatments can greatly improve survival, more so than previously thought.

Aetiologies of chronic liver disease are changing, with non-alcoholic fatty liver disease superseding alcohol as the primary pathology in the UK, with increasing prevalence of metabolic syndrome. The complexity of the organ itself having an important role in metabolic pathways, detoxification, protein manufacture, and immune surveillance means that when the liver malfunctions, it does so in colourful ways and often affecting multiple organs. A close relationship with the Intensive Care Unit is therefore vital as well, always asking the question: 'which direction is this person's liver disease heading?' If the only direction is towards deterioration, then transplantation needs to be considered, the survival outcomes of which are very good in orthotopic liver transplantation.

The aim of this chapter is to help you with your preparation with your medical school exams and raise awareness and your working practical knowledge of gastroenterology and hepatology. It would hopefully also provide you with the inspiration to read this subject further, in preparation for starting your first jobs in the hospital to make approaching the diagnosis and treatment of the unwell gastroenterology or hepatology patient less daunting.

QUESTIONS

1. A 42-year-old woman has developed dysphagia <u>simultaneously</u> to both liquids and solids for the last <u>3 months.</u> It is constant and there is no odynophagia. She has regular central chest pain and regurgitates undigested food on most occasions but does not suffer from acid reflux. She has lost nearly 3 or 4 kg over 6 months. Which is the *single* most likely diagnosis? ★

A Achalasia

B Benign oesophageal stricture

C Bulbar palsy

D Diffuse oesophageal spasm

E Oesophageal malignancy

2. A 74-year-old man has had retrosternal pain, nocturnal cough, and belching for 8 weeks. He has had no loss of appetite or weight loss. He has recently been started on some new medication and feels that this may be the cause of his symptoms. Which is the *single* most likely cause of his symptoms? ★

A Alendronic acid

B Bisoprolol

C Codeine phosphate

D Digoxin

E Quinine sulfate

3. A 63-year-old man has lost 10 kg in weight in recent months and become increasingly jaundiced over the last 4 weeks. He has no abdominal discomfort, but his urine has become very dark and his stools pale in colour. He drinks 15 units of alcohol per week. An ultrasound scan of the liver shows a dilated common bile duct. Which *single* set of liver function test results would fit best with the likely underlying diagnosis? ★

A Bilirubin 60 mmol/L, alkaline phosphatase (ALP) 240 IU/L, aspartate aminotransferase (AST) 30 IU/L, gamma-glutamyl transpeptidase (GGT) 30 IU/L

B Bilirubin 60 mmol/L, ALP 30 IU/L, AST 28 IU/L, GGT 35 IU/L

C Bilirubin 100 mmol/L, ALP 470 IU/L, AST 60 IU/L, GGT 415 IU/L

D Bilirubin 100 mmol/L, ALP 210 IU/L, AST 2020 IU/L, GGT 645 IU/L

E Bilirubin 20 mmol/L, ALP 130 IU/L, AST 2020 IU/L, GGT 630 IU/L

4. A 72-year-old man has vomited more than five times over the past 24 hours. He has also begun passing very frequent loose stools. He feels weak, dizzy, and slightly confused. He is on a disease-modifying agent for rheumatoid arthritis and has type 2 diabetes. He does not smoke, drinks 20–30 units of alcohol a week, and has not travelled abroad recently.

T 37.1°C, HR 100 bpm, BP 95/50 mmHg lying, 76/45 mmHg sitting.

His abdomen is soft, with tenderness at the epigastrium. A digital rectal examination reveals an empty rectum. Which is the *single* most appropriate course of action? ★

A Computed tomography (CT) scan of the abdomen

B Flexible sigmoidoscopy

C Insertion of a nasogastric tube

D Intravenous (IV) fluids

E Loperamide

5. A 53-year-old man has been troubled by recurrent bouts of epigastric pain associated with nausea and sweating. He has recently moved house and feels the pain has been worse, as he has needed to carry lots of heavy boxes up and down stairs. He has tried omeprazole 20 mg oral (PO) once daily, with no improvement, over the last 3 weeks. His body mass index (BMI) is 33 kg/m².

HR 82 bpm, BP 155/85 mmHg.

Which is the *single* most appropriate initial management? ★

A Barium meal

B Chest X-ray

C Computed tomography (CT) scan of the abdomen

D Electrocardiogram (ECG)

E Oesophagogastroduodenoscopy (OGD)

6. A 62-year-old man has had worsening acid reflux over the last 4 months. He attributes his symptoms to a poor diet, following the recent death of his wife. He uses a salbutamol inhaler for asthma when required but otherwise has no medical problems. Which *single* additional factor in his history would warrant an urgent referral for endoscopy? ★

A Family history of oesophageal cancer

B Progressively worsening shortness of breath

C Smoker of 20 cigarettes per day

D Weight loss

E Vomiting

7. A 37-year-old man has had upper abdominal pain and belching for the last 2 weeks. Over the last month, he has been taking regular diclofenac since dislocating his shoulder playing rugby. His bowels are opening normally, and his stools are normal in colour. He smokes ten cigarettes per day and drinks 25 units of alcohol per week. Which is the *single* most appropriate next step? ★

A Advise to reduce alcohol intake and stop smoking

B Advise to stop taking diclofenac tablets

C Empirical *Helicobacter pylori* treatment

D Stool antigen test for *H. pylori*

E Urgent referral for oesophagogastroduodenoscopy (OGD) within 2 weeks

8. A 60-year-old man is experiencing pain on swallowing. Over the last 3 months, it has been worsening, such that he can no longer tolerate food unless it is pureed. He has had chronic reflux symptoms, but no other medical problems. He has smoked 20 cigarettes a day for 40 years. Which *single* further feature is most likely to support the diagnosis? ★

A Coughs on swallowing

B Neck bulges on drinking

C Pain is intermittent

D Regurgitates oral intake

E Weight loss

9. A 66-year-old man has fallen three times in a day. He is delirious and jaundiced and is responding to things that are not there.

T 36.5°C, HR 110 bpm, BP 85/60 mmHg.

Haemoglobin (Hb) 85 g/L, mean corpuscular volume (MCV) 105 fL, international normalized ratio (INR) 1.7, albumin 26 g/L, platelets 60 × 10⁹, bilirubin 60 micromol/L, sodium (Na) 120 mmol/L.

His abdomen is distended and tense, with shifting dullness. There are spider naevi present. Which is the single most appropriate course of action? ★

A Abdominal paracentesis

B Lactulose three times daily (tds)

C Packed red cells 2 U

D Propranolol 80 mg

E Spironolactone 100 mg

10. A 62-year-old woman has an increasingly painful and swollen abdomen. She has suffered these problems many times in the past, but this time it is impairing her breathing. She has a history of poorly controlled type 2 diabetes. The palms of her hands are flushed pink and the digits are oedematous, with white nails. Her abdomen is markedly distended, with a palpable non-tender liver edge 4 cm below the costal margin. Shifting dullness is demonstrated. There is bilateral ankle oedema, pitting to the mid calf. Which *single* factor is most likely to be responsible for this woman's peripheral oedema? ★

A Concurrent nephrotic syndrome

B Hepatic vein thrombosis

C Non-alcoholic steatohepatitis (NASH) cirrhosis and portal hypertension

D Ovarian fibroma

E Right heart failure

11. A 58-year-old woman has felt increasingly lethargic over the past 3 or 4 years and has noticed that her eyes look 'yellow'. She has recently been diagnosed with hypothyroidism, for which she takes replacement therapy. She has no previous medical history but occasionally takes chlorphenamine. Which *single* autoantibody is most consistent with the diagnosis? ★

A Anti-centromere

B Anti-double-stranded DNA

C Anti-mitochondrial

D Anti-phospholipid

E Anti-smooth muscle

12. A 54-year-old woman has been dizzy and nauseated for 1 day. Prior to this, she had 3 days of epigastric pain and vomiting. She has type 2 diabetes and had a pituitary tumour excised 20 years previously, for which she remains on steroid replacement therapy. She is pale. Her abdomen is soft, with epigastric tenderness. Digital rectal examination finds tar-like liquid stool in the rectum. Which is the *single* most likely diagnosis? ★

A Angiodysplasia

B Bleeding peptic ulcer

C Diverticulitis

D Gastric carcinoma

E Mallory–Weiss tear

13. A 78-year-old woman has had epigastric pain for 1 week and had one episode of passing tarry stool. She has cognitive impairment, with a mini-mental state examination (MMSE) score of 12/30. The medical team plan to investigate her symptoms with an oesophagogastroduodenoscopy (OGD). When seeking her consent, it is noted that she does not seem to understand the explanations and cannot retain information or weigh up the risks and benefits, but the medical team feel it is in her best interests to proceed with the OGD. Which is the *single* most appropriate course of action for the medical team? ★

A Gain verbal consent from the woman's next of kin

B Gain written consent from the woman's next of kin

C Get one of the doctors to sign for consent as a proxy

D No consent is needed for such a minor procedure

E Postpone the procedure

14. A 34-year-old woman undergoes an ileo-caecal resection for Crohn's disease. The operation is uneventful, and she is discharged 1 week later. The patient asks the junior doctor whether she will need any supplementation as a result of the operation. Which is the *single* most likely supplementation she will need? ★

A Bile salts

B Folic acid

C Intrinsic factor

D Vitamins A and D

E Vitamin B12

15. A 70-year-old woman has had three bouts of haematemesis. She is dizzy, confused, and hallucinating. She is a non-smoker but admits to heavy alcohol use since her husband died 15 years previously.

T 36.5°C, HR 120 bpm, BP 85/55 mmHg.

Her abdomen is distended and tense and demonstrates shifting dullness. Which is the *single* most likely diagnosis? ★

A Bleeding gastric ulcer

B Erosive oesophagitis

C Mallory–Weiss tear

D Oesophageal carcinoma

E Oesophageal varices

16. A 42-year-old woman has had difficulty swallowing for the last 18 months. From the beginning, she has been struggling to tolerate both solids and fluids. She often regurgitates her oral intake and has lost over 5 kg. She is a non-smoker and has no other medical problems. Which *single* investigation is most likely to support the diagnosis? ★

A Abdominal X-ray

B Chest X-ray

C Endoscopic ultrasound scan

D Oesophageal manometry

E Oesophagogastroduodenoscopy (OGD)

17. A 44-year-old man has experienced acid reflux over the last 2 months and describes some difficulty swallowing. Some blood tests are taken, and he is awaiting an urgent endoscopy in the next 2 weeks. He smokes 20 cigarettes a day, and his body mass index (BMI) is 31 kg/m^2. Which is the *single* most appropriate piece of advice to give before the endoscopy? ★

A Advise him to lose weight and stop smoking

B Start a proton pump inhibitor (PPI)

C Start an alginate antacid

D Start an H2-receptor antagonist

E Start triple therapy to eradicate *Helicobacter pylori*

18. A 22-year-old woman presented to her outpatient dietician clinic with a new diagnosis of coeliac disease. She requested advice on what she could drink on her upcoming 23rd birthday celebration. Which is the *single* most appropriate response? ★

A Ale

B Beer

C Cider

D Lager

E Stout

19. A 47-year-old woman vomits repeatedly, with dark red specks visible throughout. She is initially confused but settles while being attended to in the emergency department. She has signs of chronic liver disease, including ascites. Pending an endoscopy, it is decided to control the bleeding with some medical therapy. The patient is sceptical and refuses the treatment. Which is the *single* most appropriate explanation of how this treatment works? ★★

A Constricts the vessels supplying dilated veins in the oesophagus and stomach

B Increases the levels of vitamins that encourage clot formation

C Prevents the formation of proteins that break down clots

D Reduces gastrointestinal (GI) acid secretion

E Replaces the body's lost stores of protein

20. A man with alcohol-related liver cirrhosis, who has been abstinent for 6 months, has recurrent ascites despite maximal diuretics. He has no evidence of encephalopathy. Prothrombin time: normal. Bilirubin 50 micromol/L. He is referred for transplant assessment, and a United Kingdom Model for End-Stage Liver Disease (UKELD) score is calculated. Which *single* pair of additional variables should be used to grade his risk? ★★

A Age + urea

B Alanine aminotransferase (ALT) + amylase

C ALT + albumin

D Creatinine + sodium

E Platelet count + ferritin

21. A 49-year-old man has had retrosternal burning pain for the last 2 months. He has no ALARM symptoms (see answer to question 6) and does not take any regular medications. He initially took a proton pump inhibitor (PPI) but returned to his doctor 1 month later with no improvement in symptoms. He subsequently tested positive for *Helicobacter pylori* and was given eradication therapy for 1 week. He has returned 10 days later with persisting symptoms. Which is the *single* most appropriate next step? ★★

A Metoclopramide 10 mg oral (PO) three times daily

B Omeprazole 40 mg twice daily

C One-week course of second-line *H. pylori* eradication therapy

D Refer to secondary care

E Urgent endoscopy

22. A 44-year-old woman has had diarrhoea for 2 days. It has progressed, such that she has passed 15 liquid motions in the last 12 hours. Seven days previously, she completed her second cycle of chemotherapy for breast cancer.

T 38.4°C, HR 110 bpm, BP 105/75 mmHg.

Which is the *single* most appropriate next step? ★ ★

A Await stool and blood cultures before starting antibiotics

B Do not consider antibiotics so soon after chemotherapy

C Start antibiotics if temperature (T) >38°C and heart rate (HR) >90 bpm for 12 hours

D Start broad-spectrum antibiotics

E Start loperamide 4 mg oral (PO) four times daily

23. A 33-year-old woman has a medical assessment prior to a new job. She has been well, apart from some mild coryzal symptoms the previous week.

Bilirubin 42 mmol/L, alkaline phosphatase (ALP) 60 IU/L, aspartate aminotransferase (AST) 28 IU/L, gamma-glutamyl transpeptidase (GGT) 30 IU/L.

Urine dipstick: no bilirubin detected.

Which is the *single* most likely explanation for these results? ★ ★

A Crigler–Najjar syndrome

B Epstein–Barr virus

C Gilbert's syndrome

D Hepatitis B virus infection

E Rotor syndrome

24. A 48-year-old man has an endoscopy for dyspepsia, which shows a duodenal ulcer. He is homeless and drinks >100 units of alcohol per week. He has no allergies and takes no regular medications. His *Campylobacter*-like organism (CLO) test is positive, and the doctor wants to start *Helicobacter pylori* eradication therapy. Which is the *single* most appropriate next step? ★ ★

A Amoxicillin 1 g twice daily, clarithromycin 500 mg twice daily, and omeprazole 20 mg twice daily for 1 week

B Amoxicillin 1 g twice daily, metronidazole 400 mg twice daily, and omeprazole 20 mg twice daily for 1 week

C Bismuth subcitrate 120 mg four times daily, tetracycline 500 mg four times daily, omeprazole 20 mg twice daily, and amoxicillin 1 g twice daily for 2 weeks

D Bismuth subcitrate 120 mg four times daily, tetracycline 500 mg four times daily, omeprazole 20 mg twice daily, and metronidazole 400 mg twice daily for 2 weeks

E Clarithromycin 500 mg twice daily, metronidazole 400 mg twice daily, and omeprazole 20 mg twice daily for 1 week

25. A 28-year-old woman has been admitted with abdominal pain and profuse vomiting and diarrhoea. Nursing staff call the on-call junior doctor and report that she has rolled her eyes back and is unable to prevent the protrusion of her tongue. She is currently being treated with a number of different medications for presumed gastroenteritis. Which *single* drug is most likely to have caused these symptoms? ★ ★

A Cyclizine

B Hyoscine butylbromide

C Metoclopramide

D Omeprazole

E Ondansetron

26. A 50-year-old woman has taken 70 paracetamol tablets and is acutely unwell in hospital. She says that she did not want to be found and wants to die. Her arterial pH after 24 hours is 7.23, creatinine 180 micromol/L, and prothrombin time (PT) 85 s; she is slightly confused. She is on an *N*-acetylcysteine infusion. Which is the *single* most appropriate course of action? ★ ★

A Acute liver screen bloods

B Continue *N*-acetylcysteine

C Psychiatric evaluation

D Refer to a transplant centre

E Ultrasound scan of the liver and portal vessels

27. A 48-year-old male was admitted to hospital with jaundice, ascites, and fever. He consumes 20 units of alcohol per day. On examination, a 6-cm tender hepatomegaly was found.

T 37.9°C, HR 85 bpm, BP 135/90 mmHg.

His Maddrey's discriminant function is 38. Which is the next most appropriate step in his management? ★★

A Ascitic tap

B Corticosteroids

C *N*-acetylcysteine

D Pentoxifylline

E Spironolactone

28. A 60-year-old man is weak, lethargic, and confused. He has been deteriorating gradually over many months and has just finished a 3-day alcoholic binge. He has long-standing alcohol misuse and chronic pancreatitis. He is tremulous and cachectic, with dry mucous membranes. The attending doctor plans to rehydrate him with 1 L of 5% glucose intravenous (IV). Which *single* medication should be given beforehand? ★★

A Chlordiazepoxide 30 mg oral (PO)

B Omeprazole 40 mg IV

C Pancreatin 10 000 U

D Vitamin B + C ampoules I and II

E Vitamin B Compound Strong two tablets PO

29. A 66-year-old man with a previous cholecystectomy has been passing loose stools for the past 2 weeks. They are light in colour and resistant to being flushed away. He also has generalized abdominal pain that has never really improved since its onset some years ago, and he has continued to lose weight. What is the next most appropriate investigation? ★★

A Colonoscopy

B Computed tomography (CT) pancreas

C Dietician review

D Faecal elastase

E Stool culture

30. A 55-year-old woman had a stroke 3 days ago. She fails a swallowing assessment carried out by the speech and language therapist. The decision is made to commence her on enteral feeding via a nasogastric feeding tube. The tube is inserted, and the junior doctor on call has been asked to confirm the position of the tube prior to commencing feeding. Which is the *single* most reliable way to confirm that the tube is in the correct position? ★★★

A Aspirate yellow/green-coloured fluid

B Listen over the stomach as air is passed through the tube

C Measure the length of tube left externally

D Percuss over the stomach as air is passed through the tube

E Test the pH of the aspirate with graduated pH paper

31. A 38-year-old man has felt increasingly tired and lethargic over the last 4 weeks. He has not noticed any change in his bowels recently and normally passes a small amount of blood with his motions, which he says has not changed. He was diagnosed with ulcerative colitis 15 years ago and takes mesalazine enteric-coated (EC) 800 mg oral (PO) twice daily. His abdomen is soft and non-tender. On digital rectal examination, no masses are felt and there is a small amount of fresh blood on the finger.

Haemoglobin (Hb) 106 g/L, mean corpuscular volume (MCV) 75.6 fL, ferritin 10 ng/mL.

Which is the *single* most appropriate management? ★★★

A Increase mesalazine EC to 800 mg three times daily

B Reassure that this is to be expected in ulcerative colitis

C Start a 5-day course of prednisolone 40 mg PO once daily

D Start ferrous sulfate 200 mg PO three times daily

E Urgent 2-week referral to Gastroenterology outpatient clinic

32. A 57-year-old man has vomited >350 mL of fresh blood. He is dependent on alcohol and has consumed in excess of 200 units of alcohol over the last 4 days.

T 36.2°C, HR 112 bpm, BP 105/60 mmHg.

Intravenous (IV) fluids and a dose of vitamin K are given. A request is made for packed red cells and fresh frozen plasma (FFP). As the registrar opens the endoscopy suite, he asks the junior doctor to reduce the portal venous pressure. Which is the *single* most appropriate initial management? ★★★

A Furosemide

B Glyceryl trinitrate

C Octreotide

D Propranolol

E Terlipressin

33. A 62-year-old man has been passing small amounts of blood with his bowel movements for 2 months. He is not sure whether it is mixed with the stool, but the blood is bright red in colour and he thinks it is getting less. He has always been troubled by constipation, but he has not noticed any change in his bowels recently. He has osteoarthritis and takes regular diclofenac for symptomatic relief. He has no family history of bowel cancer. Which is the *single* most appropriate management? ★★★

A Add omeprazole 40 mg oral (PO) once daily

B Commence regular lactulose 20 mL PO twice daily

C Routine referral to surgical outpatient clinic

D Send a full blood count and review whether he is anaemic

E Urgent 2-week referral to surgical outpatient clinic

34. A 63-year-old woman has had intermittent lower abdominal pain and felt bloated, despite eating less than normal, over the last 2–3 months. She is passing urine more often and feels it is more difficult to hold on to her urine after getting the feeling she needs to go. She denies any change in her bowels or weight loss. Abdominal examination is unremarkable. What is the *single* most appropriate next step? ★★★

A Blood for CA125 levels and ultrasound scan (USS) abdomen/pelvis

B Dietary advice and mebeverine

C Faecal *Helicobacter pylori* and trial of omeprazole

D Stool microscopy and sigmoidoscopy

E Urine microscopy and cytology

35. A 68-year-old man has passed a large amount of melaena over the last 2 hours and has also vomited some altered blood. He is not currently bleeding and, having been resuscitated by a junior doctor in the emergency department, is now being assessed for his predictive risk of rebleeding and death using the Rockall scoring system. Which *single* factor in the history would have the greatest effect on predicting his risk? ★★★★

A 40 units of alcohol per week

B Aged 68 years

C Chronic kidney disease

D Ischaemic heart disease

E Oesophageal carcinoma

36. A 44-year-old homeless man has developed difficulty breathing and has palpitations. He has been recovering in hospital for several days, following an alcoholic binge of around 100 units, and had been encouraged to eat and drink normally prior to discharge. He is very unkempt. His body mass index (BMI) is 19 kg/m².

T 36.7°C, HR 95 bpm, BP 115/80 mmHg, SaO₂ 98% on 4 L oxygen.

Which *single* pair of tests is the most appropriate next step? ★★★★

A Chest X-ray + arterial blood gases

B Electrocardiogram (ECG) + troponin level

C Full blood count + sputum sample

D Liver function tests + calcium

E Urea and electrolytes + phosphate

37. A 64-year-old man is jaundiced and confused. Two years ago, he underwent surgery for a colonic carcinoma but refused adjuvant chemotherapy on the basis that he felt well. Imaging shows disseminated metastatic disease, with most of the liver parenchyma being replaced by tumour. The intrinsic and extrinsic hepatic ducts are dilated, and an attempt to stent the common bile duct fails. His family asks the doctor to do everything possible. Which is the *single* most appropriate next step? ★★★★

A Attempt percutaneous drainage of the obstructed biliary duct

B Debulk the hepatic tumour to reduce the obstruction

C Focus on symptom relief using a palliative care approach

D Start chemotherapy to reduce the size of the obstructing tumour

E Try to stent the biliary duct again during another endoscopic retrograde cholangiopancreatography (ERCP)

38. A 55-year-old man has just been told he has oesophageal cancer with liver metastases. He currently spends >50% of the time in bed or lying down and is capable of only limited self-care. As a result, he has a World Health Organization (WHO) performance status of 3. He feels very positive about enjoying the time he has got left with his family and asks how much longer he has to live. Which is the *single* most appropriate response? ★★★★

A Less than a week

B 1–3 months

C 6–12 months

D 1–2 years

E More than 2 years

39. A 23-year-old woman has had intermittent loose stool with urgency over the last 8 months. She feels very bloated, particularly after eating, and can sometimes pass mucus, but opening her bowels usually relieves her symptoms. Her weight is stable. The doctor is confident of the diagnosis and gives her some dietary advice. Which *single* most appropriate dietary change should be advised? ★★★★

A Golden linseed or oats

B More than 5 pieces of fruit, as well as vegetables, per day

C Muesli containing high amounts of bran

D Reheated potato or corn

E Sweetcorn or green bananas

40. A 57-year-old man with ulcerative colitis was admitted to hospital with bloody diarrhoea 15 times per day. He has a past medical history of tuberculosis (TB) and hypertension. On day 3 of treatment with intravenous (IV) hydrocortisone, his bloods show a C-reactive protein (CRP) of 50 and temperature of 37.6°C, and he is opening his bowels nine times per day. His abdominal film shows no evidence of megacolon. What is the *single* most appropriate next step in his management plan? ★★★★

A Continue IV steroids for another 3 days

B Computed tomography (CT) scan

C Flexible sigmoidoscopy

D Start biologic therapy

E Subtotal colectomy

ANSWERS

1. A ★   OHCM 10th ed. → p. 250

This is achalasia where degeneration of ganglion cells in the oesophageal body and lower oesophgeal sphincter leads to loss of peristalsis of the oesophageal body and failure of relaxation of the lower oesophageal sphincter. This results in collection of undigested food in a dilated oesophagus and regurgitation of this.

B. Usually a history of progressive dysphagia to solids followed by liquids.

C. This involves lower motor neurones (LMN) IX–XI, often slurred speech, nasal regurgitation of food, difficulty chewing, and choking on liquids. Signs include tongue fasciculation and absence of a gag reflex.

D. This involves unco-ordinated peristaltic contractions such as the 'nut-cracker oesophagus' where the distal contractions are of excessive amplitude and cause severe intermittent chest pain, which is often mistaken for cardiac chest pain.

E. Again usually a history of progressive dysphagia to solids, followed by liquids, making malignancy less likely in this scenario, although with weight loss, malignancy should be excluded with imaging and upper gastrointestinal (GI) endoscopy.

2. A ★   OHCM 10th ed. → p. 250

The most common reaction to bisphosphonates is irritation, inflammation, or ulceration of the oesophagus. As a precaution, therefore, it should be taken 30 minutes before food (usually breakfast) and the patient should not lie down for at least 30 minutes after taking the medication.

3. C ★   OHCM 10th ed. → p. 272

The scenario suggests a diagnosis of cholestatic jaundice, compatible with biliary obstruction, likely due to a pancreatic mass. This does not usually cause significant transaminitis.

A. Raised alkaline phosphatase (ALP), but with normal gamma-glutamyl transpeptidase (GGT), suggests another source for the cholestatic liver function tests (LFTs)—think bone and haematological causes (malignancy, haemolysis).

B. This indicates Gilbert's syndrome.

D. This is a mixed hepatitic–cholestatic picture.

E. This is in keeping with a hepatitic/transaminitis picture.

Liver enzymes are often useful in trying to interpret the pattern of inflammation affecting the liver, but they can also just confuse matters. It is always important to interpret these alongside other investigations such as imaging and to remember that not all liver enzyme abnormalities are from the liver itself—consider right-sided heart failure/congestive heart failure, haematological malignancies/malignant infiltration, and sepsis as other causes.

4. D ★ OHCM 10th ed. → p. 258

Whilst the majority of patients with diarrhoea do not attend hospital, if it occurs in the elderly or immunocompromised, or if it is severe, then it can be an indication for hospital admission. Although this man is not feverish and has not passed any blood, he is weak, confused, tachycardic, and hypotensive. The priority therefore is intravenous (IV) rehydration. The most likely cause is viral gastroenteritis, but he would need admission to an isolation room in the first instance for fluid and electrolyte replacement. Stool cultures should be sent and, as he is >60 years old and immunocompromised, he is classified as high risk by the British Infection Society and should be considered for antibiotics on admission (usually ciprofloxacin orally). If there is a recent history of antibiotic use, then *Clostridium difficile*-associated diarrhoea may well be the cause, in which case metronidazole or vancomycin should be used.

A. This is only indicated if other pathologies are suspected such as malignancy or bowel obstruction.

B. This should be considered if the diarrhoea is not settling within 1 week, in view of his immunosuppression, to exclude pseudomembranous colitis or inflammatory colitis.

C. There is no suggestion of bowel obstruction here and so no need to decompress the stomach.

E. Anti-motility agents can be used to slow motions down, as long as obstruction and infection have both been excluded and this would aid fluid resuscitation. To be used with caution in the elderly due to its anticholinergic effects.

5. D ★ OHCM 10th ed. → p. 254

Epigastric pain, in association with nausea and sweating, should not automatically be attributed to a gastrointestinal cause. Instead, cardiac disease such as angina needs to be ruled out, especially in a man with risk factors and no response to proton pump inhibitors.

6. D ★ OHCM 10th ed. → p. 252

Weight loss and persistent/unexplained symptoms of dyspepsia in anyone over 55 years should prompt an urgent referral for endoscopy. This should happen, regardless of whether any ALARMS symptoms are present. ALARMS symptoms are: Anaemia, Loss of weight, Anorexia, Recent onset of progressive symptoms, Melaena or haematemesis, and Swallowing difficulty.

Indications for urgent upper gastrointestinal (GI) endoscopy (emergency or 2-week wait) include:

- Haematemesis or melaena, dysphagia, >55 years old, weight loss, and any of the following:

- Upper abdominal pain
- Reflux
- Dyspepsia.

National Institute for Health and Care Excellence (2015). *Suspected cancer: recognition and referral*. NICE guideline [NG12].

→ www.nice.org.uk/guidance/NG12

7. B ★   OHCM 10th ed. → p. 254

This man has symptoms of dyspepsia, but there are no 'red flags' present. He has a recent history of non-steroidal anti-inflammatory drug (NSAID) use with diclofenac and these commonly cause gastric irritation. There is no reason to test for, or empirically eradicate, *Helicobacter pylori*. The offending medication should be stopped. If the pain continues, he could be given a proton pump inhibitor. If no improvement, then *H. pylori* testing with stool antigen, and then further investigation.

8. E ★   OHCM 10th ed. → p. 250

Odynophagia (painful swallowing) is a concerning symptom. In someone with a background of reflux disease (and smoking), if progressive and associated with weight loss, it likely signals either squamous cell carcinoma or adenocarcinoma of the oesophagus. One in five occurrences is in the upper part of the oesophagus.

A. Coughing mid-swallow indicates difficulty in making the movement, as in, for example, a bulbar palsy.

B. This is suggestive of a pharyngeal pouch.

C. Intermittent pain is likely to be due to abnormal contractions of the oesophagus, as occurs in oesophageal spasm.

D. Regurgitation is symptomatic of a motility disorder (e.g. achalasia), as opposed to a mechanical blockage (e.g. a malignant stricture).

9. B ★   OHCM 10th ed. → p. 276

The clinical findings and blood results are suggestive of decompensated chronic liver cirrhosis with portal hypertension; the history of repeated falls and strange responses should be interpreted as hepatic encephalopathy (HE). This is defined as a disturbance in brain functioning due to nitrogenous substances derived from the gut that are ineffectively detoxified or bypass the diseased liver, causing inflammation of astrocytes and swelling. The aims in this situation are therefore:

1. Nutritional management
2. Reduction in the 'nitrogenous load': this can be achieved via bowel cleansing (regular enemas) and non-absorbable disaccharides (lactulose is the first-line pharmacological treatment of HE). The target is 2–4 soft bowel motions per day
3. Exclude sepsis: this is the most common trigger of decompensation—perform an ascitic tap, blood cultures, a chest X-ray (CXR), and a

urine dip. Antibiotics are often commenced in the absence of typical sepsis features if there is a rising bilirubin level or deteriorating synthetic function
4. Look for signs of gastrointestinal (GI) bleeding
5. Exclude intracranial bleeding.

A. This can be used for symptomatic tense, refractory, or recurrent ascites.

C. This man is anaemic, but not critically; transfusing him is not the priority at this stage. Higher haemoglobin levels can precipitate variceal bleeding by increasing portal wedge pressures.

D. This is used in the prevention of variceal haemorrhage, as it reduces the cardiac output and vasoconstricts.

E. This is a first-line treatment of ascites, but his sodium level is too low and reducing it further can worsen the encephalopathy. Cautious fluid replacement can be used to slowly bring sodium levels up by interrupting the overactive renin–angiotensin system drive that occurs in progressive liver cirrhosis (increasing peripheral vasodilatation and renal vasoconstriction due to increased nitric oxide release as cirrhosis and portal hypertension progresses).

10. C ★   OHCM 10th ed. → p. 276

This woman has decompensated non-alcoholic steatohepatitis (NASH) cirrhosis with ascites and peripheral oedema. Ascites has developed, in this case most likely as a complication of liver cirrhosis and portal hypertension. Impaired synthetic function leads to hypoalbuminaemia, the effects of which are seen in increasing peritoneal fluid, peripheral fluid distribution, and leuconychia.

11. C ★   OHCM 10th ed. → p. 282

This is primary biliary cholangitis, with anti-mitochondrial antibodies detected in up to 98% of cases. Interlobular bile ducts are damaged by chronic granulomatous inflammation, which leads to progressive cholestasis, cirrhosis, and portal hypertension. Often this is diagnosed after finding a raised alkaline phosphatase (ALP) level during routine blood examination and, as in this case, lethargy and pruritus can precede the jaundice by a number of years. It affects women in 90% of cases, and fatigue is the most common and debilitating symptom.

A. This occurs in up to 30% of limited systemic sclerosis.

B. This occurs in 60–75% of systemic lupus erythematosus (SLE).

D. This occurs in SLE and anti-phospholipid syndrome.

E. This occurs in 70% of autoimmune hepatitis.

12. B ★   OHCM 10th ed. → p. 256

Symptoms of hypotension and melaena in someone on long-term steroid therapy are highly suspicious for a bleeding ulcer. The key, however, is to discover the melaena, because the patient will not always do it themselves. In this case, for example, the presenting complaint was nausea and dizziness—in someone with an endocrine history, it would be easy to be distracted by thoughts of an Addisonian crisis. It is vital, however, to keep it simple and work through the common causes of dizziness first; among other things, this means performing a digital rectal examination.

A. This is a less common cause of upper gastrointestinal (GI) bleeding.

B. This also causes fresh bleeding that is usually sudden and painless.

C. This is more likely to present with vomiting, dysphagia, and weight loss after several weeks of non-specific symptoms.

D. This is probably the next best answer, as 3 days of vomiting could be enough to cause a tear in the oesophagus, resulting in altered blood per rectum and symptoms of hypotension. However, as this woman is at high risk because of the steroid use, peptic ulceration would be more likely.

13. C ★ OHCM 10th ed. → p. 15

The scenario suggests that the woman does not have capacity. The procedure is important to investigate the gastrointestinal bleeding, but her next of kin cannot consent on her behalf. The team need to sign a form stating this, with one of them acting as a proxy consent giver, explaining why the procedure is necessary. This should be after a formal capacity assessment has been carried out and after a best interests decision has been made and documented.

14. E ★ OHCM 10th ed. → p. 268

Loss of the terminal ileum results in an inability to absorb the intrinsic factor–vitamin B12 complex. If there has been extensive surgery to the small bowel, folic acid and fat absorption (and hence fat-soluble vitamins) may be reduced, requiring additional supplementation. Impaired bile salts absorption can be compensated by an increase in their synthesis.

15. E ★ OHCM 10th ed. → pp. 256–7

Given that this woman is hallucinating (encephalopathy) and has fluid in her abdomen (ascites), it is likely that her heavy alcohol use has caused liver cirrhosis and portal hypertension. She is now bleeding from the dilated collateral variceal veins that have developed at sites of portosystemic anastomoses in response to portal hypertension.

A. This can cause both coffee-ground haematemesis and melaena but does not fit with the clinical scenario.

B. This causes dysphagia, retrosternal pain, and hoarseness.

C. This does present with haematemesis, but usually after some violent vomiting has caused an oesophageal tear in the first place. It is a reasonable differential but is less likely, given the background of alcoholic liver disease.

D. This usually presents with burning retrosternal pain and dysphagia, with no features of alcoholic liver disease.

16. D ★   OHCM 10th ed. → p. 250

The history of difficulty swallowing solids and liquids from the start is that of a motility disorder. In disorders like achalasia (in which the lower oesophageal sphincter cannot relax due to degeneration of the myenteric plexus), oesophageal manometry can be used to perform more specific diagnostics and show features such as the resting pressure of the sphincter and the exact pattern of oesophageal peristalsis.

A. In the setting of dysphagia, this does not offer much extra to an erect chest film.

C. This is a useful, although non-specific, first step in dysphagia but may clearly show a hiatus hernia.

D and E. These can be used together—an oesophagogastroduodenoscopy (OGD) to rule out a tumour at the gastro-oesophageal junction and an endoscopic ultrasound scan for further visualization if a tumour is detected.

17. B ★   OHCM 10th ed. → p. 252

Symptom control with proton pump inhibitors (PPIs) should be a priority in this scenario and is secondary to concerns over affected biopsy results. Endoscopy is primarily used to exclude malignancy and to look for benign peptic strictures, the initial treatment of which is PPI before considering balloon dilatation. Eosinophilic oesophagitis can also present with mild oesophageal dysphagia or food bolus and requires a trial of PPI before oesophageal biopsies are taken.

Lifestyle advice regarding his weight and current smoking is appropriate but will not affect the result or interpretation of the endoscopy.

18. C ★   OHCM 10th ed. → p. 266

All the other alcoholic drinks, apart from cider, contain gluten.

19. A ★★

This describes how vasopressin and its analogues (including terlipressin) work in this situation, i.e. an upper gastrointestinal bleed in someone with likely chronic liver disease, and thus bleeding oesophageal varices. Terlipressin, along with intravenous antibiotics, has been shown to improve mortality in this situation. It acts via V1 receptors, causing vasoconstriction of splanchnic vessels, thus reducing portal inflow.

B. This describes the effects of vitamin K.

C. This is the method of action of tranexamic acid.

D. This describes how proton pump inhibitors (PPIs) work.

E. This is the effect of treatment with human albumin solution.

20. D ★★   OHCM 10th ed. → p. 277

Prioritization in the United Kingdom for liver transplant listing is based on the United Kingdom End-Stage Model for Liver Disease (UKELD) score, based on creatinine, sodium, international normalized ratio (INR), and bilirubin.

Most transplant centres require a patient to be abstinent from alcohol for at least 6 months before being considered, although there is significant controversy over the rationale for this. This patient's liver has not recovered despite abstinence, which should get us starting to think about transplantation.

21. C ★★   OHCM 10th ed. → p. 252

The man has tried 1 month of proton pump inhibitor (PPI) treatment and has been tested for, and eradicated of, *Helicobacter pylori* infection. However, he still has symptoms and if this is the case, the guidelines recommend second-line eradication before referral to secondary care.

To retest for *H. pylori* infection, the patient must stop the PPI for 14 days and be 28 days from last taking the antibiotic and is tested via carbon urea breath testing.

National Institute for Health and Care Excellence (2014). *Gastro-oesophageal reflux disease and dyspepsia in adults: investigation and management*. Clinical guideline [CG184].

→ www.nice.org.uk/guidance/cg184

22. D ★★   OHCM 10th ed. → p. 528

This woman has a systemic inflammatory response (temperature >38°C, heart rate >90 bpm), with potentially infective diarrhoea. As she is potentially septic so soon after completing a course of chemotherapy, this is febrile neutropenia. She should therefore be treated following the hospital neutropenic sepsis regimen. This may differ from trust to trust but will always stipulate that, in the presence of systemic inflammatory response syndrome (SIRS), or sepsis in this situation, broad-spectrum antibiotics need to be instituted, even before any culture results have been received. This is due to the potential severity and rapid progression of sepsis in a patient with neutropenia.

23. C ★★   OHCM 10th ed. → p. 700

Although not serious, Gilbert's syndrome is common, with up to 2% prevalence. It is often detected incidentally, as in this case. It causes unconjugated hyperbilirubinaemia, thus differentiating itself from rotor syndrome (**E**), which causes conjugated hyperbilirubinaemia and is therefore urine-positive for bilirubin. The enzyme deficit that causes the bilirubin rise in Gilbert's syndrome is heightened in intercurrent illnesses (as suggested here by the recent viral symptoms) and fasting.

A. This is a more extreme form of Gilbert's syndrome (the enzyme is totally absent) that usually presents in the neonatal period and requires liver transplantation.

24. A ★★   OHCM 10th ed. → p. 252

Treatment for *Helicobacter pylori* is a week-long course of dual antibiotic therapy with a high-dose proton pump inhibitor (PPI). In a man who drinks excessive amounts of alcohol, it would be a bad idea to give him a metronidazole-based eradication therapy (disulfiram-like reaction). First-line eradication therapy should be a PPI-based triple therapy for a week, either with clarithromycin or metronidazole. Second-line treatment is another 7-day course, with the antibiotic choice dependent on penicillin allergy and previous exposure to clarithromycin, metronidazole, or quinolones.

National Institute for Health and Care Excellence (2014). *Gastro-oesophageal reflux disease and dyspepsia in adults: investigation and management*. Clinical guideline [CG184].

→ www.nice.org.uk/guidance/cg184

25. C ★★

This is an oculogyric crisis caused by blockade of the D2 receptor by the centrally acting antiemetic metoclopramide.

A. This is an antihistamine that can cause drowsiness and dry mouth.

B. This is an anti-spasmodic that largely causes anti-muscarinic side effects such as dry mouth and blurred vision.

D. This is a proton pump inhibitor (PPI) that can cause headache and gastrointestinal upset.

E. This is an antiemetic that can cause headache and constipation.

26. D ★★   OHCM 10th ed. → p. 275

This question is testing knowledge of the Kings College Criteria in acute liver failure:

- Paracetamol-induced liver failure:
  - Arterial pH <7.3 24 hours after ingestion
  - Or all of: prothrombin time (PT) >100 s, creatinine >300 micromol/L, grade 3 or 4 encephalopathy.
- Non-paracetamol liver failure:
  - PT >100 s.
- Or three out of five of the following:
  - Drug-induced
  - Age <10 or >40 years
  - >1 week from jaundice to developing encephalopathy
  - PT >50 s
  - Bilirubin >300 micromol/L.

Acute liver failure: you will hear the term 'acute liver failure' used commonly during your general medical career. However, it is a term that is often misunderstood and misused. Understanding the definition is important, as it affects management [including referral to a liver transplant centre; acute liver failure patients are assessed and listed on the NHS Blood and Transplant (NHSBT) super urgent list], as well as prognosis. Acute liver failure is a rare condition in which rapid deterioration in liver function results in altered mental status (encephalopathy) and coagulopathy *without any evidence of pre-existing liver disease*. The clinical picture is vastly different to a patient whose liver is failing and has chronic significant fibrosis or cirrhosis, and importantly survival rates pre- and post-transplant are worse.

27. A ★★   OHCM 10th ed. → pp. 280–1

The history is in keeping with alcoholic hepatitis with cirrhosis and portal hypertension. His discriminant function meets the criteria for steroid treatment. However, in view of the fever, starting steroids could cause rapid deterioration in the context of a possible infection. A full septic screen, including an ascitic tap looking for a neutrophil count of >250, would be most appropriate, along with supportive management, as described previously. The STOPAH trial showed a non-significant trend towards benefit with steroids and no benefit with pentoxifylline. There is a role for steroids in carefully selected patients. There is insufficient evidence at present for *N*-acetylcysteine (NAC) in this situation.

28. D ★★   OHCM 10th ed. → p. 280

The key here is to realize that giving glucose—both for rehydration and for correcting hypoglycaemia—to a potentially thiamine-deficient patient can precipitate Wernicke's encephalopathy. This man has incipient Wernicke's encephalopathy and should be treated initially with two doses of vitamins B + C (i.e. Pabrinex® ampoules I + II) intravenous (IV) three times daily. All of the other drugs may be given, but not necessarily before the fluids. Pabrinex® includes thiamine, riboflavin, pyridoxine, nicotinamide, and ascorbic acid.

A. This is a benzodiazepine given for symptoms of alcohol withdrawal.

B. This is often used for alcoholic gastritis.

C. This is a pancreatic enzyme supplement.

E. This is reasonable in the acute setting if the patient is low risk and is a good idea for almost all patients once they are discharged.

National Institute for Health and Care Excellence (2010). *Alcohol-use disorders: diagnosis and management of physical complications*. Clinical guideline [CG100].

→ www.nice.org.uk/guidance/CG100

29. B ★★   OHCM 10th ed. → p. 270

This man has steatorrhoea—indicative of fat malabsorption—and acute-on-chronic abdominal pain likely secondary to chronic pancreatitis due to a history of gallstones. Continued weight loss may be caused by general malabsorption due to an atrophic pancreas causing pancreatic exocrine insufficiency; however, pancreatic malignancy, pseudocyst, and superior mesenteric vein (SMV) and portal vein thrombus would need to be excluded. Computed tomography (CT) would be the most appropriate next test. Faecal elastase is a marker of absorption and, if abnormal, can suggest pancreatic insufficiency.

30. E ★★★   OHCM 10th ed. → p. 759

A patient with an aspirate with pH of between 0 and 5.5 can safely be started on enteral feeding. There are no known reports of pulmonary aspirates at or below this figure. If the pH of the aspirate is >6, the patient should be left for an hour before retesting the aspirate. If the aspirate pH is still above 6, consider replacing the tube or checking the position by X-ray. Never commence feeding until tube placement is confirmed by someone with experience in doing so, as feeding down a misplaced nasogastric tube (into the lungs) is a never event associated with a very high mortality.

National Patient Safety Agency (2005). *Reducing harm caused by the misplacement of nasogastric feeding tubes.* Updated 2011.

→ www.npsa.nhs.uk/nrls/alerts-and-directives/alerts/nasogastric-feeding-tubes

31. E ★★★   OHCM 10th ed. → pp. 262–3

A man of any age with inflammatory bowel disease (IBD) and unexplained iron deficiency anaemia and a haemoglobin level of 110 g/L or below should be urgently referred to rule out a malignant cause. He is at an increased risk of bowel cancer with his co-diagnosis of ulcerative colitis. Initial surveillance colonoscopy is performed at 10 years from the initial diagnosis, and the frequency of subsequent surveillance endoscopy depends on the histology and distribution of disease.

32. E ★★★   OHCM 10th ed. → pp. 256–7

This man is haemodynamically compromised, following his variceal bleed, and should be given terlipressin to reduce his portal venous pressure. Terlipressin use in variceal bleeding has been shown to produce a 34% relative risk reduction in mortality and is the only vasoactive agent that has been shown to reduce mortality.

A and B. These are indicated in the acute management of pulmonary oedema and angina.

C. Octreotide causes a reduction in portal pressures but is not as effective as terlipressin. In view of its lower cardiac side effect profile, it can be considered in a patient with significant ischaemic heart disease.

D. Propranolol is used in the prophylaxis of variceal bleeding, rather than acute management.

Gøtzsche PC and Hróbjartsson A. Somatostatin analogues for acute bleeding oesophageal varices. *Cochrane Database Syst Rev.* 2008;**3**:CD000193.

→ www.cochrane.org/CD000193/LIVER_somatostatin-analogues-for-acute-bleeding-oesophageal-varices

Ioannou G, Doust J, and Rockey DC. Terlipressin is a safe and effective treatment for bleeding from oesophageal varices which is a life threatening complication of cirrhosis of the liver. *Cochrane Database Syst Rev.* 2003;**1**:CD002147.

→ www.cochrane.org/reviews/en/ab002147.html

Tripathi D, et al. UK guidelines on the management of variceal haemorrhage in cirrhotic patients, *Gut.* 2015;**64**:1680–704.

---

33. E ★★★   OHCM 10th ed. → p. 616

In those over the age of 60 years, a history of fresh rectal bleeding of >6 weeks' duration should not be attributed to diclofenac or haemorrhoids. Regardless of whether there is any change in bowel habit, an urgent referral should be made to be seen within 2 weeks in a surgical outpatient clinic. Guidance states that, when referring, all that is required is an abdominal and rectal examination and a full blood count, so as to not delay specialist assessment.

National Institute for Health and Care Excellence ICE (2015). *Suspected cancer: recognition and referral.* NICE guideline [NG12].

→ www.nice.org.uk/guidance/ng12

---

34. A ★★★   OHCM 10th ed. → p. 521

These symptoms could fit with irritable bowel syndrome (IBS). However, this lady is well over 50 years old and unlikely to develop it beyond this age. Suspicion has to be raised for a possible ovarian cancer with these symptoms, and if her CA125 is >35 IU/mL, she should undergo an ultrasound scan (USS) to assess her ovaries.

C. There is no mention of reflux-type symptoms.

D. There is no change in the stool.

E. Urinalysis would form part of the workup of this lady but is not the most appropriate step here.

National Institute for Health and Care Excellence (2011). *Ovarian cancer: recognition and initial management.* Clinical guideline [CG122].

→ www.nice.org.uk/guidance/cg122

---

35. C ★★★★   OHCM 10th ed. → p. 257

Rockall defined a number of independent risk factors that predict death, using four factors: age, co-morbidities, shock, and endoscopic findings. A score of >8 is associated with a high risk of death.

Rockall TA, Logan RF, Devlin HB, and Northfield TC. Risk assessment after acute upper gastrointestinal haemorrhage. *Gut.* 1996;**38**:316–21.

36. E ★★★★ OHCM 10th ed. → p. 587

In prolonged starvation, the lack of dietary carbohydrate means insulin secretion is reduced. As fat and protein stores are preferentially catabolized for energy, there is a loss of intracellular electrolytes, especially phosphate. When food becomes available again, a shift from fat back to carbohydrate metabolism and the resultant rise in insulin stimulate cellular uptake of phosphate. Features of refeeding syndrome can occur if this leads to profound hypophosphataemia (<0.5 mmol/L). Early features are often non-specific, but patients can go on to develop cardiorespiratory failure, arrhythmias, rhabdomyolysis, seizures, coma, and sudden death. Magnesium, glucose, and thiamine can also be low.

A and B. These are useful in patients with cardiorespiratory signs/symptoms but are not the most appropriate here.

C. This would be useful if this were a chest infection.

D. This might show changes consistent with alcoholic excess.

Hearing SD. Refeeding syndrome. *BMJ.* 2004;**328**:908–9.

37. C ★★★★ OHCM 10th ed. → p. 532

This man has metastatic colonic carcinoma, with tumour spread to the adrenals, liver, and lung. The endoscopic retrograde cholangiopancreatography (ERCP) stenting failed and, considering the degree of intrinsic and extrinsic obstruction, this was unlikely to improve symptoms radically. Percutaneous drainage would have similar effects and has significant mortality rates (20%) in this cohort. This man now has end-stage metastatic disease; the aim of treatment now should be to limit his suffering. It would be reasonable, in view of the biliary obstruction, to treat for sepsis if present, with strict ceilings of care regarding escalation and length of treatment, but it is good practice to involve the palliative care team not only to ensure that all is done to control symptoms, but also to aid communication with the family who may have expectations that are at odds with the evolving clinical situation—as in this case.

38. B ★★★★

This is not core knowledge, but it is useful to understand the concept, which is likely to be discussed in multidisciplinary team meetings you may sit in on as a junior doctor. With metastatic cancer and a performance status of 3 (>50% of the time in bed/lying down, capable of only limited self-care), the prognosis in this case is <3 months. The World Health Organization (WHO) performance status assesses general health and grades from 0 (fully active) to 4 (almost fully dependent).

Cancer Research UK (2005). *Gold Standards Framework Programme, England 2005.*

→ www.cancerresearchuk.org/cancer-help/about-cancer/cancer-questions/performance-status

39. A ★ ★ ★ ★ OHCM 10th ed. → p. 266

Ten to 20% of all people will, at some stage in their life, have symptoms of irritable bowel syndrome (IBS). She would meet criteria for a diagnosis of IBS—>6 months of: abdominal pain or discomfort, bloating, and change in bowels, as long as there are no 'red flags'—unintentional. It is necessary to establish the quantity and quality of pain or discomfort—a fixed site would be more in keeping with cancer.

IBS symptoms: pain or discomfort relieved by defecation or associated with altered bowel frequency or stool form, along with at least two of four out of: bloating, altered stool passage, symptoms made worse with eating, and passage of mucus.

She should have some blood tests—full blood count (FBC), C-reactive protein (CRP), coeliac screen—to exclude other differentials. A food diary may help her make a link with particular foods, allowing avoidance of the triggers and thereby improving her pain and symptoms. She should restrict her intake of tea or coffee to three times/day, limit to three portions of fruit/day, reduce alcohol intake and fizzy drinks, and reduce food with resistant starches.

B. She should limit her intake of fruit to no more than three portions per day and make up the rest with vegetables.

C, D, and **E.** These are high in resistant starches, which are not completely digested by the body and so ferment and produce gas, worsening symptoms of bloating and wind.

National Institute for Health and Care Excellence (2008). *Irritable bowel syndrome in adults: diagnosis and management.* Clinical guideline [CG61].

→ www.nice.org.uk/guidance/cg61

40. E ★ ★ ★ ★ OHCM 10th ed. → pp. 262–3

This question is testing knowledge of the Truelove and Witt criteria and management of acute severe ulcerative colitis. A tricky question, but the key is to be aware of escalation criteria (Travis criteria).

On day 3 of intravenous (IV) steroids, C-reactive protein (CRP) >45 or >6 motions/day has an 80% chance of predicting the need for colectomy.

Rescue therapy with infliximab or ciclosporin can be considered, but in this case, the previous history of tuberculosis could cause deterioration in the patient and would be delaying the inevitable. Excluding the presence of other infective causes of diarrhoea is paramount, such as *Clostridium difficile*, and repeat endoscopy can be used to reassess the bowel, although this should always only be flexible sigmoidoscopy in acute flares, due to the risk of perforation, as well as patient discomfort associated with colonoscopy. If perforation is a concern (rising CRP and haemodynamic compromise despite treatment with steroids), then computed tomography (CT) scan should be performed.

Chapter 5

Renal medicine

William White

The kidney causes problems for medical students and junior doctors alike—the convoluted journey from plasma to urine, the conundrum of what is reabsorbed and excreted where, and the tangled web of the glomerulonephritides are traditionally learnt, rather than actually understood.

As in all clinical medicine, a good place to start is with the fundamentals of the organ in question. Passage from plasma to urine follows the pathway:

- Blood
- Glomerulus
- Tubules
- Collecting duct
- Ureter
- Bladder
- Urethra.

The primary functions of the kidney are:

- Removal of toxins
- Electrolyte homeostasis
- Maintenance of acid–base balance
- Activation of vitamin D
- Stimulation of erythropoiesis
- Maintenance of blood volume.

The challenge then is to implement these basics by being sensitive to deviations from normal physiology: recognizing the accumulation of any potential toxins (hyperkalaemia, uraemia, and acidosis) or the lack of any synthetic products (hypocalcaemia and anaemia), suggesting triggers for such deviations, and pinpointing the specific parts of the anatomy that may be malfunctioning in some way so as to cause impairment.

Despite its bad reputation, the kidney reveals more about itself than any other organ and, in theory, should be the easiest to monitor. It achieves this through its *raison d'être*: urine. Its presence, absence, contents, smell, and colour offer a running commentary on the activity of the renal tract at any given point in time—it is the internal, intangible workings of specialized cells made physical, measurable, and dippable. So, far from being those much-feared Objective Structured Clinical Examination (OSCE) stations, the dipstick and the catheter are our friends. Or they should be, for it is our ability to harness the information that they provide, allied to the series of numbers on the oft-requested 'U&Es' (urea and electrolytes), against a background of wide-ranging symptoms that will make us sensitive to the running of the kidney. This—not just our ability to regurgitate the three types of renal tubular acidosis—is what is at stake in this chapter. Indeed, as the span of questions that follow confirms, it is the urinary tract infections, blocked catheters, stones, and hypovolaemic failures that are our bread and butter. Identify and treat these successfully, and the interstitial nephritides, Fanconi's syndrome, and even glomerulonephritis will seem less daunting and may even start to make sense.

QUESTIONS

1. You receive a phone call from the biochemistry lab confirming that a patient on your ward has a potassium level of 7.1 and an acute kidney injury (AKI) with a creatinine level that has risen from 130 to 450 in 72 hours. A nurse has performed an electrocardiogram (ECG) (Figure 5.1). What is the *single* most appropriate next step? ★

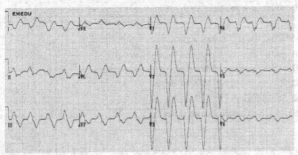

Figure 5.1
Reproduced with permission from Wilkinson I.B, Raine T., Wiles K. et al, *Oxford Handbook of Clinical Medicine*, Tenth edition, figure 7.4, p. 301. Copyright (2017) with permission from Oxford University Press.

A 10 mL of 10% calcium chloride intravenous (IV)

B 250 mL of crystalloid fluid IV

C Insert a dialysis line

D Insert a urinary catheter

E Repeat the urea and electrolytes (U&Es)

2. A 70-year-old man with stage 4 chronic kidney disease (CKD) [estimated glomerular filtration rate (eGFR) 28] due to diabetes requires a coronary angiogram following a non-ST-elevation myocardial infarction. His lisinopril is held. Which *single* intervention will help protect his kidneys from contrast-induced nephropathy (CIN)? ★

A Fluid restriction

B Furosemide 40 mg intravenous (IV) post-procedure

C Haemodialysis post-procedure

D IV fluid

E *N*-acetylcysteine 600 mg oral (PO) twice daily for a day before and after the scan

3. A 70-year-old man attends his local hospital for a blood test, having started taking lisinopril 10 mg oral (PO) once daily 2 weeks previously. His doctor contacts him with the results (Table 5.1):

Table 5.1 Blood results pre- and post-lisinopril

	Pre-lisinopril	2 weeks later
Estimated glomerular filtration rate (eGFR) (mL/min)	50	40
Creatinine (micromol/L)	150	180

Which is the *single* most appropriate management? ★

A Admit the man to hospital for investigations

B Halve the dose of lisinopril

C Repeat the test in 10 days' time

D Stop lisinopril immediately

E Switch to bendroflumethiazide 2.5 mg oral (PO) once daily

4. A 66-year-old man has had a right femoral–popliteal bypass. He received 2.5 L of Hartmann's solution during the procedure. He has been oliguric for the last 3 hours.

T 36.5°C, HR 72 bpm, BP 105/65 mmHg, RR 14/min.

What is the *single* most appropriate next step? ★

A Abdominal examination

B Catheter insertion

C Fluid challenge

D Mixed venous saturation from the central venous pressure (CVP) line

E Turn off the epidural

5. A 76-year-old man has been unwell for several days. He has been feverish, coughing, and vomiting.

Sodium 131 mmol/L, potassium 6.3 mmol/L, urea 46 mmol/L, creatinine 522 micromol/L.

He is treated aggressively with intravenous fluids for 12 hours. Which *single* factor would most indicate the need for emergency renal replacement therapy? ★

A Creatinine increased by >25%

B Hyperglycaemia

C Pulmonary oedema

D Systolic blood pressure dropped to <90 mmHg

E Urine output <10 mL/hour

6. A 30-year-old man has had intermittent abdominal pain for the past 3 days. It begins on his left side and travels down into his groin. He has also felt nauseated and is finding it difficult to lie still. His renal function is normal. Which is the *single* most appropriate analgesic agent? ★

A Codeine phosphate 60 mg oral (PO)

B Diclofenac 75 mg intramuscular (IM)

C Morphine 10 mg PO

D Pethidine 150 mg IM

E Tramadol 100 mg PO

7. An 82-year-old man has been confused and coughing for the past week. He is admitted to hospital and started on intravenous antibiotics, as his renal function is markedly worse than usual.

Urea 22 mmol/L, creatinine 210 micromol/L.

Which of his *single* drug from his regular medications would it be most appropriate to withhold? ★

A Aspirin

B Calcium 600 mg/colecalciferol 10 micrograms

C Levothyroxine

D Ramipril

E Tamsulosin

8. A 48-year-old woman has felt increasingly lethargic and nauseated over the last few weeks and undergoes blood tests via her general practitioner (GP).

Creatinine 630 micromol/L, alkaline phosphatase (ALP) 45 IU/L, calcium 2 mmol/L, haemoglobin (Hb) 7 g/L, potassium 6.5 mmol/L, phosphate 1.8 mmol/L.

Which *single* blood test result supports a diagnosis of chronic kidney disease? ★

A ALP

B Calcium

C Hb

D Phosphate

E Potassium

9. A 78-year-old man has a painfully distended lower abdomen that has developed over the past 2 days, and he has not passed urine during this time. He has benign prostatic hypertrophy and has had this problem before. A urinary catheter is placed. Which is the *single* most appropriate course of action? ★

A Abdominal X-ray

B Digital rectal examination

C Intravenous (IV) antibiotics

D IV fluids

E Ultrasound scan of the kidneys

10. A 40-year-old woman is admitted from the psychiatric unit, as the staff are concerned she has become drowsy and dehydrated.

Sodium 156 mmol/L, potassium 5.5 mmol/L, urea 18 mmol/L, creatinine 116 micromol/L.

Which further feature would be most useful in the assessment of her renal function? ★

A Full drug history

B Haemoglobin

C Protein:creatinine ratio

D Urine output

E Weight

11. An 88-year-old man is admitted to hospital, having been found on the floor by his carer one morning. There are no signs of infection. He is treated with intravenous fluids.

Urea 17 mmol/L, creatinine 368 micromol/L.

Which *single* further test would support the most likely diagnosis? ★

A Calcium

B Creatine kinase

C Erythrocyte sedimentation rate (ESR)

D International normalized ratio (INR)

E Troponin

12. A 72-year-old Afro-Caribbean man has a routine check-up. At the end of the consultation, it is suggested that he provides a urine sample and go for blood tests to look for kidney disease. His body mass index (BMI) is 33 kg/m^2.

Blood pressure (BP) 135/90 mmHg.

Fasting venous blood glucose 6.4 mmol/L.

Which *single* factor should have prompted the doctor to suggest these tests? ★

A Age

B Ethnicity

C Fasting glucose

D Gender

E None of the above

13. A 25-year-old man has had intermittent right-sided abdominal pain for the last 5 days. It has struck several times for short periods, always focused on the right side of his back before moving into his groin. When it comes, it is severe—enough to wake him from sleep on one occasion—and causes him to roll around to try to get comfortable.

T 36.6°C, HR 90 bpm, BP 125/80 mmHg.

Which *single* pair of investigations would be most likely to support the diagnosis? ★

A Amylase + computed tomography (CT) scan of the abdomen

B Digital rectal examination + abdominal X-ray

C Full blood count + laparotomy

D Liver function tests + liver ultrasound scan

E Urine dipstick + CT kidneys, ureters, and bladder (KUB)

14. A 76-year-old man has become increasingly confused over the last 3 days. He has not opened his bowels in the last 48 hours.

T 37.8°C, HR 100 bpm, BP 135/80 mmHg, SaO$_2$ 97% on air.

His chest is clear. His abdomen is distended, with suprapubic dullness to percussion.

Which is the *single* most appropriate immediate management? ★

A Give a phosphate enema

B Pass a urinary catheter

C Request an abdominal X-ray

D Request a urinalysis

E Start broad-spectrum antibiotics

15. An 82-year-old female has had a laparoscopic repair of a femoral hernia. Two days after surgery, she appears quite dehydrated and is still taking metformin. She is vomiting and breathing rapidly.

What *single* investigation would be likely to support the diagnosis? ★

A Blood gases

B Chest X-ray

C Full blood count

D Random capillary blood glucose

E Urea and electrolytes

16. A 72-year-old man is recovering from major colorectal surgery. Two days after the operation, his urine output tails off. There is no history of renal disease. His abdomen is not distended; there is no bladder palpable, and he appears well hydrated. There is a catheter *in situ* that remains patent on flushing.

Urea 16 mmol/L, creatinine 323 micromol/L.

Which is the *single* most appropriate initial management? ★

A Change the catheter

B Insert a central venous pressure (CVP) line

C Request an ultrasound scan of the bladder and kidneys

D Start cefuroxime 1.5 g intravenous (IV) three times daily

E Start furosemide 40 mg oral (PO) once daily

17. A 55-year-old woman is listed for a Nissen's fundoplication. She has type 2 diabetes with nephropathy. She is prescribed a sliding-scale insulin regime and requires thromboprophylaxis. Her creatinine clearance is calculated at 14 mL/min. Which is the *single* most appropriate management? ★

A Aspirin 75 mg oral (PO) once daily

B Reduced-dose low-molecular-weight heparin subcutaneous (SC)

C Rivaroxaban 10 mg PO once daily

D Thromboembolic disease stockings

E Thromboprophylaxis is contraindicated in severe renal impairment

18. A 77-year-old man has been confused for the past 48 hours. The staff at his nursing home report that he has not been communicating or behaving as normal.

T 37.2°C, HR 110 bpm, BP 90/66 mmHg.

Urea 25 mmol/L, creatinine 395 micromol/L.

Which *single* further finding would indicate the need for aggressive resuscitation with intravenous (IV) fluids? ★

A Absent jugular venous pressure (JVP)

B Capillary refill time 2 s

C Clear chest

D Gallop heart rhythm

E Reduced Glasgow Coma Scale score

19. A 52-year-old man had an open cholecystectomy 3 days ago. The surgical team are concerned, as he has a persistently fast heart rate. He is thirsty and in pain and, over the last 12 hours, has had several dark-coloured vomits.

T 37.2°C, HR 130 bpm, BP 90/45 mmHg.

His blood results 2 and 3 days post-surgery are shown in Table 5.2.

Table 5.2 Blood results post-surgery

	Two days post-surgery	Three days post-surgery
Haemoglobin (Hb) (g/L)	116	114
Urea (Ur) (mmol/L)	7.2	15.4
Creatinine (Cr) (micromol/L)	57	62

Which is the *single* most likely diagnosis? ★

A Dehydration

B Intra-abdominal collection

C Lower respiratory tract infection

D Pulmonary embolism

E Upper gastrointestinal bleed

20. A 66-year-old man attends diabetes outpatient clinic. He remains asymptomatic and continues to control his blood sugars with metformin 850mg PO twice daily.

T 36.6°C, HR 75 bpm, BP 135/95 mmHg.

Albumin:creatinine ratio 4.9 mg/mmol.

His chest is clear; heart sounds are normal, and there is no peripheral oedema. Which is the *single* most appropriate next step in management? ★

A Bendroflumethiazide 2.5 mg oral (PO) once daily

B Gliclazide 80 mg PO once daily

C Lisinopril 5 mg PO once daily

D Long-acting insulin subcutaneous (SC) once at night

E No alteration to management required

21. A 72-year-old woman has urinary sepsis and severe acute kidney injury. She is a nursing home resident with severe frontal dementia and is clutching her lower abdomen and writhing around in pain. Clinical examination suggests urinary retention. During her admission, she has repeatedly pulled out her urinary catheter and now tells the junior doctor that she does not want them replaced. During discussions, she is unable to retain information and cannot weigh up the relevant risks and benefits in order to formulate a decision. Which would be the *single* most appropriate next step? ★

A Contact her next of kin before making a decision

B Insert a catheter, as passive euthanasia is illegal

C Insert a catheter in her best interests, as she has no capacity to refuse

D Withhold treatment, as it is in her best interests to die

E Withhold treatment, as passive euthanasia is legal

22. A 75-year-old man presents with a 2-month history of persistent nasal and sinus congestion and, in the last fortnight, coughing up increasing amounts of blood.

Blood pressure (BP) 140/90 mmHg.

Urea 12 mmol/L, creatinine 570 micromol/L (85 micromol/L 6 weeks ago), albumin 37 g/L.

Urine dipstick: protein 2+, blood 2+.

Which is the *single* most likely diagnosis? ★★

A Hypertensive nephropathy

B Minimal change disease

C Myeloma

D Rapidly progressive glomerulonephritis

E Tubulointerstitial nephritis

23. A 17-year-old woman has noticed her face becoming very puffy, particularly around the eyes, and her legs swelling over the past 6 weeks. She has noticed that her urine is frothy. She has no other symptoms or medical problems.

Urea 4 mmol/L, creatinine 60 micromol/L, albumin 12 g/L.

Urine protein:creatinine ratio (PCR) 1200 mg/mmol.

Which is the *single* most likely diagnosis? ★★

A Immunoglobulin A (IgA) nephropathy

B Membranous nephropathy

C Minimal change disease

D Rapidly progressive glomerulonephritis

E Tubulointerstitial nephritis

24. A 21-year-old man has noticed his urine is red for the second time. He recovered quickly after the first episode but was unwell with a sore throat beforehand.

Urine dipstick: blood 3+.

Which is the *single* most likely explanation for the urine dip results? ★★

A Antibodies binding the kidney's basement membrane

B Congenitally enlarged cystic kidneys

C Immune complex deposition within the glomerulus

D Inflammation of the bladder wall

E Necrotizing granulomatous inflammation in Bowman's capsule

25. A 45-year-old Congolese man presents with uncomfortable lower limb swelling. He has previously tested positive for human immunodeficiency virus (HIV) but has taken no medications for this in the past 18 months.

Blood pressure (BP) 135/95 mmHg.

Urea 18 mmol/L, creatinine 410 micromol/L (110 micromol/L 2 years previous), albumin 19 g/L.

Urine dipstick: protein 3+, blood 1+.

Which is the *single* most likely diagnosis? ★★

A Focal segmental glomerulosclerosis (FSGS)

B Minimal change disease

C Rapidly progressive, necrotizing glomerulonephritis

D Thin basement membrane nephropathy

E Tubulointerstitial nephritis

26. A 68-year-old man with a 70 pack-year smoking history, type 2 diabetes, and hypertension presents with a 3-month history of worsening lower limb, scrotal, and abdominal swelling. A chest X-ray (CXR) shows a suspicious lesion in his right lung.

Urea 9 mmol/L, creatinine 102 micromol/L, albumin 16 g/L.

Urine dipstick: protein 3+.

Which is the *single* most likely diagnosis? ★★

A Diabetic nephropathy

B Membranous nephropathy

C Minimal change disease

D Thin basement membrane nephropathy

E Tubulointerstitial nephritis

27. A 30-year-old woman has been passing minimal amounts of concentrated urine for the past 3 days. She is feeling tired but, prior to this, had been well other than receiving a short course of oral antibiotics for an infection.

Blood pressure (BP) 140/90 mmHg.

Urea 9.2 mmol/L, creatinine 105 micromol/L, albumin 38 g/L.

Urine dipstick: protein 1+, blood 2+.

Which is the *single* most likely diagnosis? ★★

A Acute tubular necrosis

B Interstitial nephritis

C Nephritic syndrome

D Nephrotic syndrome

E Renovascular disease

28. An 82-year-old man has had a series of heavy nosebleeds. These started yesterday and occur whenever he exerts himself or leans forward. Three days ago, he started an antibiotic for a urinary infection. He has atrial fibrillation, for which he takes warfarin. His international normalized ratio (INR) is 6.4. Which *single* antibiotic has he been taking? ★★

A Amoxicillin

B Cefalexin

C Ciprofloxacin

D Co-amoxiclav

E Nitrofurantoin

29. A 35-year-old man is worried that his urine has been slightly red in colour over the last few days. He is a keen runner and usually exercises three times a week but has been off work for the last few days with a cough and sore throat.

T 37.1°C, HR 85 bpm, BP 125/60 mmHg.

Urine dipstick: leucocytes −, nitrites −, protein 1+, blood 3+.

Which is the *single* most likely diagnosis? ★★

A Bladder carcinoma

B Immunoglobulin A (IgA) nephropathy

C Nephrotic syndrome

D Renal calculi

E Urinary tract infection

30. A 31-year-old man has had a sore throat for 3 days. Over the last 12 hours, he has become concerned that he has blood in his urine because it has become a pale red colour. He has no previous medical history.

What is the *single* most likely pathological process occurring? ★★

A Diffusely thickened glomerular basement membrane

B Focal scarring of the glomerulus

C Fusion of the podocytes

D Inflammatory reaction in mesangial and endothelial cells

E Mesangial proliferation with immunoglobulin A (IgA) and complement deposits

31. A 28-year-old woman is referred to the nephrology clinic, having been diagnosed with polycystic kidney disease. Her brother is also affected. She says her father also had polycystic kidneys and died when she was quite young from 'a bleed on the brain'. Her renal function and blood pressure are normal, and her urine dip contains no blood, protein, or evidence of infection.

Which *single* investigation would you perform next? ★★

A A 24-hour urine collection for protein

B Computed tomography (CT) kidneys, ureters, and bladder (KUB)

C CT brain

D Magnetic resonance angiography (MRA) brain

E Serum cholesterol

32. A 28-year-old woman is referred to hospital as an emergency, with the following blood results, having not passed any urine in 2 days, despite drinking good amounts.

Urea 40 mmol/L, creatinine 1500 micromol/L, potassium 8 mmol/L, haemoglobin 11 g/L.

She has no previous medical history and was entirely well until this episode. She has no palpable bladder nor flank pain.

What is the *single* most likely diagnosis? ★★

A Anti-glomerular basement membrane (GBM) disease

B Chronic kidney disease

C Dehydration

D Obstructive nephropathy

E Renal infarction

33. A 22-year-old woman has long-standing intermittent joint pain, rashes, and hair loss. She has had a renal biopsy and a course of immunosuppressive therapy.

T 37.8°C, HR 90 bpm, BP 135/95 mmHg.

Urine dipstick: protein 3+.

Which *single* site within the kidney is most likely to be responsible for her proteinuria? ★★★

A Collecting duct

B Distal tubule

C Glomerulus

D Interstitium

E Proximal tubule

ANSWERS

1. A ★   OHCM 10th ed. → p. 301

Hyperkalaemia is a medical emergency that requires immediate treatment. A potassium level >6.5 mmol/L or with electrocardiogram (ECG) changes (request an ECG if >6 mmol/L) should be treated. In this case, we have no reason to suspect the high potassium level is spurious (e.g. due to haemolysis) and there are ECG changes which mean cardiac arrest is not far away. Calcium chloride (or calcium gluconate) is the immediate treatment but will only stabilize the myocardium temporarily and buy time for further treatment. Insulin and salbutamol will only shift potassium into the cells and levels will rebound. Definitive treatment is removal from the body, and in the absence of renal function, this may require renal replacement therapy (dialysis or filtration).

2. D ★   OHCM 10th ed. → pp. 319, 748

There is ongoing debate about the true existence of contrast-induced nephropathy (CIN), but patients at risk of CIN include those undergoing high-volume or intra-arterial iodinated contrast procedures, those with chronic kidney disease (CKD) and an estimated glomerular filtration rate (eGFR) <60 (especially with diabetic nephropathy), those over 75 years old, and those who are septic, dehydrated, and exposed to nephrotoxins (such as aminoglycosides). All patients should be resuscitated to euvolaemia, nephrotoxins and angiotensin-converting enzyme (ACE) inhibitors held, and then volume-expanded as above if at high risk. The volume of contrast used should be kept to a minimum and low- or iso-osmolar contrast used. Renal function should be monitored to 72 hours after the procedure. There is no evidence for a protective effect of N-acetylcysteine (NAC) or post-contrast haemodialysis or filtration. Metformin should be withheld for 48 hours after intravenous (IV) contrast administration because of the risk of lactic acidosis.

→www.londonaki.net/downloads/LondonAKInetwork-ContrastInduced NephropathyProphylaxis.pdf

3. C ★   OHCM 10th ed. → p. 114

The National Institute for Health and Care Excellence (NICE) guidance is that if the fall in the estimated glomerular filtration rate (eGFR) is <25% and the rise in serum creatinine is <30%, then the results can be re-checked within 2 weeks without altering the dose of the angiotensin-converting enzyme (ACE) inhibitor. If the fall is more precipitous, then other causes of acute renal failure (hypovolaemia, other drug side effects) need to be excluded. If no other cause can be found, then the ACE inhibitor should be stopped, with an alternative antihypertensive added if required.

→ www.nice.org.uk/guidance/cg182/chapter/1-recommendations#ph armacotherapy

4. A ★   OHCM 10th ed. → p. 763

Hopefully, this is an obvious measure to take, but if in a rush on call, a reflex response to oliguria may be a quick fluid challenge (C) before rushing to another ward. However, before it can be assumed that the patient is not producing urine because of dehydration, a blocked catheter must be excluded. If examination of the abdomen reveals dullness to percussion up to the umbilicus, then the catheter itself and its patency need to be checked.

B. This would be the route to go down if abdominal examination reveals a full bladder and the catheter seems patent but does not fill on flushing.

D. Mixed venous saturations >75% and a central venous pressure (CVP) >8–10 cmH$_2$O would suggest that the patient was well filled, but central lines are rarely used for fluid balance these days and never outside critical care environments.

E. Epidural analgesia typically lowers the blood pressure, but switching it off is not the answer in suspected dehydration.

5. C ★   OHCM 10th ed. → p. 301

Renal replacement therapy is ideally planned for and started on an elective basis for people with deteriorating chronic kidney disease. However, emergency dialysis or filtration is occasionally needed for acutely unwell patients whose renal function rapidly drops off with severe acute kidney injury. The main indications for acute dialysis are resistant hyperkalaemia, uraemic pericarditis, severe acidosis, and pulmonary oedema.

6. B ★   OHCM 10th ed. → p. 638

Intramuscular non-steroidal anti-inflammatory drugs (NSAIDs) have been demonstrated to provide the best and most sustained analgesia for renal colic in the emergency room, with the fewest side effects. Tramadol has many side effects and should be avoided where possible.

Pathan SA, Mitra B, Straney LD, et al. Delivering safe and effective analgesia for management of renal colic in the emergency department: a double-blind, multigroup, randomised controlled trial. *Lancet.* 2016;**387**:1999–2007.

7. D ★   OHCM 10th ed. → p. 298

As well as ensuring patients admitted to hospital are started on the appropriate emergency treatment, it is vital to rationalize their existing prescriptions in light of their new problems. In those presenting with acute kidney injury, this entails withholding any potentially nephrotoxic drugs. The most common culprits in these scenarios are angiotensin-converting enzyme (ACE) inhibitors, diuretics, and non-steroidal anti-inflammatory drugs (NSAIDs). It is also worth considering which drugs may have accumulated in renal failure such as digoxin.

8. C ★   OHCM 10th ed. → p. 315

Phosphate may rise in acute kidney injury (AKI), and hyperphosphataemia and hypocalcaemia are particularly exaggerated in AKI due to rhabdomyolysis and tumour lysis syndrome. In chronic kidney disease, persistently low calcium and high phosphate levels cause parathyroid hormone levels [and alkaline phosphatase (ALP)] to rise (which would be suggestive of chronic disease). Hyperkalaemia can occur in both acute and chronic disease. In the absence of another explanation, anaemia would be very suggestive of long-standing kidney disease, although AKI with microangiopathic haemolytic anaemia (MAHA) in, for example, haemolytic uraemic syndrome (HUS) needs to be considered.

9. D ★   OHCM 10th ed. → p. 762

In the acute phase after relief of an obstruction, the kidneys kick back into action by producing a lot of urine. It is therefore essential to provide concurrent rehydration therapy to avoid immediate dehydration. During this phase of diuresis, sodium and bicarbonate will also be lost in large quantities, so it is also important to keep a close eye on electrolyte levels and replace where necessary.

If the catheter does not relieve his distended abdomen, then imaging would be required (**A** and **E**). Given his chronic prostate problem, it would also be important to perform a rectal examination, but also to exclude constipation as a cause of acute urinary retention (**B**). One-off doses of antibiotics (**C**) can be given at the time of catheterization as prophylaxis but should not be continued without good reason.

10. E ★   OHCM 10th ed. → p. 669

Serum creatinine requires consideration in the context of body mass; this is especially important in those with minimal muscle bulk (such as patients with eating disorders or the elderly). Glomerular filtration rate (GFR), calculated using a formula that takes weight into account such as Cockroft–Gault, or a calculated creatinine clearance gives a better reflection of renal function than an isolated creatinine or an estimated GFR. A creatinine level of 115 micromol/L may produce a creatinine clearance within the normal range for a muscular young man who weighs 100 kg, but in this woman with an eating disorder who weighs only 30 kg, it actually reflects significant renal impairment.

11. B ★   OHCM 10th ed. → p. 319

This unfortunately is an all too common scenario in clinical practice. A fall with subsequent prolonged immobility is enough to cause considerable muscle breakdown in an older person. This can be measured via serum creatine kinase (CK) on a standard biochemistry blood test. One of the breakdown products of muscle—myoglobin—is particularly harmful to kidneys and in a poorly hydrated older person who may already be unwell— hence the fall—is highly likely to precipitate an acute kidney injury. If the renal failure can be directly attributed to the raised CK, the diagnosis is rhabdomyolysis.

A serum troponin will be hard to make sense of, as it will be falsely elevated in renal failure. If in the setting of diarrhoea and renal failure, then it is important to consider clotting and platelet function, as haemolytic uraemic syndrome (HUS) and thrombotic thrombocytopenic purpura (TTP) are both rare, but important, diagnoses not to miss. Erythrocyte sedimentation rate (ESR) would add little to this case. In all cases of acute renal failure, it is important to measure and correct electrolytes, but the level of calcium does not hold the key to the diagnosis here.

12. **C** ★ OHCM 10th ed. → p. 302

In the absence of risk factors for chronic kidney disease (hypertension, diabetes, cardiovascular disease, structural renal tract disease, or multi-system disease with renal involvement), age (**A**), gender (**D**), and ethnicity (**B**) should not be used as independent risk markers. An often forgotten risk factor for kidney disease, however, is metabolic syndrome, which is defined as:

- Central obesity or body mass index (BMI) >30 kg/m^2, plus two of the following:
  - Triglycerides >1.7 mmol/L
  - High-density lipoprotein <1.03 mmol/L
  - Blood pressure (BP) >130/85 mmHg
  - Fasting glucose >5.6 mmol/L.

→   www.nice.org.uk/guidance/cg182/chapter/1-Recommendations#investigations-for-chronic-kidney-disease-2

13. **E** ★ OHCM 10th ed. → p. 310

This is a typical history of colic in the distribution of the right ureteric system. Supportive evidence should be sought via haematuria on urinalysis and non-contrast computed tomography (CT) of the kidneys, ureters, and bladder (KUB). Occasionally, where CT is not readily available, an X-ray KUB is done instead, though it is less sensitive and will not reveal other causative pathology, e.g. appendicitis.

A. This is used to diagnose acute pancreatitis.

B. This should be performed in most cases of an acute abdomen, particularly in suspected bowel obstruction.

C. After basic blood tests and a convincing history, the only way to diagnose an acute appendicitis is to proceed to theatre.

D. This is useful for biliary colic or cholecystitis.

14. **B** ★ OHCM 10th ed. → p. 260

This man has features of urinary retention. This is the first thing to treat, as it may explain all of the symptoms (abdominal distension, delirium, and be caused by constipation). Once the catheter has been passed, it would be sensible to send the urine for culture (D), but to treat with antibiotics (E) *only* if there were other signs of infection (fever, raised inflammatory markers, preceding dysuria). Constipation should be addressed with oral laxatives plus enemas/suppositories, as appropriate, as this may well have been the precipitant for the retention (A and C).

15. A ★   OHCM 10th ed. → p. 208

The consultant is concerned that his patient has been receiving metformin whilst her kidneys are potentially poorly perfused—it is in this setting that the drug is very occasionally known to cause lactic acidosis (displayed by the laboured Kussmaul breathing, which tries to blow off the excess acid). A blood gas (venous is sufficient) should be performed immediately, with the anion gap calculated (lactic acidosis causes metabolic acidosis with a raised anion gap). Of the others, (E) would have the most merit, given the concern over poor renal perfusion in a diabetic, whilst (D) would also be useful.

16. C ★   OHCM 10th ed. → p. 298

Why does this man have acute kidney injury (AKI)? The usual causes—hypovolaemia and distal obstruction—are not to blame. However, the absence of a palpable bladder does not rule out a more proximal obstruction as the cause, which could be shown by an ultrasound scan. When confronted with acute renal failure, it is the junior doctor's job to rule out the most likely causes, which will often involve arranging imaging of the renal tract.

A. This is sensible if a catheter appears patent in the setting of a palpable bladder but is still not draining.

B. Central venous pressure (CVP) lines are occasionally used for monitoring fluid balance (which is not a concern here) in acutely ill patients.

D. There is no suggestion that there is an infective precipitant.

E. Diuretics are not part of the management of acute renal failure, especially in someone who is well hydrated.

17. B ★   OHCM 10th ed. → p. 350

Current advice is to give low-molecular-weight heparin, with the dose adjusted to renal function. Whilst monitoring of factor Xa levels is commonly advocated, there is no consensus as to what represents safe and effective levels. Aspirin (A) has been shown to be less effective than anticoagulation in certain types of surgery (particularly major joint operations). Direct-acting oral anticoagulants (DOACs) (C) are not licensed for use in patients with severe renal impairment. Compression stockings (D) are often used in conjunction with other forms of thromboprophylaxis.

→ bestpractice.bmj.com/best-practice/monograph/1087/treatment/step-by-step.html

18. A ★   OHCM 10th ed. → p. 32

Before resuscitating, it is important to assess a patient's fluid status—
are they euvolaemic or over- or underfilled? Blood pressure (especially
lying and sitting or standing), weight, jugular venous pressure (JVP),
heart sounds, auscultation of the lung bases, and assessment for oedema
and signs of global perfusion should provide the answer. This man is in
acute pre-renal failure, most likely due to hypovolaemia from sepsis. He
is probably delirious, secondary to dehydration, and will improve with
intravenous (IV) fluids.

B. This is a normal finding and is suggestive of adequate tissue perfusion.

C. This is reassuring prior to starting aggressive fluid therapy but needs
to be monitored, especially in those known to have cardiac impairment.

D. This is indicative of heart failure, and therefore the need for careful
fluid therapy.

E. This may also be a reason to start IV fluids but does not inform about
fluid balance.

19. E ★   OHCM 10th ed. → p. 256

Tachycardia is common after surgery and, in the early stages, can be
attributable to pain. However, if persistent, then investigations need to
be performed. In this case, given the vomiting and the rapid increase in
urea levels, a gastrointestinal (GI) bleed is the most likely cause. Although
a rising urea level usually represents dehydration (**A**), this would normally be accompanied by a rising creatinine level. The fact that it rises on
its own suggests an increase in circulating protein levels, i.e. by digested
blood, rather than failure of the kidneys. Even without a past medical
history of gastro-oesophageal reflux disease (GORD) or stomach ulcers, GI bleeds are common after periods of physiological stress such
as surgery or time in intensive care. Although the haemoglobin level is
stable, it often takes longer for this to fall than it does for the urea level
to rise. However, she needs to be cross-matched for blood and listed
for an endoscopy.

Most surgical teams would be keen to perform a computed tomography (CT) abdomen in this situation, as a post-operative collection (**B**)
would necessitate further emergency surgery or at least a radiologically
inserted drain. Both pulmonary emboli (**D**) and chest infections (**C**) are
common after surgery, but other than the tachycardia, there are no real
indications of either in this case.

20. C ★   OHCM 10th ed. → p. 304

Microalbuminuria should be tested every 6 months in type 2 diabetes
for two reasons: it gives an early warning of impending renal disease
and it is an independent risk factor for cardiovascular disease. Therefore,
regardless of the blood pressure, those who have it should start immediately on an angiotensin-converting enzyme (ACE) inhibitor. These

days, it can be accurately assessed by sending a *single* urine sample for albumin:creatinine ratio testing.

→ www.nice.org.uk/guidance/ng28

21. C ★ OHCM 10th ed. → p. 15

This is a difficult, but common, scenario. As the woman has no capacity, she cannot refuse treatment (unless there is formal documentation in the form of an advance directive). The doctors need to weigh up what is in her best interests. In the short term, that should normally include relieving pain and discomfort by the minimal restraint possible; in this case, this may entail giving low-dose sedation in order to insert the catheter—which will relieve the obstruction, and therefore provide pain relief. In the medium term, (A) comes into play—to guide the doctors as to what may more generally be in the woman's best interests, it would be useful to know how she had been over the preceding months, whether she had expressed thoughts about medical interventions, whether she was depressed or indeed suicidal, and how likely she is to recover with treatment. Armed with this information, a best interests decision might instead opt to switch to supportive palliative care or limit the interventions which she does not find distressing. In this scenario, assuming full active treatment without a second thought, although commonly done, should be carefully considered in the context of the patient.

22. D ★★ OHCM 10th ed. → p. 311

This gentleman's symptoms and investigations are suggestive of a vasculitic process, specifically granulomatosis with polyangiitis (formally known as Wegener's), resulting in rapidly progressive glomerulonephritis and pulmonary haemorrhage. This is a medical emergency and requires urgent treatment with corticosteroids and plasma exchange, and immunosuppression with cyclophosphamide and rituximab.

23. C ★★ OHCM 10th ed. → p. 312

This lady demonstrates nephrotic syndrome, most likely due to minimal change disease. This is more common in children than adults and is often idiopathic. It presents with (often massive) oedema. The glomerulus looks unremarkable on light microscopy, hence 'minimal change'. It carries an excellent prognosis if promptly treated with corticosteroids but relapses in 30–70% of cases.

24. C ★★ OHCM 10th ed. → p. 311

Immunoglobulin A (IgA) nephropathy is the most common primary glomerulonephropathy in high-income countries and occurs due to overproduction of IgA (classically in response to a streptococcal throat infection), which then forms immune complexes that lodge in mesangial cells. In older patients with microscopic or macroscopic haematuria, a urological malignancy must be excluded prior to consideration of glomerular disease.

A. This is the process behind Goodpasture's (anti-glomerular basement membrane) disease, which is rare and may also present with haemoptysis (as antibodies may also bind to alveolar membranes).

B. This occurs in polycystic kidney disease, which more commonly presents via screening of relatives of affected patients.

D. Cystitis is more common in women and would be more likely to present with frequency and dysuria, as well as haematuria.

E. This would be the biopsy finding in rapidly progressive glomerulonephritis. It would present with acute renal failure, following either vasculitic or infective processes.

25. A ★★   OHCM 10th ed → p. 313

This man with currently untreated human immunodeficiency virus (HIV) infection is presenting with advanced kidney impairment and likely nephrotic syndrome. In the setting of HIV, collapsing focal segmental glomerulosclerosis is known as HIV-associated nephropathy (HIVAN), a serious complication of HIV that rapidly progresses to end-stage renal disease without treatment. The mainstay of treatment is initiation of appropriate highly active anti-retroviral therapy (HAART).

26. B ★★   OHCM 10th ed. → p. 313

Membranous nephropathy is one of the most common causes of nephrotic syndrome in adults and may be primary or 'idiopathic' (70% of which result from an autoantibody to the phospholipase A2 receptor present in podocytes) or secondary (due to infections, autoimmune disease, drugs, or as in this case malignancy). Angiotensin-converting enzyme (ACE) inhibitors/angiotensin receptor blockers (ARBs) should be used in all cases of membranous nephropathy. Idiopathic membranous nephropathy may require immunosuppression, whilst secondary membranous nephropathy is treated by removal/treatment of the causative 'agent'.

27. C ★★   OHCM 10th ed. → p. 310

Nephritic syndrome is proteinuria, haematuria, oliguria, and hypertension, with rising urea and creatinine levels. In this case, it is most probably due to post-streptococcal glomerulonephritis.

A. Acute tubular necrosis is due to ischaemia, drugs, or toxins, and presents as acute kidney injury and renal failure.

B. Interstitial nephritis can occur secondary to drugs or infections and presents with either progressive renal impairment, acute renal failure, or hypertension.

D. Nephrotic syndrome is the triad of proteinuria, hypoalbuminaemia, and oedema, occurring most commonly in the wake of glomerular damage.

E. If renovascular disease occurs in a 30-year old, it is most likely due to fibromuscular dysplasia, which presents gradually with resistant hypertension. In those >50 years old, it is most likely due to atherosclerosis.

28. C ★★ OHCM 10th ed. → p. 757

This is an enzyme inhibitor and potentiates the effects of warfarin. It is sometimes used in the treatment of urinary tract infections, although its use is restricted now due to a high risk of *Clostridium difficile* infection. Although studies have failed to demonstrate an interaction with coumarin anticoagulants (such as warfarin) and penicillins, experience from anticoagulant clinics suggests that the international normalized ratio (INR) can be altered by broad-spectrum antibiotics such as amoxicillin.

29. B ★★ OHCM 10th ed. → p. 293

This man is describing visible or macroscopic haematuria. Any one *single* episode of macroscopic haematuria should be considered significant. It is important to rule out transient causes (urinary tract infection or drug side effects) and then to test for urea and electrolytes and the urinary protein:creatinine ratio before referring to either a urologist or a nephrologist. He has developed haematuria soon after what sounds like an upper respiratory tract infection—this is classical for immunoglobulin A (IgA) nephropathy, in which overproduction of IgA leads to immune complexes that deposit in mesangial cells.

A. If this man were older, then bladder carcinoma would be the most likely diagnosis. It presents with painless macroscopic haematuria and becomes more likely with age, especially if certain environmental risk factors are in place (smoking and amines in some dyes, paints, solvents, and textiles). It would need to be excluded in this case (via an ultrasound scan and cystoscopy) but is not the most likely diagnosis.

C. Nephrotic syndrome is, by definition, proteinuria (>3 g/24 hours), hypoalbuminaemia (<30 g/L), and oedema—this man has none of these. Berger's disease can, however, cause the nephritic syndrome—haematuria with proteinuria and hypertension.

D. Stones do cause haematuria, but this man has no pain to suggest that they are present.

E. This man has no urinary symptoms and is afebrile and not tachycardic, and his urine is nitrite-negative, although urine dipsticks have a very poor sensitivity and specificity for investigation of urinary tract infections (UTIs) and should not usually be used. As part of the initial investigations, however, it would be important to send off a urine sample for microscopy, culture, and sensitivity.

30. E ★★ OHCM 10th ed. → p. 313

This man has described visible haematuria—which should be considered significant. It is important to rule out transient causes such as a urinary tract infection or a drug side effect, before testing urea and electrolytes and the urinary protein:creatinine ratio and ordering an ultrasound scan of his urinary tract. Any further concerns should prompt referral to a nephrologist.

This man has developed haematuria after an upper respiratory tract infection, a classical way for immunoglobulin A (IgA) nephropathy or Berger's disease—the most common primary glomerulonephritis in the western world, characterized by IgA deposition in the mesangium—to present. In older patients, haematuria should trigger investigations for a urological malignancy.

31. D ★★   OHCM 10th ed. → p. 320

Autosomal dominant polycystic kidney disease (ADPKD) is associated with intracranial aneurysms that can cause subarachnoid haemorrhage (SAH). Screening with magnetic resonance angiography is recommended for patients <65 years with a personal/family history of SAH.

32. A ★★   OHCM 10th ed. → pp. 310–11

Anti-glomerular basement membrane (GBM) disease (previously known as Goodpasture's disease) is a rare condition caused by autoantibodies to type IV collagen present in glomerular and alveolar basement membranes. It presents with oliguric/anuric acute kidney injury (AKI), and often, though not always, with pulmonary haemorrhage. Dialysis dependence and significant damage on biopsy predict a poor chance of recovery. Diagnosis is by anti-GBM antibodies in circulation or deposited in the kidney.

Treatment is by plasma exchange, corticosteroids, and immunosuppression (often cyclophosphamide).

There are, in fact, very few conditions that present with abrupt and unheralded anuria, this being one. The others are obstruction and infarction/thrombosis, neither of which this young woman appears to have.

33. C ★★★   OHCM 10th ed. → p. 314

The skeleton history, along with the urine dip result, is suggestive of systemic lupus erythematosus (SLE) with concurrent lupus-induced nephritis. In cases such as this, where there is proteinuria, it is the glomerular filtrating apparatus that has been damaged, leading to a chronic leak of protein and/or blood. Treatment is threefold: to reduce proteinuria with angiotensin-converting enzyme (ACE) inhibitors (and/or angiotensin II receptor blockers), to manage hypertension (proteinuria is an independent risk factor for hypertension), and to slow the renal disease process via immunosuppression (steroids +/− mycophenolate or azathioprine +/− cyclophosphamide).

Chapter 6

Haematology

Dan Furmedge and Rudy Sinharay

Tackling haematology is never easy. Revision can be a struggle, as it may not always be obvious which topic areas will be directly relevant to clinical practice. We still, however, benefit from an understanding of these areas and an appreciation of how to do and interpret the basics and when more expertise is required. Sometimes the answers require a trip right back to the stem cell (Figure 6.1).

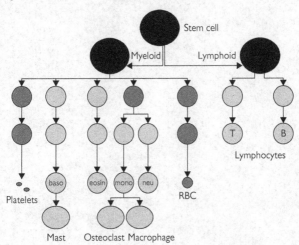

Figure 6.1

A junior doctor's most frequent contact with haematology is in interpreting a full blood count. In this task, the core skills of the chapter come to the fore—in response to an anaemia, we should be able to explore the possibilities of iron deficiency, vitamin deficiency, and haemolysis. On seeing a thrombocytopenia or an abnormal clotting profile, we should be able to make a clinical assessment and perform further appropriate tests, with a view to suggesting differential diagnoses. The questions in this chapter aim to build confidence in these tasks.

There is a lot more to haematology, however, than a blood count. As a junior doctor, there will be regular practical challenges such as prescribing and altering anticoagulation therapy, overseeing the safe delivery of a blood transfusion, and managing acute situations such as sickle-cell crises. The way forward is to be able to master these basics and start to see the bigger picture. This means developing a feel for the more subtle symptoms and signs of haematological disease and becoming proactive in the face of abnormal blood results.

As with all of the chapters in this book, it is a way of thinking that is crucial—one that allows confident management of common situations and recognition of potentially catastrophic conditions, but also one that encourages creativity and initiative. When faced with a clinical conundrum, we should have the knowledge and confidence to ask appropriately: 'Is the answer in the blood?'

QUESTIONS

1. A 55-year-old man is receiving a transfusion of packed red cells during his recovery from colorectal surgery. He has developed a fever 30 minutes into the transfusion.

T 38.3°C, HR 90 bpm, BP 125/70 mmHg, SaO₂ 98% on air.

The transfusion has been stopped.

Which *single* additional development should make the junior doctor most wary about restarting the transfusion? ★

A Pruritus

B Shivering

C Systolic BP <100 mmHg

D Temperature >38.5°C

E Urticaria

2. A 23-year-old woman has been feeling tired and lethargic for the past 18 months. She occasionally feels dizzy on standing and is generally weak.

Haemoglobin (Hb) 95 g/L, mean corpuscular volume (MCV) 69 fL.

Which is the *single* most appropriate further investigation to confirm the diagnosis? ★

A Hb electrophoresis

B HbA2 level

C Serum iron + ferritin

D Thyroid function tests

E Vitamin B12 + folate levels

3. A 72-year-old woman has been breathless and unwell for the past week. She is admitted to hospital and started on intravenous (IV) antibiotics for a chest infection. She has atrial fibrillation and is on warfarin 2 mg daily. The on-call junior doctor is asked to check her blood results after she is moved to the medical ward. Her international normalized ratio (INR) is 6.6. There is currently no evidence of bleeding.

Which is the *single* most appropriate management? ★

A Fresh frozen plasma (FFP) 2 U IV

B Reduce the warfarin dose to 0.5 mg

C Stop antibiotics

D Vitamin K 5 mg IV

E Withold warfarin

4. A 68-year-old woman has had a swelling in her neck, weight loss, and night sweats for 6 months. Her GP refers her for investigations as an inpatient. After 72 hours on the ward, she asks one of the doctors if she can read through her medical notes. Which is the *single* most appropriate response to her request? ★

A Allow the patient to take the notes whenever she likes

B Copy the parts of the notes that would be relevant to the patient

C Discuss the request with the hospital's information guardian

D Refuse as all medical notes are confidential

E Write a summary of the notes for the patient, but withhold the original

5. A 52-year-old man has been feeling lethargic over the past year. He has had intermittent abdominal pain and has lost 5 kg. His initial blood results are:

Haemoglobin (Hb) 106 g/L, mean corpuscular volume (MCV) 106 fL, vitamin B12 305 ng/L, folate 1.4 mg/L, ferritin 110 mg/L.

Which is the *single* most appropriate further investigation to establish the diagnosis? ★

A Anti-endomysial antibodies

B Anti-gastric parietal cell antibodies

C Liver function tests

D Peripheral blood film

E Thyroid function tests

6. A 75-year-old man has had lower back pain for over a year. It has got progressively worse, and he has now noticed new pains in his right thigh and left arm. He is normally fit and well but has recently suffered repeated chest infections.

Creatinine 164 IU/L, urea 8.4 mmol/L.

Which *single* set of investigations would be the most likely to support the underlying diagnosis? ★

A Bone marrow aspirate + immunoglobulin profile

B Digital rectal examination + prostate-specific antigen (PSA)

C Erythrocyte sedimentation rate + rheumatoid factor

D Full blood count + vitamin B12 and folate + ferritin

E Liver function tests + calcium

7. A 42-year-old woman has been increasingly tired over the past 6 months. She has felt faint on exertion, with occasional palpitations. She admits to feeling irritable and rather low. Her skin and conjunctivae are pale.

Haemoglobin (Hb) 92 g/L, mean corpuscular volume (MCV) 102 fL.

Film: hypersegmented polymorphs.

Which is the *single* most likely cause of the woman's symptoms? ★

A Alcoholism

B Liver disease

C Myxoedema

D Pernicious anaemia

E Pregnancy

8. A 66-year-old man has felt increasingly tired over the past 18 months. He has also been intermittently dizzy and complains of a sore tongue. He is pale and has a swollen red tongue.

Haemoglobin (Hb) 99 g/L, mean corpuscular volume (MCV) 105 fL, white cell count (WCC) 6.2 × 10⁹/L, platelets 265 × 10⁹/L.

Which *single* pair of investigations is most likely to confirm the diagnosis? ★

A Ferritin + total iron-binding capacity

B Folate + thyroid function tests

C Lactate dehydrogenase + reticulocytes

D Peripheral blood film + bone marrow aspirate

E Vitamin B12 + anti-gastric parietal cell antibodies

9. A 19-year-old woman has been in severe pain for the past 12 hours. It started in her left hip and has moved down her thigh. She is doubled over in agony and confined to bed. She has experienced similar episodes intermittently over the years. Paracetamol and codeine do little to relieve the pain, and it is only after morphine 20 mg subcutaneous (SC) that there is any improvement.

Haemoglobin (Hb) 77 g/L, mean corpuscular volume (MCV) 86 fL.

Which is the *single* most appropriate explanation for her pain? ★

A Infarction of the bone marrow

B Localized tissue hypoxia due to anaemia

C Pathological bone fracture

D Pooling of red blood cells in the liver and spleen

E Sudden reduction in bone marrow production of red blood cells

10. A 72-year-old man has a sudden onset of pain in the right side of his chest. He recalls no trauma to the area and is surprised when he is told he has fractured ribs. He also has pain in his lower back and has had two admissions to hospital in the past 6 months with chest infections. Which *single* cell type is most likely to be proliferating? ★ ★

A Germinal centre B cell

B Immunoglobulin M (IgM)-secreting cell

C Mature B lymphocyte

D Myeloid cell

E Plasma cell

11. A 54-year-old woman has had bleeding from her gums daily for the past 2 weeks. She has also suffered four nosebleeds during this time. Over the past month or so, she has had burning pain in her hands and feet, with throbbing in the tips of her fingers and toes, as well as intermittent headache. Which *single* cell type is most likely to be proliferating? ★ ★

A Blast cell from marrow myeloid

B Immunoglobulin M (IgM)-secreting cell

C Lymphoid progenitor cell

D Megakaryocyte

E Plasma cell

12. A 62-year-old woman has had a high temperature for the past 3 hours. Other than a slightly sore throat and a general feeling of tiredness, she has no real symptoms of note. Eight days previously, she completed her first cycle of chemotherapy for carcinoma of the breast.

T 38.4°C, HR 110 bpm, BP 95/65 mmHg.

Blood and urine samples are sent for culture.

Which is the *single* most appropriate next stage in her treatment? ★ ★

A Await the results of the blood tests before starting any treatment

B Discharge home and contact if the cultures grow anything

C Discharge home on oral antibiotics

D Observe for 24 hours on intravenous fluids

E Start broad-spectrum intravenous antibiotics

13. A 72-year-old woman has been feeling tired and lethargic for the past 2 years. Her doctor performs a range of blood tests, the majority of which are within normal limits. However, she is referred to the haematologists due to the presence in her serum of a 'monoclonal protein'. Which *single* additional feature should offer the most reassurance that the condition is not yet serious? ★★

A Bone marrow concentration of monoclonal plasma cells >10%

B Clotting profile is within normal limits

C Lactate dehydrogenase (LDH) is within normal limits

D Monoclonal protein is of immunoglobulin M (IgM) type

E Serum concentration of monoclonal protein <30 g/L

14. A 62-year-old man has felt generally unwell for the past 3 months. His main problem is widespread, intractable itch, but he has also lost his appetite, and >5 kg in weight. He is lethargic and low in mood, and suffers from intermittent fevers with sweats at night. There is an enlarged, rubbery left cervical lymph node that is non-tender to palpation. Which is the *single* most likely cause of this man's symptoms? ★★

A B-cell malignancy

B Bone marrow malignancy

C Myeloid cell malignancy

D Plasma cell malignancy

E T-cell malignancy

15. A 33-year-old man has a routine pre-employment medical examination. He is asymptomatic but has sickle-cell disease.

T 36.7°C, HR 65 bpm, BP 122/78 mmHg.

Haemoglobin (Hb) 81 g/L, mean corpuscular volume (MCV) 88 fL.

His chest is clear, and heart sounds are normal. Which is the *single* most appropriate explanation for why he is not short of breath? ★★

A Due to chronic haemolysis, Hb is diluted and actually much higher

B His cardiac output has been able to increase over time to compensate

C His MCV is within normal limits

D His oxygen dissociation curve is shifted to the right

E His vital capacity has been able to increase over time to compensate

16. A 24-year-old man with known HBSS sickle-cell anaemia is brought to the Emergency Department. He describes severe bony pain in his arms, lower back, and chest. He feels unwell and is short of breath. He is writhing in pain. On examination, his chest has diffuse wheeze.

T 37.4°C, BP 131/76 mmHg, HR 110 bpm, RR 22/min, SaO$_2$ 90% on 6 L O$_2$.

What is the *single* most important definitive treatment? ★★

A Antibiotics

B Exchange transfusion

C High-flow oxygen

D Opiate analgesia

E Salbutamol nebulizer

17. A 39-year-old woman has received her second course of chemotherapy for a recently diagnosed acute myeloid leukaemia. She is a Jehovah's Witness and has a witnessed signed document stating that she would not accept supportive blood products at any stage. She has become breathless, weak, and confused.

Haemoglobin (Hb) 36 g/L.

The medical team caring for her feel that if she is not transfused with blood now, she will not survive.

Which is the *single* most appropriate next step? ★★★

A Apply for a court order to allow transfusion to go ahead

B As she is now confused, then transfuse her in her best interests

C Gain consent for the proposed transfusion from her next of kin

D Reassess her capacity to decline the proposed transfusion

E Respect her earlier wishes and withhold transfusion

18. A 27-year-old woman is being treated in hospital for a chest infection. She has been switched to oral antibiotics, with a view to completing the course at home. All her blood indices are improving, but her haemoglobin (Hb) levels have dropped by >40 g/L in the 5 days she has been in hospital. The registrar asks for a *single* blood test to assess the cause. Which is the *single* most appropriate explanation of the 'test' to which the registrar refers? ★★★

A Assessment of the ability to absorb vitamin B12

B Assessment of red cell fragility by placing in acid

C Detection of levels of methaemalbumin

D Examination of a smeared drop of blood on a slide

E Identification of red cells coated with antibody or complement

19. A 41-year-old woman has had pain in her lower chest for 3 hours. It began while at rest and has been constant since. It is focused over the sternum and lower left ribs, with radiation to under the left scapula. There is no associated breathlessness. In the preceding 2 weeks, she has experienced episodes of severe localized pain, most notably in her neck and shoulders, but also in her thighs. She has also had several nosebleeds.

Haemoglobin (Hb) 95 g/L, mean corpuscular volume (MCV) 82 fL, white cell count (WCC) 2.9 × 10⁹/L, platelets 85 × 10⁹/L.

Which *single* investigation would be most likely to confirm the diagnosis? ★ ★ ★

A Autoantibodies

B Haemoglobin electrophoresis

C Peripheral blood film

D Rheumatoid factor

E Vitamin B12, folate, and ferritin

20. A 22-year-old woman attends an antenatal booking appointment. She has previously had three miscarriages at <24/ 40 weeks. She has recently had mouth ulcers and intermittent joint pain, which is being investigated by the rheumatologists. Which *single* pair of results is most likely to confirm the underlying cause of her symptoms? ★ ★ ★

A ↑ activated partial thromboplastin time (aPTT) + ↓ platelets

B ↑ erythrocyte sedimentation rate (ESR) + ↑ rheumatoid factor

C ↓ haemoglobin (Hb) + ↓ mean corpuscular volume (MCV)

D ↓ Hb + ↑ reticulocytes

E ↑ lactate dehydrogenase (LDH) + ↑ bilirubin

21. A 72-year-old man has had an acute non-ST-elevation myocardial infarction. He is being treated in hospital with a range of new medications. His renal function is moderately impaired, and so he is given unfractionated heparin and monitored for signs of an adverse immune reaction.

Which *single* subsequent episode is most likely to signal a reaction? ★ ★ ★

A Epistaxis

B Syncope

C Venous thrombosis

D Visual disturbance

E Widespread blanching rash

22. A 71-year-old man has noticed a change in sputum colour from clear to green and an increase in sputum volume over a 5-day period. He is started on 28% oxygen, antibiotics, steroids, and regular nebulizers. He has chronic obstructive pulmonary disease (COPD) and takes warfarin for atrial fibrillation. His international normalized ratio (INR) is normally well controlled within the target range of 2–3. However, on the fourth day of his hospital stay, his INR is reported as 5.4. Which *single* drug is most likely to have caused his increased INR? ★★★

A Amoxicillin

B Clarithromycin

C Ipratropium

D Prednisolone

E Salbutamol

23. A 48-year-old man has a right inguinal hernia repair. A few days later, his right leg becomes tender and swollen, and he is started on a treatment dose of subcutaneous low-molecular-weight heparin (LMWH). A Doppler ultrasound confirms deep vein thrombosis (DVT) and he is started on warfarin, as he has renal impairment and a direct-acting oral anticoagulant (DOAC) is contraindicated. He asks why he needs to have both an injection and a tablet if the warfarin is replacing the LMWH on discharge. Which is the *single* most appropriate way to explain this strategy to the patient? ★★★

A Warfarin and the injection initially work together to give a greater clot-busting effect

B Warfarin can make the blood too thin too quickly, but the injection reduces the chances of this happening

C Warfarin initially increases the ability of the blood to clot, so the injection is needed to keep the blood thin

D Warfarin takes a long time to reach a steady concentration in the blood, which is reduced by the injection

E Warfarin was started after the injection, so it has to be built up as the injection is weaned down

24. A 62-year-old man has had a headache, coupled with dizziness, intermittently for the past 6 months. He has also noticed an unpleasant burning sensation in his hands and feet. Both the hallux and first toe of his right foot are dusky in colour and tender to touch. Which *single* pathological process is most likely to be the cause of his symptoms? ★★★

A Bone marrow failure

B Chronic haemolysis

C Myeloproliferation

D Plasma cell proliferation

E Thrombophilia

25. A 21-year-old man has had severe chest pain for the last 4 hours. It is persistent and throbbing and has not been relieved by co-dydramol. It is typical of his sickle-cell disease, of which he has frequent crises.

T 37.1°C, HR 110 bpm, BP 105/70 mmHg, SaO₂ 95% on air.

As per his analgesia protocol, he is prescribed morphine 10 mg. Which is the *single* most appropriate route of administration? ★★★

A Intramuscular (IM)

B Intravenous (IV)

C Oral (PO)

D Per rectum (PR)

E Subcutaneous (SC)

26. A 52-year-old man has noticed increasing abdominal fullness over the past 18 months. He has no other symptoms. His abdomen is distended. There is a notched edge palpable in the right iliac fossa that moves further towards the anterior superior iliac spine on inspiration. There is dullness to percussion over the umbilicus. Which is the *single* most likely cause of the abdominal mass? ★★★

A Chronic myeloid leukaemia

B Idiopathic thrombocytopenic purpura (ITP)

C Myelodysplasia

D Polycythaemia rubra vera

E Portal hypertension

27. A 64-year-old man has had an increasingly full abdomen for the past year. He has felt lethargic but otherwise has been well. Initially, his blood results were normal. At his latest haematology appointment, he has the following blood results:

Haemoglobin (Hb) 77 g/L, white cell count (WCC) 1.8×10^9/L, platelets 76×10^9/L.

A bone marrow aspirate was reported as normal. Which is the *single* most likely explanation for the blood results? ★★★

A The bone marrow has stopped making cells

B Cells are trapped in the spleen's reticuloendothelial system

C DNA damage to a pluripotent haematopoietic stem cell

D Failure of normal differentiation of haematopoietic stem cells

E Immunoparesis due to monoclonal proliferation of plasma cells

28. A 77-year-old man is being treated for a chest infection. He has had multiple pulmonary emboli in the past and takes warfarin 4 mg once daily. His last international normalized ratio (INR) was 3.1 (target 3–3.5) 3 days ago. He is self-medicating on the ward, but following his evening medications, he is unsure whether or not he has taken his warfarin tonight. The nursing staff ask the junior doctor on call for advice. Which is the *single* most appropriate advice to give in this situation? ★★★

A Give the appropriate warfarin dose tonight + repeat the INR tonight

B No more warfarin tonight + request an INR for tomorrow

C No more warfarin tonight + send an urgent INR tonight

D Take 2 mg warfarin tonight + request an INR for tomorrow

E Take 4 mg warfarin tonight + request an INR for tomorrow

29. A 52-year-old woman on weekly methotrexate has had 5 days of dysuria and urinary frequency. She is treated for a presumed urinary tract infection (UTI) with empirical antibiotics. She returns to her doctor a week later with recurrent bleeding of her gums. What is the *single* most likely antibiotic that has been used? ★★★

A Amoxicillin

B Cefalexin

C Co-amoxiclav

D Nitrofurantoin

E Trimethoprim

30. A 78-year-old man is diagnosed with multiple myeloma. As part of the workup, his haematologist decides to order a test which may help prognosticate.

Which *single* test listed is the most likely to help prognosticate in myeloma? ★★★

A Beta-2 microglobulin

B Calcium

C Haemoglobin

D Lactate dehydrogenase

E Serum free light chains

31. A 36-year-old woman has had intermittently heavy periods over the past 18 months. When they are heavy, they are no more painful than normal, but she does feel very weak and dizzy during them. She has also had nosebleeds at least two or three times a week for the past 6 months. There are numerous purple nodules on her buttocks, which do not disappear with pressure. Which is the *single* most likely explanation for this woman's symptoms? ★★★★

A Antibodies directed against the platelet membrane

B Bone marrow has been infiltrated

C Bone marrow has been suppressed

D Chronic haemolysis due to vitamin B12 deficiency

E Delayed hypersensitivity reaction to an unknown precipitant

32. A 56-year-old man has been admitted, following three large episodes of haematemesis. He has been resuscitated with 2 L of intravenous crystalloids and cross-matched for 4 units of packed red blood cells. Each unit of blood has been prescribed to be transfused over 1 hour. The nurse in charge contacts the junior doctor on call with concerns that the patient is having a reaction to the blood, which started 15 minutes ago. What is the *single* most worrying feature of the reaction the nurse has described? ★★★

A Bibasal crepitations

B Increased respiratory rate

C Rapid rise in temperature

D Severe generalized itching

E Widespread urticarial rash

33. A 42-year-old woman has complained of having a swollen neck for the past month. He is found to have bilateral swollen parotid glands. A full blood count (FBC) showed a white cell count (WCC) of 50×10^9, and a subsequent blood film showed multiple immature blasts. A diagnosis of acute lymphoblastic leukaemia (ALL) is suspected, and he is referred on to the haematology team for further investigation and management.

Which *single* association from the following options is associated with a poor prognosis? ★ ★ ★ ★

A Female sex

B Haemoglobin (Hb) 120 g/L

C Philadelphia chromosome

D T-cell ALL

E WCC >50 × 10⁹

34. A 62-year-old man presents with a swollen right calf, which is subsequently found to be deep vein thrombosis (DVT). On examination, he is also found to have facial plethora and splenomegaly. His blood tests reveal a haematocrit of 60, haemoglobin (Hb) level of 180 g/L, white cell count (WCC) of 13×10^9/L, and platelets of 550×10^9/L. He has never smoked and does not have any other chronic health problems.

Which *single* genetic mutation from the list below is most likely associated with the patient's condition? ★ ★ ★ ★

A *BRCA2*

B *BCL2*

C *JAK2*

D *MYC*

E Philadelphia chromosome (*BCR–ABL1* fusion)

ANSWERS

1. C ★   OHCM 10th ed. → p. 348

Increasing hypotension (with fever) is the most worrying sign, as it heralds a severe systemic inflammatory response syndrome (SIRS) reaction and possible sepsis (i.e. bacterial contamination) or an acute haemolytic reaction and warrants stopping the transfusion and urgent discussion with a haematologist and a microbiologist. As his temperature is already raised, it would be the fall in blood pressure, rather than a specific temperature, that would be the most worrying development.

A and E. These most likely represent allergic reactions; in these cases, the transfusion could be slowed with the addition of chlorphenamine 10 mg intramuscular (IM)/intravenous (IV) and close monitoring.

B. Shivering is seen with fever in non-haemolytic reactions and can be treated by slowing the transfusion, giving paracetamol, and monitoring.

2. C ★   OHCM 10th ed. → p. 324

It is not enough to know that a patient is anaemic. Before presenting such a finding on a ward round, it is vital to know what 'type' of anaemia it is. The first step to doing this is to look at the mean corpuscular volume (MCV). Different MCVs suggest different reasons behind the anaemia and so prompt the next stage in investigations:

- A raised MCV (>100 fL) should be followed up with thyroid function tests (**D**), liver function tests, reticulocytes, and vitamin B12 and folate levels (**E**). Of course, an MCV can be raised for a different reason (alcohol excess, certain drugs) in a patient with anaemia of a different aetiology.
- A normal MCV should prompt examination of the rest of the blood count, including platelets, along with renal function. For example, a normal MCV with a raised red cell distribution width (RDW) can indicate a mixed anaemia.
- A low MCV (<75 fL) is most commonly indicative of iron deficiency, especially—as in this case—where it may be associated with menorrhagia. Low serum iron and ferritin, with a raised total iron-binding capacity (TIBC) and transferrin, would seal the diagnosis. If there is no convincing source of iron loss, then it is important to investigate the gastrointestinal tract—an incidental microcytic anaemia is a common way in which a tumour of the caecum or ascending colon presents and should not be overlooked.

A. Haemoglobin (Hb) electrophoresis would also be useful in the exploration of a possible thalassaemia trait, as it would in the diagnosis of sickle-cell disease. Whilst thalassaemia minor can present with minor symptoms, it would be very unlikely for sickle-cell disorders to do so (admittedly the sickle-cell trait might, but usually acutely in specific precipitating situations, such as hypoxic environments, rather than the more gradual presentation in this case).

B. HbA2 is one of the three main types of Hb in adult blood. If iron studies were inconclusive in this case, then this may be a reasonable test to run, as high levels of HbA2 against a backdrop of a microcytic anaemia can occur in the relatively benign beta-thalassaemia minor.

3. E ★   OHCM 10th ed. → p. 351

This is a common dilemma for the junior doctor. With such a high international normalized ratio (INR), it may be tempting to reverse it, but in the absence of bleeding, the British Society of Haematology guidelines state that readings <8 just need to be watched whilst warfarin is withheld. If the INR is >8 and/or there is minor bleeding, then the agent of choice for reversal is vitamin K 0.5 mg intravenous (IV) or 5 mg oral (PO). If there is major bleeding, vitamin K 5–10 mg and prothrombin complex concentrate may be needed, and this should always be discussed with a haematologist due to variations in local protocols (E).

A. Fresh frozen plasma (FFP) has only a partial effect, is not the optimal treatment, and should never be used for the reversal of warfarin over anticoagulation in the absence of severe bleeding.

B. Warfarin should be stopped and restarted once the INR is <5.

C. Some antibiotics do indeed interfere with the INR [ciprofloxacin and macrolides, e.g. erythromycin (enzyme inhibitor) and rifampicin (enzyme inducer)], but this patient is in hospital for treatment of sepsis and it is warfarin that should be stopped.

→ www.bcshguidelines.com/documents/warfarin_4th_ed.pdf

4. C ★

A patient has a right of access to their medical notes under the Data Protection Act 1998. There is no reason for this patient not to be allowed access to her notes, and this should be made clear to her. It is also, however, important to weigh her right with the Caldicott principles. These were put in place to ensure maximum safety of confidential information. In order to implement these principles, every hospital should have a designated Caldicott Guardian.

A Caldicott Guardian is a senior person responsible for protecting the confidentiality of patient and service user information and enabling appropriate information sharing. The Guardian plays a key role in ensuring that the National Health Service (NHS), Councils with social services responsibilities, and partner organizations satisfy the highest practicable standards for handling patient-identifiable information.

In this case, therefore—as with all such cases—it is sensible to contact the Guardian for a brief discussion of the situation or review your local trust guidance, whilst reassuring the patient that their rights will be respected.

Department of Health. *UK Caldicott Guardian Council.*

→ www.gov.uk/government/groups/uk-caldicott-guardian-council

5. A ★ OHCM 10th ed. → p. 332

This man is anaemic due to folate deficiency. In this age group, without a significant history of alcohol abuse, dietary deficiency is less likely and it is important to exclude malabsorption, specifically coeliac disease, as the cause.

B. The presence of these antibodies is seen in pernicious anaemia, in which there is a lack of intrinsic factor, and thus an inability to absorb vitamin B12 in the terminal ileum.

C. These are useful but would not be diagnostic.

D. This is more useful in the investigation of pancytopenia than folate deficiency.

E. Hypothyroidism can cause symptoms of lethargy and macrocytic anaemia but is not related to vitamin deficiencies.

6. A ★ OHCM 10th ed. → p. 368

This man has worsening back pain with other bony pains, along with the suggestion of immunosuppression and renal impairment. C, D, and E would all provide useful, but not diagnostic information for this presentation. A would be desirable in the diagnosis of myeloma, whilst B would detect the majority of prostate malignancies. It is difficult to find reasons that totally exclude prostate cancer as the cause here, but the lack of urinary symptoms would certainly be one. The other would be that the history is textbook for a myeloma (unexplained backache + pathological fractures + recurrent bacterial infections + renal impairment). The workup of this patient should, however, certainly include a digital rectal examination and a blood test for prostate-specific antigen (PSA), but the diagnosis would be confirmed by finding increased plasma cells on bone marrow aspiration. Indeed, a myeloma screen should be considered in any patient with anaemia, renal impairment and hypercalcaemia.

7. D ★ OHCM 10th ed. → p. 334

When anaemia with a high mean corpuscular volume (MCV) is detected, the important tests to run include thyroid function tests, vitamin B12 and folate levels, and reticulocytes. Added to these, a peripheral blood film can provide important information about the individual cells. Although all of the options given can cause macrocytic anaemia, only D would show hypersegmented polymorphs on a blood film (all other options cause non-megaloblastic macrocytic anaemias, i.e. liver disease showing 'target cells' on the blood film). The characteristic appearance of these polymorphs—large with multiple segments—is because the rate at which the nucleus develops is slower than the rate at which the cytoplasm develops. The delay in the nucleus developing is due to a lack of folate and/or vitamin B12, which are necessary for DNA synthesis. When these cells are detected in the bone marrow, they are referred to as megaloblasts.

Pernicious anaemia is the most common cause of macrocytosis with a megaloblastic bone marrow. Symptoms stem from the inability of the gut to absorb vitamin B12, due to a lack of secretion of intrinsic factor (following an autoimmune atrophic gastritis). Treatment is therefore to replenish stores of the vitamin by intramuscular (IM) injections.

8. E ★   OHCM 10th ed. → p. 334

A, B, C, and E would all be reasonable and useful investigations into anaemia, although only B and E are targeted specifically at macrocytic anaemia (A would be useful in iron deficiency. Whilst reticulocytes do cause macrocytosis, this is usually in response to other events such as haemolysis and haemorrhage). Given the specificity of the clinical signs (a 'swollen red tongue'), the diagnosis would be confirmed by low vitamin B12 levels and the antibodies to gastric parietal cells that characterize pernicious anaemia. Only D would be inappropriate in this instance—it would be indicated in a case of pancytopenia to explore the possibility of a haematological malignancy.

9. A ★   OHCM 10th ed. → p. 340

This woman is having a painful crisis, common to sickle-cell disease (SCD). For some reason (often idiopathic, but can be due to hypox-aemia, dehydration, cold, or infection), the microvasculature becomes occluded by a backlog of abnormally shaped (sickled) red blood cells. This results in ischaemia, and then infarction of the red bone marrow, and the characteristic deep-seated bone pain that can only be relieved by high-dose opioids. E refers to an aplastic crisis, whilst D refers to a sequestration crisis—both complications of SCD in which much more severe anaemia than in this case would be expected.

10. E ★★   OHCM 10th ed. → p. 368

Osteolytic bone lesions can cause unexplained backache with patho-logical fractures. Immunoparesis from monoclonal proliferation of plasma cells and marrow infiltration can lead to intermittent infections. Both of these features are suggestive of myeloma.

A. This is Hodgkin's/non-Hodgkin's lymphoma.

B. This is Waldenström's macroglobulinaemia.

C. This is B-cell lymphoma.

D. This is acute/chronic myeloid leukaemia.

11. D ★★   OHCM 10th ed. → p. 366

This woman is suffering with bleeding and the symptoms of microvascular occlusion. This is due to essential thrombocythaemia (high levels of platelets that are derived from a clonal proliferation of megakaryocytes and so do not function normally).

A. This is acute/chronic myeloid leukaemia.

B. This is Waldenström's macroglobulinaemia.

C. This is acute/chronic lymphoblastic leukaemia.

E. This is myeloma.

12. E ★★   OHCM 10th ed. → p. 528

Between 7 and 10 days post-chemotherapy is when the bone marrow is likely to be at its 'nadir'. A fever occurring at this time—even before the results of the full blood count are known—should be treated as neutropenic sepsis, even if symptoms are mild or even absent. Treatment is to send off all cultures and to start immediate broad-spectrum intravenous antibiotics.

13. E ★★   OHCM 10th ed. → p. 370

It is very common to find a monoclonal protein in the serum of those over 50 years old. However, in the absence of end-organ damage (anaemia, hypercalcaemia, lytic bone lesions, renal failure, hyperviscosity), if the concentration is low (<30 g/L), it is described as an asymptomatic plasma cell dyscrasia and labelled as monoclonal gammopathy of uncertain significance (MGUS). However, if the concentration is high, if the bone marrow concentration of monoclonal plasma cells is >10%, and as end-organ damage appears, it transforms into something more malignant—depending on the class of protein involved, either multiple myeloma, amyloid, or Waldenström's macroglobulinaemia. Consequently, MGUS does need to be followed up, but infrequently and by serial measurements of the serum monoclonal protein concentration.

14. A ★★   OHCM 10th ed. → p. 360

The symptoms described are classical B-cell symptoms. These are found in malignancies of lymphocytes, such as lymphoma and chronic lymphocytic leukaemia (CLL), and generally involve B cells more than T cells.

15. D ★★   OHCM 10th ed. → p. 340

The oxygen dissociation curve illustrates the relationship between the partial pressure of oxygen in arterial blood (PaO_2) and the arterial oxygen saturation (SaO_2) (Figure 6.2). The standard curve is calculated for normal adult HbA. The curves for fetal HbF and HbSS in sickle-cell disease (SCD) occupy different positions.

In SCD, the dissociation curve is shifted to the right, indicating that haemoglobin (Hb) has a lower affinity for oxygen and can therefore more easily release it to the tissues. As a result, lower levels of Hb can be well tolerated.

A. There is chronic haemolysis in SCD, but this does not cause haemodilution; rather, it causes a rise in bilirubin and reticulocytes.

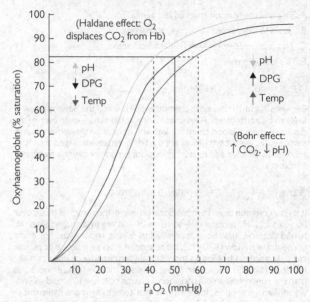

Figure 6.2

B. An increase in cardiac output is seen in some conditions (e.g. hyperthyroidism, Paget's disease, and multiple myeloma) as a response to increased demands, but not in SCD.

C. Having a 'normal' mean corpuscular volume (MCV) does not preclude breathlessness.

E. If anything, a man this age with SCD is likely to have a restrictive lung defect due to recurrent episodes of pulmonary vaso-occlusion.

Sylvester KP, Patey RA, Milligan P, et al. (2004). Pulmonary function abnormalities in children with sickle cell disease. Thorax. 2004;**59**:67–70.

→ thorax.bmj.com/cgi/content/abstract/59/1/67

16. B ★★   OHCM 10th ed. → p. 340

This man is seriously unwell. Not only does he have an acute painful sickle crisis, but he also has features of a severe acute chest crisis with wheeze and significant hypoxia [90% on 6 L oxygen should prompt urgent escalation, discussion with a haematologist and intensive therapy unit (ITU) involvement]. Whilst all of the options are appropriate, the only option which offers definitive treatment of the crisis (by removal of the sickled cells) is exchange transfusion. A haematologist would expect to be called urgently at any time if this man presented to the emergency department and will often come and support the exchange transfusion themselves.

17. E ★ ★ ★   OHCM 10th ed. → pp. 14, 568

This woman has made an advance decision to refuse a particular treatment, based on some strongly held personal beliefs. When the proposed treatment is life-sustaining, the advance decision—as in this woman's case—needs to be 'formally' recorded; under the Mental Capacity Act 2005, this means that she needs to have signed it and to have been witnessed doing so by a responsible healthcare professional. This then overrides any change in the patient's capacity or any desire for the medical team to treat her in her best interests.

18. E ★ ★ ★   OHCM 10th ed. → p. 338

The registrar is referring to the possibility of an autoimmune haemolytic anaemia (AIHA) as a complication of a *Mycoplasma pneumoniae* infection. The test he has in mind is the Coombs' test, which would confirm the presence or absence of a direct anti-globulin reaction characteristic of AIHAs. AIHAs are mediated by autoantibodies and are most commonly idiopathic but can occur following infections (e.g. *Mycoplasma* or Epstein–Barr virus) and cause extravascular haemolysis and spherocytosis.

A. This is the basis of the Schilling test. It is used in megaloblastic macrocytic anaemias to determine whether a low serum vitamin B12 level is due to reduced absorption at the terminal ileum or to decreased secretion of intrinsic factor.

B. This describes the Ham's test for paroxysmal nocturnal haemoglobinuria (PNH), in which acidified serum activates an alternative complement pathway, which induces lysis of erythrocytes (the diagnosis of choice is now flow cytometry). PNH causes chronic intravascular haemolysis, with pancytopenia and an increased risk of thrombosis.

C. Methaemalbumin is formed when haemoglobin (Hb) is broken down to haematin which then combines with albumin. It is raised in severe intravascular haemolysis.

D. This is a basic description of how a peripheral blood film is performed. Although it often provides useful information in cases where any of the cell lines are depleted, it is not the specific test referred to here.

19. C ★ ★ ★   OHCM 10th ed. → p. 354

With a presenting complaint of chest pain, it would be right at first to exclude a cardiac cause. This would involve taking some routine bloods. When these reveal pancytopenia, the recent history of aches, pain, and epistaxis becomes important. This woman's problems stem from decreased cell counts across the lineages; the first diagnostic test would be a peripheral blood film before the haematologists proceed to bone marrow aspiration and immunophenotyping.

A. This would be reasonable, based on the history of pain, which is suggestive of some kind of chronic inflammatory process. Conditions such as systemic lupus erythematosus (SLE) can also suppress some of the cell lines. A rheumatological disease probably comes in second place as the likely cause in this scenario.

B. This is useful in diagnosing haemoglobinopathies but would not explain the lymphopenia and thrombocytopenia.

D. This would be an unusual presentation of the disease, which, although it may cause anaemia of chronic disease over time, would be more likely to raise the platelets in response to chronic inflammation.

E. These are useful in most anaemias and would certainly be part of the workup in this case, but are unlikely to explain the complex set of symptoms.

20. A ★★★   OHCM 10th ed. → pp. 374, 554

The history is suggestive of anti-phospholipid syndrome, which most commonly occurs on its own but can occur—as here—with systemic lupus erythematosus (SLE). As well as the presence of the anti-cardiolipin antibodies and lupus anticoagulant, results also show thrombocytopenia and a paradoxically prolonged activated partial thromboplastin time (aPTT) (as a result of a reaction between the lupus anticoagulant and phospholipids involved in the coagulation cascade).

B. These are most commonly raised together in rheumatoid arthritis.

C. This woman may have microcytic anaemia, but this would not be the confirmatory finding in the search for a diagnosis.

D and E. These are suggestive of haemolytic anaemia [↑ haemoglobin (Hb), ↑ lactate dehydrogenase (LDH), bilirubin = increased red cell breakdown, ↑ reticulocytes = increased red cell production).

21. C ★★★   OHCM 10th ed. → p. 350

The reaction to heparin referred to is heparin-induced thrombocytopenia (HIT) and the platelet count falls, although not usually enough for bleeding to occur. The most common symptom is enlargement of a pre-existing blood clot or the development of a new one. This reaction takes a minimum of 4 days to develop—this is how long it takes for antibodies against heparin to be produced, which then bind to the molecule and cause platelet activation and subsequent thrombosis. As well as monitoring symptoms, it is important to take serial full blood counts over the first week to 10 days of the initiation of heparin therapy.

When HIT is suspected clinically, heparin treatment needs to be stopped immediately and a HIT antibody screen sent to the lab. However, this alone does not halt the fall in platelets or reduce the risk of thrombosis. To achieve this, treatment with non-heparin anticoagulants that do not cross-react with the HIT antibodies is required to dampen the storm of thrombin, as well as a more protracted course (2–3 months) of warfarin to prevent the recurrence of thrombosis.

A. This is unusual in HIT, as platelet levels tend not to drop far enough.

B. This would be more suggestive of orthostatic hypotension due to decreased blood volume following haemorrhage.

D. Rather than thrombocytopenia, this would be more suggestive of a hyperviscosity syndrome such as polycythaemia rubra vera or myeloma.

E. A proportion of patients who suffer HIT will develop a rash, but this would be a non-blanching petechial rash caused by the low platelet count.

22. **B** ★★★ OHCM 10th ed. → p. 689

As warfarin is metabolized via the cytochrome P450 system, any concurrent drugs that inhibit this system will potentiate anticoagulation [increase the international normalized ratio (INR)], whilst those that induce the system will impair anticoagulation (decrease the INR). Of the drugs listed, only clarithromycin has been shown to definitely act as an enzyme inhibitor. Prednisolone has been shown to both induce and inhibit, whilst the others have no effect.

23. **C** ★★★ OHCM 10th ed. → p. 350

Warfarin is a vitamin K antagonist which has become less popular since the more widespread use of direct-acting oral anticoagulants. The level of protein S is dependent on vitamin K activity and, because it acts as a co-factor for protein C, there is a reduction in the breakdown of factors Va and VIIIa. This causes the clotting cascade to favour the formation of clots and produces a transient prothrombotic state. To cover this period, low-molecular-weight heparin (LMWH) is employed as an anticoagulant and can be discontinued once the warfarin has been through its prothrombotic state and the international normalized ratio (INR) is within target range.

24. **C** ★★★ OHCM 10th ed. → p. 366

The symptoms described—headaches and erythromelalgia—could be due to either hyperviscosity (as in polycythaemia rubra vera where there are excess red and white blood cells and platelets) or microvascular occlusion (as in essential thrombocytosis where there is a persistently high platelet count). The other myeloproliferative disorders—myelofibrosis and chronic myeloid leukaemia—tend to present with general symptoms of lethargy or the discomfort of an enlarged spleen.

A. This describes what happens in aplastic anaemia, which would be more likely to present with anaemia, bleeding, or infection.

B. This occurs in, for example, sickle-cell disease.

D. This is the process behind myeloma, which, due to marrow infiltration, can also present with anaemia, bleeding, or infection, but also with backache and pathological fractures.

E. Although thromboses are features of myeloproliferative disorders, this is due to thrombocytosis (i.e. the sheer number of platelets), rather than thrombophilia (an innate tendency towards clotting due to defects in the coagulation pathway).

25. E ★★★   OHCM 10th ed. → p. 341

According to the British Committee for Standards in Haematology, subcutaneous (SC) is probably the route of choice in sickle-cell crises. Although absorption is slightly unpredictable, it is safest for the short- and long-term health of the patient. Sites should be varied between the abdomen and upper arms and legs.

A. This route used to be widely used, particularly in the administration of pethidine. However, due to the risk of muscle fibrosis, this is now contraindicated.

B. The intravenous (IV) route allows rapid absorption, but in a patient who has regular crises, access may be a problem; indeed, repeated attempts may continue to compromise this, which could become a very serious problem if a lifesaving transfusion were ever needed.

C. The oral route is used for moderate pain or once pain has been controlled by other means.

D. The rectal route is used for non-steroidal anti-inflammatory drugs (NSAIDs) in ureteric and pelvic pain but is not commonly used to administer opioids.

26. A ★★★   OHCM 10th ed. → p. 63

When confronted with a vague history, it is important to perform a rigorous examination. The findings elicited here suggest that the mass palpated in the abdomen is the spleen. The fact that its notched edge is felt in the right iliac fossa confirms this as a case of massive splenomegaly.

As chronic myeloid leukaemia (CML) presents insidiously, the finding of the enlarged spleen often predates any symptoms. In 50% of cases, it extends >5 cm below the left costal margin at the time of first discovery, and interestingly its size actually correlates with the full blood count, i.e. patients with the largest spleens are those with the highest white cell counts.

It can be useful to think of splenomegaly as being due to three main causes:

1. Increased workload (e.g. red blood cell turnover, extramedullary haematopoiesis)
2. Infiltration (e.g. leukaemias, metabolic diseases)
3. Abnormal circulation (e.g. portal hypertension, cardiac failure).

Of the options, portal hypertension (E) is the only other option that can cause moderate to large splenomegaly, but this would be in association with hepatomegaly.

B does not increase the workload of the spleen, and although myelodysplasia (C) and polycythaemia (D) both do, they cause a more subtle splenomegaly than seen in this case of CML.

27. B ★★★   OHCM 10th ed. → p. 364

The scenario outlines splenomegaly with pancytopenia, but a normal bone marrow. Pancytopenia is due either to reduced cell production or to increased cell destruction. Only **B** refers to the increased destruction that is the hallmark of hypersplenism, whilst all of the others refer to decreased production and implicate the bone marrow in some way: aplastic anaemia (**A**), myelodysplasia (**C**), acute myeloid leukaemia (**D**), and myeloma (**E**). Hypersplenism is pancytopenia caused by splenomegaly. When a spleen is large enough, it causes sequestration of all blood groups passing through its system, and thus reduced counts. It does not exist on its own, but as a secondary process to almost any cause of splenomegaly.

28. B ★★★

This is a common dilemma for the on-call junior doctor. It can feel like a difficult decision, but really just one thing needs to be remembered—if there are any uncertainties about whether a dose of warfarin has been given, no further doses should be given on that occasion and an international normalized ratio (INR) should be taken the next day. Taking an INR on the same night would not leave long enough for any doses that had been given earlier that evening to be evident and, as a result, an extra dose may then be given.

29. E ★★★   OHCM 10th ed. → p. 757

Although this interaction is a rare cause of myelosuppression/pancytopenia in practice—about ten cases in the literature—the key learning point is that there are a number of drugs that should prompt you to think 'Will this interact?' when adding new medications to existing drug therapy. Trimethoprim is widely used as a first-line antibiotic for urinary infections, but there are many other suitable agents (**A–D**) that cause no problems when used in combination with methotrexate (MTX).

There is a theoretical risk of interaction with penicillins—it is thought that penicillin blocks MTX secretion by inhibiting cellular uptake and stimulating efflux.

30. A ★★★   OHCM 10th ed. → p. 368

Beta-2 microglobulin is a protein component of major histocompatibility complex (MHC) class I molecules. It is a standard part of the workup for patients with multiple myeloma, as it is a key prognostic indicator.

31. A ★★★★   OHCM 10th ed. → p. 345

The scenario describes menorrhagia, epistaxis, and purpura—collectively evidence of platelet dysfunction. In this demographic, the most likely cause is idiopathic thrombocytopenic purpura (ITP). ITP is a relatively common autoimmune disorder in which platelets that are coated in antibody are removed from the reticuloendothelial system, thus reducing their lifespan to a few hours. The purpuric rash is as a result of thrombocytopenia causing the breakdown of capillaries and bleeding into the skin. This type of rash (as well as petechiae and ecchymoses, which are just smaller and larger versions, respectively) is due to disorders of platelets or the vasculature. Coagulation disorders (including deficiencies of any factors—factor VIII here in haemophilia A) are more likely to cause bleeding into joints (haemarthrosis) or muscle.

B. This occurs, for example, in acute leukaemias, lymphoma, myeloma, and myelodysplasia, all of which would be most likely to present with more symptoms than just those due to platelet dysfunction.

C. The most extreme example of this is aplastic anaemia, a rare stem cell disease in which the bone marrow becomes hypoplastic and stops making cells, therefore affecting all cell lineages.

D. This refers to the lemon tinge that those with vitamin B12 deficiency can acquire; they are anaemic but do not suffer with platelet dysfunction and the symptoms that accompany it.

E. This refers to a non-specific haemolytic anaemia that, although it could present with platelet dysfunction, would also present with symptoms of anaemia.

32. C ★★★

A rapid rise in temperature (>1.5° C from baseline) should prompt you to think about whether this could be features of an acute haemolytic reaction or a bacterial contamination. Although it is more common to see contamination of transfused platelets (they are stored at 22°C), it does occur. The transfusion should be stopped, and a full blood count (FBC)/urea and electrolytes (U&Es)/clotting/culture should be sent to the lab together with the unit.

A. At the prescribed rate of 1 unit (about 280 mL) over 1 hour, he has received too little blood in the 15 minutes for a reaction to be due to fluid overload.

B. Although an increase in the rate is not a concern in isolation, respiratory difficulty/distress should prompt a search for other features of transfusion-related acute lung injury (TRALI). This is non-cardiogenic pulmonary oedema of uncertain cause associated with hypoxia and pulmonary infiltrates.

D and E. These could be seen in allergic reactions and are both quite common reactions. The transfusion should be slowed/stopped, and the patient given chlorphenamine; the blood transfusion can be started again after 30 minutes if there is no further reaction.

The important lesson is that if you are in any doubt that a change in your patient's condition could be a result of a treatment you are giving, stop the treatment and reassess.

33. C ★★★★ OHCM 10th ed. → p. 354

Acute lymphoblastic leukaemia (ALL) is a malignancy of lymphoid cells, affecting B- or T-lymphocyte cell lineages. The maturation of lymphoid cell lines is halted, and uncontrolled proliferation of immature blast cells occurs. The blood film characteristically shows immature blast cells, and the white cell count (WCC) is usually high. Patients often present with signs of bone marrow failure, opportunistic infections, or signs of infiltration such as lymphadenopathy, hepatosplenomegaly or central nervous system (CNS) involvement. Factors associated with a poor outcome include: being an adult, male sex, Philadelphia chromosome, decreased haemoglobin (Hb), WCC >100 × 10⁹, and B-cell ALL.

34. C ★★★★ OHCM 10th ed. → p. 366

This patient has clinical features of polycythaemia, which is confirmed by the results of his full blood count (FBC) [raised haematocrit and haemoglobin (Hb), as well as white cell count (WCC) and platelets]. In the absence of any obvious causes of secondary polycythaemia, polycythaemia rubra vera is the most likely diagnosis. This is associated with a mutation in *JAK2* in >95% of cases.

A. This mutation causes defective stem cell repair and chromosomal fragility. It is associated with Fanconi anaemia and breast cancer.

B. This mutation is commonly associated with follicular lymphoma.

D. This mutation is commonly associated with Burkitt's lymphoma.

E. The Philadelphia chromosome is present in >80% of cases of chronic myeloid leukaemia (CML).

Chapter 7

Infectious diseases

Doug Fink

Infectious diseases are global and local. They impact health and disease in every country, but protean factors—cultural, geographical, and political—determine their particular local distribution. Every single patient is globally colonized by microorganisms, but singular behaviours, genetics and co-morbidities significantly determine what organisms cause disease in any individual. The practice of infectious diseases medicine necessarily demands an understanding of the person and the world in which they live. This chapter will emphasize the importance of context in assessing patients for infectious diseases.

In terms of global mortality, communicable diseases remain the leading causes of mortality. Despite the evocative epithet of 'infectious diseases', these are not all caused by creatures that creep and crawl. Cosmopolitan diseases (i.e. universally distributed infections such as influenza or bacterial pneumonia) represent a huge burden wherever medicine is practised. However, it is important to note that in high-resource settings, infection imported by travel and migration is increasing. In particular, the international traffic of emerging infections, such as Zika virus, and antimicrobial resistance (AMR) are already major healthcare problems. As the world shrinks and the climate changes, the distribution of infectious diseases will continue to change.

The threat of AMR no longer looms—it is a present and real danger. In the time it will take for disciples of this text to reach the end of their specialty training, AMR will account annually for more deaths than cancer. The delivery of almost all interventional, surgical, and immunomodulatory therapies depends on our ability to provide effective anti-microbial prophylaxis and rescue. The ability of organisms to adapt rapidly to novel iatrogenic selection pressures means that the treatment of human immunodeficiency virus (HIV), tuberculosis (TB), malaria, and manifold other pathogens will be compromised, not simply anti-bacterial agents. The future of modern medicine depends on the global healthcare community sharing both concern and responsibility. This chapter will include cases pertaining to the management of AMR.

QUESTIONS

1. A 22-year-old engineering student returned from 3-month travel in South East Asia. He flew back from Bangkok, Thailand 7 days ago. Of note, he went on a trek in the hills around Chiang Mai, Thailand 3 weeks ago and went river-tubing in Vang Vieng 5 days before his flight. He has a 2-day history of fever, headache, and myalgia. He has a palpable spleen, muscle tenderness, and subconjunctival haemorrhages. His blood tests show that he is thrombocytopenic, with a mild transaminitis. His rapid diagnostic test for malaria antigen is negative, pending reporting of his blood film.

What is the *single* most likely test to diagnose the infection at this stage? ★

A Blood culture

B Bone marrow culture

C Polymerase chain reaction (PCR)

D Serology

E Urine culture

2. A 74-year-old woman attends her general practice with a 4-day history of progressive lower left leg pain, with enhancing redness. She grazed her left shin while cleaning her fireplace at home. She has ischaemic heart disease and varicose veins. She feels generally unwell, but not febrile. Her general practitioner identifies a large area of non-purulent, tender erythema and associated swelling on her left lower leg. She is able to mobilize. He prescribes her first-line antibiotics and considers investigations.

What is the *single* most likely means of diagnosing this condition? ★

A Blood culture

B Clinical examination

C Leg X-ray

D Skin microscopy, culture, and sensitivity (MC&S)

E Skin punch biopsy

3. A 22-year-old woman attends her second antenatal appointment for her first pregnancy. Besides blood test screening for hepatitis B virus (HBV), hepatitis C virus (HCV), human immunodeficiency virus (HIV), rubella, and syphilis infections, she also provides a routine urine sample. She is well and has no past medical history of note. Her midwife phones to report that her urine specimen has grown *Escherichia coli*. On direct questioning, Stacey denies any urinary symptoms at all and reports no history of urine infections. What is the *single* most likely management plan for this patient? ★

A High vaginal microscopy, culture, and sensitivity (MC&S)

B No intervention

C Provide emergency antibiotic supply for use, should she become symptomatic

D Repeat urine MC&S

E Treat with appropriate antibiotics

4. A 26-year-old man attended sexual health clinic screening. His serum was reactive for human immunodeficiency virus 1 (HIV-1) antibody. His most recent previous test was negative 3 months ago. He has previously been treated for rectal gonorrhoea twice. He re-attends for post-test counselling; his CD4+ T-cell count is 512 cells/microlitre, and his viral load 312 434. His drug resistance profile shows wild-type virus. He is asymptomatic.

Which is the *single* most likely management plan for this patient? ★ ★

A Monitor his CD4+ T-cell count until it is below 350 cells/microlitre prior to starting anti-retroviral therapy (ART)

B Monitor his CD4+ T-cell count until it is below 500 cells/microlitre prior to starting ART

C Repeat drug resistance profile to assess for archived resistance prior to starting ART

D Rescreen for other sexually transmitted infections prior to starting

E Start ART immediately

5. A 34-year-old man from Masvingo province in southern Zimbabwe has been referred to the tuberculosis (TB) clinic. He is human immunodeficiency virus 1 (HIV-1) antibody positive. He describes a cough that started 3 months ago and night sweats, and he has created new notches on his belt to hold up his trousers. He is cachectic, with oral *Candida* and onycholysis of his left great toe. His chest X-ray is reported at the clinic as normal. His sputum is smear-negative for acid-fast bacilli (AFB) and GeneXpert-negative. What is the *single* most likely organism causing his symptoms? ★★

A *Cryptococcus neoformans*

B *Mycobacterium abscessus*

C *Mycobacterium tuberculosis*

D *Streptococcus pneumoniae*

E *Talaromyces marneffei*

6. A 3-year-old girl was admitted to hospital after she was found unconscious by her parents in her bedroom. She had fever and malaise for the preceding 3 days. By the time she reached hospital, her skin was diffusely discoloured and her blood pressure unrecordable. She was stabilized with anti-microbial therapy and fluid resuscitation. The next day, the microbiology registrar contacts the intensive therapy unit (ITU) to inform the clinical team that her blood cultures are growing Gram-negative diplococci. Public Health England traces her parents and two siblings. What is the *single* most likely antibiotic regimen that each household contact will receive? ★★

A One week of ampicillin

B One week of rifampicin

C Single dose of amoxicillin

D Single dose of benzylpenicillin

E Single dose of ciprofloxacin

7. A 19-year-old woman returned from her gap year volunteering as a ranger at Lake Malawi National Park 3 months ago. She has noticed her urine has been consistently darker than usual. Her general practitioner (GP) has prescribed her two courses of antibiotic, which have not helped. She self-presents to the walk-in tropical diseases clinic. She is worried about one weekend spent swimming in Lake Malawi. She took praziquantel that week as prophylaxis. She is clinically well on examination. Ova are detected in her urine sample.

Which is the *single* most likely organism to be responsible for her symptoms? ★ ★

A *Fasciola hepatica*

B *Schistosoma mekongi*

C *Schistosoma haematobium*

D *Schistosoma mansoni*

E *Schistosoma intercalatum*

8. A 34-year-old woman is 28 weeks pregnant. She presents to her general practitioner (GP) with a 12-hour history of rash that appeared overnight. Two weeks ago, she looked after her best friend's 4-year-old son for the afternoon. Two days later, he developed chickenpox. She is uncertain about her own chickenpox history and did not consult her GP at that time. Her GP examines her, and the rash is vesicular over her torso and limbs. She is afebrile, and her examination is otherwise normal.

What is the best immediate management for this patient? ★ ★

A Aciclovir intravenous (IV)

B Aciclovir oral (PO)

C No treatment

D Varicella-zoster virus antibody testing

E Varicella-zoster immunoglobulin

9. A 27-year-old man was diagnosed with human immunodeficiency virus (HIV) infection 5 years ago and initiated anti-retroviral therapy soon afterwards. He reports good treatment adherence and has had an undetectable viral load during routine follow-up. In the last 5 years, he has also been treated for syphilis twice and rectal gonorrhoea. He reports five casual partners in the last 3 months and do not always use condoms.

He has a 2-week history of rectal pain and bloody discharge. There is a small ulcer at the anal verge. He has tender palpable inguinal lymph nodes. He is afebrile and reports no recent foreign travel. McCoy cells are visible on microscopy of his rectal swab.

What is the *single* most likely organism causing his symptoms? ★★

A *Chlamydia trachomatis*

B *Haemophilus ducreyi*

C *Herpes simplex virus*

D *Klebsiella granulomatis*

E *Treponema pallidum*

10. An 80-year-old woman has been in hospital for 3 months. She has myasthenia gravis and was originally admitted with aspiration pneumonia. She received 10 days of broad-spectrum antibiotics. She developed diarrhoea shortly after completing her antibiotic course, and her stool tested positive for *Clostridium difficile* antigen and toxin. Her diarrhoea improves with metronidazole. Ten days later, she passes three unformed stools. The samples again test positive for *C. difficile* antigen and toxin. She is afebrile; her abdomen is soft and non-tender, and her blood tests are normal. What is the *single* most likely treatment? ★★

A Intravenous (IV) metronidazole

B IV vancomycin

C Oral fidaxomicin

D Oral metronidazole

E Oral vancomycin

11. A 46-year-old South African prospector is in London on business. He returned from a remote gold mine in Angola 7 days ago. During his visit, he spent time inside mines colonized by bats. He reports 24 hours of fever, severe myalgia, and headache. Clinically, he has a temperature of 38.3°C but is otherwise well, with a normal clinical examination. What is the *single* most likely haemorrhagic fever that needs to be excluded? ★★

A Crimean–Congo haemorrhagic fever

B Dengue fever

C Ebola virus disease

D Lassa fever

E Marburg

12. A 34-year-old man was admitted through the emergency department with severe breathlessness. He was subsequently diagnosed with advanced human immunodeficiency virus (HIV) infection and *Pneumocystis jiroveci* pneumonia. CD4+ T-cell count 80 cells/microlitre.

During the first week of his admission, he complains of blurring of his vision, associated with small lumps floating across his gaze and apparent flashing lights. Ophthalmology assessment describes characteristic perivascular yellow-white fluffy retinal lesions associated with haemorrhage.

What is the *single* most likely organism causing this patient's visual problems? ★★

A *Candida albicans*

B Cytomegalovirus

C Epstein–Barr virus

D Herpes simplex virus

E *Toxoplasma gondii*

13. An 89-year-old woman is seen by her general practitioner (GP) with a mild headache. She has no other symptoms. In particular, there is no dysuria, urgency or frequency of urination, back or loin pain, or fever. The practice nurse performs urinalysis.

BLO −, PRO −, KET −, LEU ++, NIT +, GLU −.

What is the *single* most appropriate treatment? ★ ★

A Give a rescue pack of antibiotics for if she develops urinary symptoms in the next week

B No further action

C Send a urine sample for microscopy, culture, and sensitivity (MC&S)

D Treat with a 3-day course of oral antibiotics, as per local anti-microbial guidelines for urinary tract infections (UTI)

E Treat with a 7-day course of oral antibiotics, as per local anti-microbial guidelines for UTIs

14. A 24-year-old nurse receives a blood splash to her eye during cannulation of an encephalopathic patient with chronic liver disease and clinical stigmata consistent with intravenous drug use. The patient's bloodborne virus serology will be available in 24 hours. The nurse has a hepatitis B surface antibody (HBsAb) titre of 118 mIU/mL, after completing a full course of hepatitis B virus (HBV) vaccination 9 months ago. What is the *single* most likely treatment plan to manage risk of HBV transmission to the nurse? ★ ★ ★

A Accelerated course of HBV vaccination

B Accelerated course of HBV vaccination and tenofovir prophylaxis

C Immediate intravenous immunoglobulin (IVIG) and accelerated HBV vaccination

D No intervention

E Single dose of HBV vaccination

15. A 66-year-old woman had a week's history of progressive breathlessness and fever. Past medical history includes atrial fibrillation, type 2 diabetes, cervical spondylosis, and mitral valve replacement surgery 10 years ago for mitral valve prolapse. Current medications are metformin, ramipril, simvastatin, tramadol, and warfarin. The admitting medical team note significant mitral regurgitation and clinical findings consistent with heart failure. These findings are not reported in her last outpatient cardiology letter from 6 months ago. After ensuring the collection of three sets of blood cultures, she is started on antibiotics for possible endocarditis, pending further investigations. Twenty minutes into the infusion, the nurse pulls the resuscitation alarm. Mary is complaining of severe chest pain and worsening breathlessness; she appears flushed with diffuse erythema. Her observations are stable. Which is the *single* most likely antibiotic to be causing her symptoms? ★★★

A Ceftriaxone

B Flucloxacillin

C Gentamicin

D Rifampicin

E Vancomycin

16. A 34-year-old mixed martial arts fighter, born in northern Cambodia, suffered a pathological fracture to his right femur and was subsequently diagnosed with high-grade non-Hodgkin's lymphoma. His chemotherapy regimen includes rituximab and dexamethasone. Within the first week of his treatment, he suffers high fevers, wheeze, and haemoptysis. He also suffers abdominal pain. His chest X-ray demonstrates diffuse reticulo-nodular changes. Two days later, blood cultures grow *Escherichia coli*. His clinical team send his stool for urgent microscopy analysis.

What is the *single* most likely organism causing his symptoms that they will find in his stool? ★★★

A *Ancylostoma duodenale*

B *Ascaris lumbricoides*

C *Necator americanus*

D *Strongyloides fuelleborni*

E *Strongyloides stercoralis*

17. A 21-year-old man, originally from rural Kurdish Iraq, has lost weight over the last 6 months and complained of a persistent cough and some pleuritic right-sided chest pain. His examination is unremarkable, although he appears underweight. He has an abnormal chest X-ray, and a computed tomography (CT) chest showed cysts in his lungs and liver.

What is the most likely organism causing these lesions? ★★★

A *Echinococcus granulosus*

B *Entamoeba histolytica*

C *Leishmania infantum*

D *Mycobacterium tuberculosis*

E *Streptococcus anginosus*

18. A 24-year-old man returned to London 3 days ago from visiting his extended family for a wedding outside of Kano in northern Nigeria. He used no anti-malarial prophylaxis. For 5 days, he has complained of fever, myalgia, headache, and diarrhoea. A blood film reports rings, trophozoites, and schizonts of *Plasmodium falciparum*. Parasitaemia is reported as 3%. His clinical examination, observations, and chest X-ray are normal. His routine serum biochemistry and haematology tests are also normal. What is most appropriate management of this patient? ★★★

A Intravenous (IV) artesunate

B IV quinine sulfate and oral (PO) doxycycline

C PO quinine sulfate and PO doxycycline

D PO artemether–lumefantrine

E PO artemether–mefloquine

19. A 38-year-old man returned 10 days ago from his company's annual hike to the Great Smoky Mountains National Park in North Carolina and Tennessee, USA. In the last 72 hours, he has complained of high fever and headache, and a rash that has spread overnight. On examination, he has a diffuse maculopapular rash. There is no meningism. His observations are normal, except for his temperature which is 37.8°C.

White cell count (WCC) 6.7, haemoglobin (Hb) 136 g/L, platelets 110.

Which is the *single* most likely organism responsible for his presentation? ★★★

A *Borrelia afzelii*

B *Borrelia burgdorferi*

C *Borrelia garninii*

D *Rickettsia conorii*

E *Rickettsia rickettsii*

20. A 65-year-old man returned from holiday in Sharm-El-Sheik, Egypt 3 weeks ago. He had a febrile jaundice illness and was diagnosed with hepatitis A virus (HAV) infection. His wife is also 65 years old and is concerned about acquiring the infection herself. She believes she was vaccinated for HAV 12 years ago when they were travelling to India for their son's wedding.

What is the *single* most appropriate management to prevent his wife from developing hepatitis A? ★★★★

A Human normal immunoglobulin (HNIG) and a single dose of monovalent HAV vaccine

B HNIG and a single dose of monovalent HAV vaccine, followed by a second dose at 6 months

C HNIG

D No treatment

E Single-dose monovalent HAV vaccine

21. A 32-year-old woman attends her first antenatal appointment. She has a history of injection drug use and is well established on methadone substitution therapy. She undergoes routine infection screening. Her results are as follows:

Anti-hepatitis B surface (HBs): positive

Anti-hepatitis B core (HBc): positive

Hepatitis B surface antigen (HBsAg): negative

Hepatitis C virus (HCV) antibody (Ab): positive

Human immunodeficiency virus 1 (HIV-1) Ab: negative

Rubella Ab: positive

Syphilis: negative.

What is the *single* most appropriate next test to perform? ★ ★ ★

A Hepatitis B virus (HBV) ribonucleic acid (RNA)

B HCV deoxyribonucleic acid (DNA)

C Hepatitis delta virus (HDV) Ab

D Rubella immunoglobulin M (IgM)

E Vaccinate against HBV

22. A 44-year-old man returned from a rural spiritual retreat in northern India 3 weeks ago. He has had a fever for at least 5 days despite paracetamol. He describes abdominal pain but denies diarrhoea or vomiting. On his abdomen are faint blanchable pink lesions. His abdomen is soft. He reports that he had a full set of vaccinations, including hepatitis A virus, hepatitis B virus, typhoid, and rabies.

What is the *single* best test to diagnose the organism at this stage of infection? ★ ★ ★

A Bone marrow culture

B Blood culture

C Stool culture

D Widal test

E Urine culture

ANSWERS

1. C ★   OHCM 10th ed. → p. 425

Leptospirosis is principally spread by soil or water contaminated by infected animal urine. River sports is a common means of acquisition for returning travellers. Incubation is between 3 and 30 days. An acute septicaemic febrile phase is followed by a second immune phase during which multi-organ failure can occur. Polymerase chain reaction (PCR) is thought to be most sensitive within the first 5 days after disease onset. Antibodies to *Leptospira* develop after 10 days. Blood cultures are insensitive, but if positive, they occur during the first 10 days of illness. Urine cultures are also insensitive but become positive later during the second week of illness and persist for up to 30 days. Bone marrow culture is not typically used for diagnosis of leptospirosis.

There is generally a weak evidence base for leptospirosis diagnostics. Detail can be found from the National Leptospirosis service at:

→ www.gov.uk/guidance/leptospira-reference-unit-services

2. B ★   OHCM 10th ed. → p. 34

Cellulitis is very common. It is a clinical diagnosis. Blood cultures are relevant if the physician suspects sepsis and bacteraemia from a skin source. There is no role for samples of cellulitic skin. It is just as likely that commensal organisms from the skin will be detected that are simple passengers, and not pathogens related to the underlying infection. Imaging is also not indicated. Empirical treatment guided towards predominantly Gram-positive bacteria is appropriate.

3. E ★

All pregnant women should be routinely screened for asymptomatic bacteriuria in early pregnancy. Approximately a third of untreated asymptomatic bacteriuria in pregnancy leads to symptomatic infection. During pregnancy, there is a higher risk of pyelonephritis, and therefore morbidity and mortality. Asymptomatic bacteriuria may also be independently associated with an increased risk of preterm birth and low birthweights. Antibiotic therapy is indicated after a single positive sample. Certain antibiotics are contraindicated during different trimesters, and in the context of increasing anti-microbial resistance, this is an area of antibiotic prescribing that is already challenging.

Public Health England have accessible summaries of infection screening in pregnancy at:

→www.gov.uk/government/collections/infectious-diseases-in-pregnancy-screening-clinical-guidance

4. E ★★ OHCM 10th ed. → p. 402

After nearly three decades of anti-retroviral therapy (ART) for human immunodeficiency virus (HIV) infection guided by immunological status (CD4+ T-cell count), there is now clear global consensus that immediate initiation of ART for individuals newly diagnosed with HIV infection has a short- and long-term survival advantage. In certain circumstances, including intercurrent anti-microbial therapy for tuberculosis and other opportunistic infections, there is evidence that a short delay before initiating ART is appropriate.

The British HIV Association (BHIVA) has excellent summaries at the start of each guideline at:

→ www.bhiva.org/HIV-1-treatment-guidelines.aspx

5. C ★★ OHCM 10th ed. → p. 393

This human immunodeficiency virus (HIV)-infected individual has advanced immunosuppression, suggested by opportunistic infections, such as oral *Candida* and fungal toenail infections, and >10% weight loss. People living with HIV have approximately 30 times greater risk of developing tuberculosis (TB), compared to populations without HIV. Nearly 80% of the world's HIV/TB co-infection occurs in sub-Saharan Africa. In individuals with TB and CD4 counts <200 cells/microlitre, chest radiographs are as likely to be normal as abnormal and HIV-infected individuals are also more likely to have smear-negative TB [no mycobacterial organisms—acid-fast bacilli (AFB) on microscopy]. In smear-negative patients, nucleic acid amplification (including the Xpert assay) has significantly reduced sensitivity for TB. In hospitalized HIV-infected individuals with CD4 counts <100 cells/microlitre, urinary antigen detection (mycobacterial lipoarabinomannan) is also an appropriate test for TB. *Mycobacterium avium* complex (MAC) might also present with similar symptoms. *Mycobacterium abscessus* is not a MAC organism. It is a rapidly growing non-tuberculous *Mycobacterium*, most commonly associated clinically with chronic lung infections in patients with cystic fibrosis and other chronic lung diseases and skin or soft tissue infections. HIV-infected individuals are at an increased risk of invasive *Streptococcus pneumoniae* disease, but an abnormal X-ray and more severe illness would be expected. *Talaromyces marneffei*, or penicilliosis, is an opportunistic organism endemic to parts of Asia that causes multi-systems infections.

6. E ★★ OHCM 10th ed. → p. 390

This patient has meningococcaemia and may or may not have meningococcal meningitis—there is insufficient detail in the stem. *Neisseria meningitidis* appears as Gram-negative diplococci on microscopy. Invasive meningococcal disease incidence peaks in children under 5 years and teenagers at around university age. A priority, even in probable cases before a confirmed microbiological diagnosis, is the public health response to identify and manage contacts. The aim of chemoprophylaxis is to reduce the risk of invasive disease by eradicating upper respiratory tract carriage of the organism from close contacts. The case is likely to have acquired the invasive meningococcal strain from a close contact, who is an asymptomatic carrier, in the week preceding disease onset. Close contacts are typically defined as individuals with prolonged contact (>8 hours) in a household setting during the 7 days before onset of illness. Close contacts also include those with transient contact if there may have been large-particle droplet exposure from the respiratory tract of the case at around the time of admission to hospital (e.g. kissing). Single-dose oral ciprofloxacin or intramuscular/intravenous ceftriaxone, or 48 hours of twice-daily rifampicin are preferred regimens. Single-dose azithromycin is also acceptable chemoprophylaxis in pregnancy.

7. C ★★   OHCM 10th ed. → p. 434

Genitourinary schistosomiasis is caused by *Schistosoma haematobium*, which can also cause intestinal or hepatosplenic schistosomiasis like the other *Schistosoma* species. *S. haematobium* and *Schistosoma mansoni* are responsible for the bulk of schistosomiasis in sub-Saharan Africa. Travellers can acquire the infection after a single exposure. Infected snails release cercariae which penetrate human skin in freshwater. These cercariae become schistosomulae in the human host and migrate through the circulation towards the liver where they become adult worms. Adult worms tend to subsequently migrate to vesical venous plexus where migration of eggs causes granulomatous inflammation in the bladder and ureters. Praziquantel is only effective against adult worms, not the larval stages, and is therefore most effective at preventing egg-mediated end-organ damage when given 4 weeks after freshwater exposure. Fascioliasis is a liver fluke pathology, which does not typically present with genitourinary symptoms.

8. B ★★   OHCM 10th ed. → p. 404

A pregnant woman presenting with vesicular rash and the appropriate clinical history is very likely to have varicella-zoster infection. The diagnosis is clinical. Once the window has been missed, as in this case, to administer post-exposure prophylaxis [i.e. varicella-zoster immuglobulin (VZIG)] to a pregnant woman with no childhood chickenpox history, then immunoglobulin, has no role in treatment. Maternal zoster can be associated with significant morbidity—complicated varicella infection most commonly presents as pneumonia but can affect multiple body systems and is a medical emergency. In terms of fetal risks, after 20 weeks' gestation, congenital varicella syndrome is unlikely. Neonatal varicella is a risk if the mother acquires varicella immediately before or after delivery. Uncomplicated maternal varicella infection should be treated with aciclovir. Intravenous therapy is indicated for complicated infection, signified by fever, respiratory symptoms, or persistent vesicle cropping after day 6.

Public Health England (PHE) publishes the *Green Book* which summarizes updated information about immunization against infectious diseases, available at:

→   www.gov.uk/government/publications/varicella-the-green-book-chapter-34

9. A ★★   OHCM 10th ed. → p. 412

Lymphogranuloma venereum (LGV) is caused by the L1, L2, and L3 serovars of *Chlamydia trachomatis*. It was historically an illness of tropical and subtropical climates but is increasingly seen in men who have sex with men (MSM) in temperate parts of the world. The vast majority of MSM who have acquired LGV are also HIV-infected (up to 76%). The primary phase is typically marked by a painless papule or ulcer at the site of inoculation. Proctitis is also common. Secondary lesions after days to weeks manifest as inguinal lymphadenitis and may lead to fistulating bubos. Late disease can behave like Crohn's disease with proctocolitis and fistulae.

Haemophilus ducreyi causes chancroid, which is epidemiologically uncommon and does not typically cause proctitis. Herpes simplex virus (HSV) can cause proctitis, but significant bleeding and lymphadenitis would be atypical. *Klebsiella granulomatis* causes granuloma inguinale (or donovanosis), which may manifest as inguinal abscess formation but is not associated with rectal disease. *Treponema pallidum* is the organism responsible for syphilis and does not cause lymphadenitis or proctitis.

The British Association for Sexual Health and HIV (BASHH) has detailed, but well-organized, guidelines available at:

→ www.bashh.org/guidelines

10. E ★★   OHCM 10th ed. → p. 411

Recurrent *Clostridium difficile*-associated disease (CDAD) occurs in 20% of individuals after the first episode and >50% individuals after their second episode. Risk is associated with advancing age and co-morbidities. Relapse is a form of recurrent disease that occurs within 2 weeks of completing anti-microbial therapy. Guidelines advise oral vancomycin 125 mg four times daily (qds) for approximately 10 days after the first recurrence. Intravenous vancomycin does not reach the gastrointestinal lumen and therefore has no role in treating any manifestation of CDAD. Fidaxomicin and faecal transplantation are other treatment options for recurrent non-severe CDAD; however, they are typically reserved for patients with multiple recurrence. Intravenous metronidazole is reserved for severe CDAD that does not respond to vancomycin. Severe CDAD is diagnosed by the presence of any of the following: white cell count >15 × 10⁹/L, high creatinine (>50% above baseline), fever, and clinical evidence of severe colitis. Oral metronidazole is used to treat mild or moderate CDAD.

11. E ★★   OHCM 10th ed → p. 426

Marburg virus is endemic across southern Africa. Bats are thought to be the main reservoir. Transmission occurs most often through mucous membranes or broken skin. It is probably shed by bats and humans through all body fluids. Dengue fever could also present with undifferentiated fever, although a diffuse maculopapular rash is typical. Also, dengue is not typically spread between humans and does not have the same mortality risk as Marburg, so it does not have the same public health implications and need for urgent diagnosis. Ebola virus may be carried by fruit bats which are not thought to be cave dwellers. The reservoir for Lassa fever is the multimammate rat and is mostly sequestered in West Africa.

12. B ★★   OHCM 10th ed. → p. 404

Cytomegalovirus (CMV) retinitis is associated with advanced immuno-suppression in human immunodeficiency virus (HIV) infection; in the pre-anti-retroviral therapy (ART) era, up to 25% of individuals with CD4 counts <200 had evidence of CMV retinitis. Symptoms of CMV retinitis may also paradoxically become more symptomatic during reconstitution of T cells during ART. Diagnosis is clinical. Treatment in most cases now entails systemic valganciclovir. After a period of induction therapy, maintenance therapy should be continued until HIV is suppressed.

Toxoplasmic chorioretinitis typically presents as eye pain, and lesions have a non-vascular retinal distribution. Epstein–Barr virus (EBV) is not usually associated with ophthalmic pathology; herpes simplex virus (HSV) is more commonly a cause of exogenous keratitis than any endogenous retinal disease. *Candida albicans* can cause endophthalmitis in immunocompromised individuals but is less common as an opportunistic infection causing visual loss in HIV-infected individuals. It is also usually associated with severely unwell patients who have a clear source of fungaemia (such as an indwelling central venous catheter).

13. B ★★   OHCM 10th ed. → p. 296

Urine dips and urinalysis are grossly overused and should only be used in the over >65s to rule out renal disease, and not infection. This is because a large proportion of older women have asymptomatic bacteriuria and this does not equate to infection. Unfortunately, swathes of frail older people are labelled with a urinary tract infection (UTI), as this is an easy clinical diagnosis to make with a 'positive urine dip'; but in congratulating themselves on this (incorrect) diagnosis, other serious pathology or causes of delirium can go unnoticed for days. Therefore, with no symptoms of a UTI, even with a positive urine dip, she is extremely unlikely to have a urine infection. If she did have genuine urinary symptoms suggestive of a UTI (not just 'off legs' and 'more confused'), then it may be appropriate to send for urine microscopy, culture, and sensitivity (MC&S) and consider starting empirical antibiotics—but again a urine dip would not give any additional information.

14. D ★★★   OHCM 10th ed. → p. 287

Healthcare workers (HCWs) undertaking exposure-prone procedures (EPPs) should receive hepatitis B virus (HBV) vaccination. Vaccination response should be assessed in HCWs at 1–3 months after completing the vaccination course. More than 90% of individuals under 40 years will be protected after the third dose of a 3-dose vaccination series. A protective response is defined by anti-hepatitis B surface (HBs) titre of >100 mIU/mL. However, international guidelines do vary, and often an adequate response is defined as >10 mIU/mL. According to UK guidelines, a HCW with a post-vaccination anti-HBs titre of 10–100 mIU/mL should receive a routine fourth dose of vaccine before undertaking EPPs. After percutaneous or mucosal membrane exposure to blood or body fluids from a donor (i.e. patient) with an unknown HBV status, a HCW with a full vaccination schedule and documented anti-HBs titre of >100 mIU/mL would require no further vaccination or prophylaxis.

Pre- and post-HBV exposure prophylaxis is summarized very effectively in:

Public Health England (2013). *Hepatitis B: the green book, chapter 18*.

→ www.gov.uk/government/publications/hepatitis-b-the-green-book-chapter-18

15. E ★★★   OHCM 10th ed. → pp. 151, 386

The patient is being treated empirically for prosthetic valve endocarditis >10 years since cardiothoracic surgery. Irrespective of her penicillin allergy, guidelines advocate gentamicin, rifampicin, and vancomycin as anti-microbial therapy. There are several types of vancomycin hypersensitivity. The most common adverse reaction is 'red man syndrome'. It is believed that vancomycin directly causes mast cells to release histamine and other vasoactive substances. It is not a true allergic reaction. Mast cell activation is thought to be more likely in the presence of opioids (tramadol in this case). It is not generally life-threatening and occurs typically during or shortly after infusion. Even in severe reactions, administering pre-medications and restarting the infusion at a slower rate is acceptable. However, immunoglobulin E (IgE)-mediated hypersensitivity is also possible with vancomycin, which would present as anaphylaxis where hypotension, urticaria, and wheeze might be expected. It can be difficult to separate these diagnoses, and if anaphylaxis is suspected, vancomycin infusions should not be restarted.

16. E ★★★   OHCM 10th ed. → p. 433

Strongyloidiasis is a threadworm infection that affects up to 100 million people worldwide. Up to 60% of inhabitants of northern Cambodia carry *Strongyloides stercoralis* in their gastrointestinal tract. The nematode is endemic to many tropical and subtropical regions. Most infected patients do not experience symptoms. Chronic gastrointestinal infection over years is perpetuated by autoinfection by the helminth offspring which continue the life cycle indefinitely. Cell-mediated immune responses reduce this level of autoinfection to a subclinical level. Hyperinfection syndrome occurs when autoinfection accelerates and larvae disseminate rapidly, typically across the bowel into the bloodstream and into small airways. Human T-lymphotropic virus (HTLV) co-infection and immuno-suppression (e.g. high-dose steroids) are both strongly associated with driving hyperinfection.

The other organisms listed are all nematodes; *Ancylostoma duodenale* and *Necator americanus* are hookworms; *Ascaris lumbricoides* is a roundworm—these organisms do potentially have a transpulmonary passage during their life cycle, but hyperinfection is not thought to occur. *Strongyloides fuelleborni* is almost only seen in Papua New Guinea.

17. A ★★★   OHCM 10th ed. → p. 435

Echinococcus granulosus is the most common cause of echinococcosis or hydatid disease. The most common clinical presentation is with isolated liver cysts, which typically only become symptomatic once larger than 10 cm and exert mass effect. Pulmonary cysts can also occur in isolation, but around 20% of patients with lung cysts also have liver cysts. Cough and chest pain are common symptoms. Cyst rupture can result in acute life-threatening hypersensitivity reactions and also secondary bacterial infections. Extra-intestinal amoebiasis caused by *Entamoeba histolytica* can also cause pulmonary disease, but this is rare compared with amoebic liver abscess. *Streptococcus anginosus* group (previously *Streptococcus milleri*) of organisms are common causes of pyogenic liver abscess and may also cause discrete thoracic infections, including abscess, pneumonia, and empyema. Along with *Mycobacterium tuberculosis* and *Leishmania infantum*, *S. anginosus* does not cause cystic disease.

18. A ★★★   OHCM 10th ed. → p. 418

More than 80% of malaria imported into the UK is from travel to Africa. Nearly three-quarters of these cases are from West Africa. Of malarial parasites, *Plasmodium falciparum* accounts for the vast majority of imported infections. Both *P. falciparum* and *Plasmodium vivax* independently can cause severe malaria. International criteria for this entails a mixture of clinical and simple blood tests, including parasitaemia >10%. However, despite not meeting these criteria, the presence of schizonts and parasitaemia of >2% means that the currently observed parasite burden is likely to increase and the patient is at high risk of severe disease. Admission to hospital and treatment with intravenous artesunate is indicated in this circumstance.

→ www.journalofinfection.com/article/S0163-4453(16)00047-5/abstract

19. E ★★★   OHCM 10th ed. → p. 422

Rickettsia rickettsii is the pathogen responsible for this classic presentation of Rocky Mountain spotted fever (RMSF): maculopapular rash, fever, and headache within 2 weeks of travel to an endemic region. Thrombocytopenia is also suggestive of rickettsial infection.

Life-threatening infection is possible and doxycycline treatment is typically indicated, pending formal diagnosis. North Carolina and Tennessee are two of five states that account for over 60% of all RMSF. The *Borrelia* species listed may present as early localized Lyme disease. Erythema migrans would be the typical rash in this instance. Fever is also less common. *Borrelia burgdorferi* is the primary North American pathogen responsible for Lyme disease, and >95% of infections occur in states along the eastern seaboard. *Borrelia afzalii* and *Borrelia garinii* are associated with Lyme disease in Asia and Europe. *Rickettsia conorii* is also a spotted fever-group rickettsia but causes Mediterranean spotted fever in regions adjoining the Mediterranean sea.

20. A ★★★★   OHCM 10th ed. → p. 278

Hepatitis A virus (HAV) is transmitted through faeco-oral contact. Vaccination against HAV is thought to be protective for 10 years. The severity of hepatitis with HAV rises with age, particularly after 60 years. In susceptible close contacts aged over 60 years, guidelines advocate human normal immunoglobulin (HNIG) administration within 14 days and a single dose of HAV vaccination. A second dose of HAV vaccination is also advised, but this is intended to provide long-term protection, rather than any protection from recent contact with an acute infection.

The *Green Book* offers detailed coverage of pre- and post-exposure prophylaxis against HAV at:

→ www.gov.uk/government/publications/hepatitis-a-the-green-book-chapter-17

21. B ★★★   OHCM 10th ed. → p. 286

All pregnant women should be screened for chronic hepatitis B virus (HBV) in order to prevent vertical transmission. Hepatitis B surface antigen (HBsAg) is an adequate screening tool for most women, but those with epidemiological risk factors (such as HBV-infected partners or previous injection drug use) should also undergo anti-hepatitis B core (HBc) and anti-hepatitis B surface (HBs) testing. Mothers without evidence of prior HBV infection (negative for all) should be vaccinated. Presence of anti-HBs and anti-HBc with negative HBsAg typically implies previous natural infection. There is no role for HBV DNA testing in this setting. Anti-HBs is usually positive alone after immunization. Hepatitis C virus (HCV) antibody (Ab) testing is only offered to mothers at high risk of chronic HCV infection. All reactive antibody tests should be followed by HCV RNA testing. Despite seroconversion, approximately 50% of adults will clear HCV spontaneously, thus reactive HCV Ab does not always represent an ongoing chronic infection, but merely previous exposure. Hepatitis delta virus (HDV) only occurs with HBV co-infection or superinfection. Rubella susceptibility testing by immunoglobulin G (IgG) should be offered to all pregnant women at some stage of their pregnancy, and those identified as being at risk of contracting rubella should be vaccinated in the postnatal period to protect future pregnancies. Chagas' disease and Zika virus screening should be offered to patients from endemic countries.

22. B ★ ★ ★   OHCM 10th ed. → p. 415

Typhoid fever is endemic globally in areas of poor sanitation. Both injectable and oral typhoid vaccines are significantly <70% protective. The incubation period is between 5 and 21 days, depending on the size of the inoculum, among other factors. Typhoid classically commences with undifferentiated fever. In week 2, abdominal pain and 'rose spots' on the abdomen and trunk may manifest. During the third week, there is a risk of gastrointestinal perforation and late neurological conditions. Constipation and diarrhoea are seen in typhoid fever, but it is common for patients to present with neither. Blood culture is the most common form of diagnosis in travellers returning to the UK and mostly from those visiting friends and relatives. Stool and urine can also isolate *Salmonella enterica* serotype Typhi but are far less sensitive. Bone marrow culture is sensitive, even after antibiotic therapy, but is rarely required and is of course unreasonably invasive. Widal's test represents non-specific serology and is not used in most high-resource settings.

Chapter 8

Neurology

Ross Paterson and Laszlo Sztriha

The face of neurology in clinical practice is changing. Neurology is no longer primarily a diagnostic specialty. As more therapeutic treatments become available in all fields from epilepsy to multiple sclerosis, early and accurate diagnosis is increasingly required so that patients can benefit from early treatment aiming to reduce the lifelong burden of neurological disease.

Diagnosis of neurological disorders is often considered by junior doctors to be highly complex and, as such, is responsible for a great deal of anxiety. One of the most difficult challenges can be determining the location of the lesion. A helpful approach to this is by analysis of the patterns that each lesion produces. Table 8.1 describes some of the common patterns seen in clinical practice, and the questions in this chapter will attempt to highlight some of the other specific presentations needed in assessing the neurology patient.

Table 8.1 Patterns of neurology depending on location of lesion

Location of lesion	Signs
Cortex	Normal or increased tone Weakness of all movements of the hand or foot 'Higher-level' dysfunction such as dyspraxia, dyscalculia, or deficits in language, visual processing, sensory perception, or alterations in behaviour or personality
Internal capsule/corticospinal tract	Contralateral hemiplegia with upper motor neurone weakness
Cerebellum	Ataxia, intention tremor, nystagmus, hypotonia. Signs ipsilateral to the lesion
Spinal cord	Para- or tetraplegia Lower motor neurone signs at the level of the lesion Upper motor neurone signs below the lesion Dissociated sensory modality loss Testable sensory level
Central spinal cord syndrome	'Cape-like' distribution of sensory loss, with preservation of distal sensation
Hemi-cord syndrome	Weakness and proprioceptive loss on the same side as the lesion, with loss of pain and temperature sensation on the opposite side
Peripheral nerve	Distal weakness (although can also be proximal weakness) Areflexia Sensory loss in a glove-and-stocking distribution (length-dependent neuropathy) or following the cutaneous pattern of one or more peripheral nerves (multiple neuropathies)

Location of lesion	Signs
Neuromuscular junction	Fatiguable weakness Reflexes slightly reduced
Autonomic nervous system	Absence of, or increase in, sweating Pupillary anomalies Cardiovascular instability; can manifest as (pre)syncope, 'coat hanger' pain, or palpitations Urinary or bowel dysfunction

QUESTIONS

1. A 60-year-old woman has lost the ability to pick up small objects with her right hand. She also finds it difficult to fasten buttons. There is no other weakness. She is unable to copy one particular movement made by the doctor examining her (Figure 8.1).

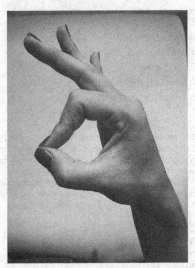

Figure 8.1

Which *single* nerve is most likely to have been compromised? ★

A Anterior interosseous

B Median

C Musculocutaneous

D Radial

E Ulnar

2. A 76-year-old man has collapsed. This has happened increasingly over the past year and tends to happen when he stands from sitting. This is not associated with any residual ill effects, but he also reports mild lower abdominal pain. He has hypertension and type 2 diabetes.

On examination, the abdomen is soft, with mild suprapubic tenderness that is dull to percussion. Digital rectal examination reveals hard impacted stool.

Which is the *single* most likely underlying cause of this man's symptoms? ★

A Accumulation of cerebrospinal fluid, with normal intracranial pressure

B Degeneration of the basal ganglia

C Disturbance of autonomic nerve function

D Permanent loss of cerebral neurones

E Temporary loss of local cerebral blood flow

3. A 66-year-old woman has awoken to find that the right side of her mouth is sagging and she has difficulty eating on that side, with food getting trapped. She has a very watery right eye; her speech is impaired, and she is hypersensitive to sounds in her right ear. The doctor assessing her feels the cause is almost certainly 'idiopathic'. Which is the *single* most likely factor in her history that influenced the doctor's judgement? ★

A Hypersensitivity to sounds

B Speech impairment

C Trapping of food

D Unilateral sagging of the mouth

E Watery eye

4. A 68-year-old man has had a worsening tremor of his hands for 9 months. He says his father and brother were troubled with the same problem and that they both noticed improvement after treatment with a beta-blocker. Which *single* additional feature in the history would be consistent with the most likely diagnosis? ★

A He uses two types of inhaler for his asthma

B His writing seems smaller than it used to be

C It disappears when he moves his hands

D It is only noticeable when his hands are still

E It seems to improve with alcohol

5. A 24-year-old woman has had a headache and double vision for 2 weeks. She is nauseated and has vomited on two occasions, but finds that her symptoms get better as the day progresses. A magnetic resonance imaging (MRI) scan of her head is normal. A lumbar puncture is performed and has an opening pressure of 36 cmH$_2$O (normal range: 0–25 cmH$_2$O). Which *single* additional feature from her history is most relevant to the likely diagnosis? ★

A Her father had chemotherapy 2 years ago for a glioma

B She drinks five or six cups of strong coffee each day

C She has a family history of migraine

D She smokes 20 cigarettes per day

E She takes orlistat 120 mg oral (PO) three times daily

6. A 49-year-old woman has weakness in her right arm and her right leg. She has been finding it increasingly difficult to find words. These symptoms have developed gradually over a 2-week period.

T 37.1°C, HR 85 bpm, BP 105/70 mmHg.

She has reduced power on the right, with brisk reflexes and upgoing plantars. Which is the *single* most likely underlying diagnosis? ★

A Cerebral infarct

B Cerebral metastases

C Hemiplegic migraine

D Subarachnoid haemorrhage

E Transient ischaemic attack

7. A 77-year-old man has felt 'muddled' for the last 5 days. He cannot put his finger on what is wrong, but neighbours say he has been talking and acting inappropriately.

T 37.8°C, HR 110 bpm, BP 95/70 mmHg, RR 26/min, SpO$_2$ 92% on air.

He is pale, clammy, and agitated, and in an abbreviated mental test, he scores 5/10. Which *single* set of investigations would be the most likely to support the diagnosis? ★

A Computed tomography (CT) of the head + carotid Doppler ultrasound scan

B CT of the head, thyroid function tests + mini-mental state examination

C Electrocardiogram (ECG), 12-hour troponin level + echocardiogram

D Full blood count, blood cultures + chest X-ray

E Random venous blood glucose + glycosylated haemoglobin (HbA1c)

8. A 50-year-old woman has had an aching pain and numbness in her right hand and arm for 5 months. She finds that shaking her arm vigorously relieves the symptoms. She takes levothyroxine, although she admits that she often forgets to take it. Which is the *single* most appropriate instruction to confirm the diagnosis? ★

A Cross your middle finger over the dorsal surface of the index finger

B Move your wrist towards the thumb laterally

C Place the thumb in a closed fist and tilt your hand towards the little finger

D Raise your thumb vertically out of an open palmar surface

E Spread your extended fingers open horizontally

9. A 48-year-old man has undergone a 10-hour intra-abdominal operation. After the operation, he has some numbness in the ring and little finger of his right hand. The doctor thinks he may have damaged a nerve and examines him to confirm the diagnosis. Which is the *single* most appropriate instruction to confirm the diagnosis? ★

A Cross your middle finger over the dorsal surface of the index finger

B Move your thumb across the palm and touch the base of the little finger

C With the palm facing downwards, bend the wrist up towards your forearm

D With the palm facing sideways, keep your hand in this position against resistance

E With the palm facing upwards, bend the wrist up towards your forearm

10. The junior doctor on call receives a bleep from a nurse during a busy night shift. A 78-year-old man has been found on the floor. He did not lose consciousness but was unable to get back on his feet, despite normally being fully independent. He is hoisted back into bed. He has no pain in his hips or wrists. He was admitted 3 days ago with a urinary tract infection and atrial fibrillation. Which is the *single* most important detail from the nurse, in isolation, that should prompt an immediate review of the patient, i.e. in the next 5 minutes? ★

A Alcohol dependence

B Headache

C Large swelling over his occiput

D Speech disturbance

E Temperature 37.7°C

11. A 58-year-old man has double vision, especially whilst reading. He has hypertension and type 2 diabetes. As he is talking, he tilts his head to the right, but when asked to straighten up, his left eye appears to be slightly higher vertically than the right. Which is the *single* most likely diagnosis? ★

A Left inferior oblique palsy

B Left inferior rectus palsy

C Left lateral rectus palsy

D Left superior oblique palsy

E Left superior rectus palsy

12. A 39-year-old man has suffered a seizure whilst out shopping. He is admitted to hospital where he is drowsy and confused. This is his third such episode in the past 6 months. He has idiopathic generalized epilepsy and has been through a variety of treatment regimens. He currently takes sodium valproate 500 mg twice daily (bd). Which is the *single* most appropriate investigation to determine the trigger? ★

A Blood levels of valproate

B Calcium and phosphate

C Computed tomography (CT) brain

D Electroencephalogram (EEG)

E Random capillary blood glucose

13. A 26-year-old man lost consciousness 30 minutes ago at work. He was found on the floor, shaking; this lasted for 10 minutes. He had a similar attack 1 month ago. He drinks only occasional alcohol and takes no medications.

T 36.1°C, HR 88 bpm, BP 142/78 mmHg, SaO_2 99% on air.

Glasgow Coma Scale (GCS) score 12/15.

A computed tomography (CT) head scan is reported as 'normal'. Which is the *single* most likely diagnosis? ★

A Cataplexy

B Drop attacks

C Epilepsy

D Non-epileptic attack disorder

E Vasovagal syncope

14. A 77-year-old woman has fallen 4.5 m from a balcony. Her cervical spine is immobilized, and she has a non-rebreather mask on, with 15 L/min of oxygen running. She is agitated and groaning and grabs the doctor's hand and opens her eyes as he rubs her sternum. She is awaiting a computed tomography (CT) scan of her head and neck, but within a few minutes, she starts to make snoring sounds and her oxygen saturation drops. Which is the *single* most appropriate next step? ★

A Head tilt and chin lift manoeuvre

B Jaw thrust

C Laryngeal mask airway

D Oropharyngeal airway

E Tracheostomy

15. A 55-year-old man has had a headache for the last 3 days. The pain is over the occipital region and associated with nausea and vomiting.

T 36.5°C, HR 80 bpm, blood pressure (BP) 150/80 mmHg.

He complains of double vision and has difficulty opening his right eye. He has grade 5/5 power in his limbs and down-going plantar reflexes. Which *single* pathological process is most likely to explain these symptoms? ★

A Demyelination

B Normal pressure hydrocephalus

C Idiopathic intracranial hypertension

D Ruptured cerebral aneurysm

E Subdural haematoma

16. A 38-year-old woman has fractured her right fibula. She says that she has some numbness on the top of her right foot. The junior doctor thinks she may have damaged a nerve and examines her to confirm the diagnosis. Which is the *single* most appropriate instruction to confirm the diagnosis? ★

A Bend your foot up towards your knees

B Make the sole of your foot into a cup

C Point your toes and place the soles of your feet together

D Stand up on your tiptoes

E While I hold your foot, bend the furthermost joints in your toes

17. A 60-year-old man has developed new headaches. He smokes 30 cigarettes per day. He describes a strictly left-sided head-ache, with eye watering and nasal stuffiness. During an attack, of which he has now had at least ten, each of which can last several hours, he paces around the room and feels like he wants to rip his eye out of its socket.

What *single* test should you do next? ★

A Computed tomography (CT) brain

B Electroencephalogram

C Lumbar puncture

D Measure central motor conduction velocites

E Trial of high-flow oxygen

18. A 42-year-old man complains of clumsy walking over the past 3 days. He describes severe back pain. Since yesterday, he has struggled to open a bottle because his hands 'don't feel right'.

On examination, his lower limb reflexes are absent. His heart rate is 110 bpm (regular), but his blood pressure is satisfactory.

What is your *single* next management step? ★

A Lumbar puncture

B Measure vital capacity

C Magnetic resonance imaging (MRI) spine

D Nerve biopsy

E Nerve conduction studies

19. A 30-year-old man has weakness of his right hand, shown in Figure 8.2. He has been involved in a road traffic collision and is being assessed for other injuries.

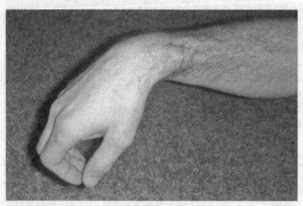

Figure 8.2

Which is the *single* most likely point of injury? ★

A Between the two heads of the pronator teres

B Epicondylar groove

C Flexor retinaculum

D Lateral to medial epicondyle

E Middle third of the humeral shaft

20. A 72-year-old woman, who is normally fit and well, loses the ability to grip and move her right arm for a 12-hour period. She is assessed overnight in hospital, and by the morning, she has no residual weakness. Which is the *single* most appropriate treatment? ★

A Aspirin 75 mg oral (PO) and dipyridamole modified release (MR) 200 mg PO twice daily

B Aspirin 300 mg PO

C Clopidogrel 75 mg PO

D Dipyridamole MR 200 mg PO twice daily

E Warfarin [variable doses, target international normalized ratio (INR) of 2–3]

21. An 80-year-old woman's speech has suddenly become slurred. She can find words without trouble but has difficulty enunciating them. A similar thing happened 2 weeks previously. She takes bendroflumethiazide 2.5 mg oral (PO) once daily. Which *single* further detail in the history would be most supportive of the likely diagnosis? ★

A Episode of urinary incontinence

B Difficulty swallowing

C Photophobia

D Symptoms followed a severe occipital headache

E Symptoms resolved after 20 minutes

22. A 72-year-old lady attends her general practitioner because her voice has changed in recent weeks. Her family say that she sounds like Donald Duck. She struggles to finish meals and avoids steak. Occasionally, she will choke on liquids. She has stopped driving, since she has started to see car headlights 'on top of one another' when driving in the dark.

What *single* investigation is most likely to confirm the diagnosis? ★

A Acetylcholine antibodies

B Anti-MuSK antibodies

C Computed tomography (CT) mediastinum

D Genetic testing

E Magnetic resonance imaging (MRI) of head and neck

23. A 66-year-old man has suffered sudden-onset weakness of his left arm and left leg. An urgent computed tomography (CT) scan of his head is performed and is suggestive of an acute ischaemic event. He is admitted to a hyperacute stroke unit where his care is handed over to the on-call junior doctor.

T 38.4°C, HR 100 bpm, BP 195/110 mmHg, SaO$_2$ 96% on air.

Random capillary blood glucose: 10.2 mmol/L.

Which *single* reading listed above warrants the most urgent attention? ★

A Blood glucose

B Blood pressure

C Heart rate

D Oxygen saturation

E Temperature

24. An 81-year-old woman is found groaning and coughing in bed. She was admitted 3 days ago, following a large left middle cerebral artery infarct.

T 39.4°C, BP 110/50 mmHg, SaO$_2$ 92% on 15L O$_2$.

Her chest has coarse crepitations bilaterally; her jugular venous pressure (JVP) is not seen, and she has no peripheral oedema. Which is the *single* most likely cause of her deterioration? ★

A Aspiration pneumonia

B Myocardial infarction

C Pleural effusion

D Pulmonary embolism

E Pulmonary oedema

25. A 30-year-old woman has had a seizure. Within 15 minutes, she has arrived at the emergency department but is still fitting. The ambulance crew have given diazepam 10 mg per rectum (PR). She is given 15 L of oxygen via a Hudson™ mask, and intravenous (IV) access is secured via a peripheral vein. Which is the *single* most appropriate next step? ★

A Arrange electroencephalogram monitoring

B Contact intensive care for intubation

C Lorazepam 4 mg IV slow bolus

D Phenytoin 15 mg/kg at 50 mg/hour IV

E Thiamine 250 mg IV over 10 minutes

26. A 55-year-old man has had muscle pain for about 2 weeks, mainly affecting his thighs and which is particularly bad when he climbs stairs. He has type 2 diabetes and high blood pressure. He started simvastatin 40 mg oral (PO) once at night a month ago. He has 5/5 power in both legs. Which is the *single* most appropriate investigation? ★

A Creatine kinase

B Erythrocyte sedimentation rate

C Lactate dehydrogenase

D Troponin

E Urea and electrolytes

27. A 23-year-old man has pain in his right shoulder after a heavy tackle whilst playing rugby. He has no neurovascular deficit of the upper limb, but he has some soft tissue swelling and tenderness over the head of the humerus. His range of movement is slightly reduced globally, and he is unable to abduct his right arm without first leaning to the right. Which is the *single* muscle most likely to have been affected? ★

A Infraspinatus

B Subscapularis

C Supraspinatus

D Teres major

E Teres minor

28. A 48-year-old man has a mid-shaft fracture of the right humerus. He has some numbness on his right hand and forearm. The junior doctor thinks he may have damaged a nerve and examines him to confirm the diagnosis. Which is the *single* most appropriate instruction to confirm the diagnosis? ★

A Move your thumb across your palm to the base of the little finger

B Resist displacement of a piece of paper between the middle and ring fingers

C Spread your fingers open, increasing the space between them

D With the palm facing downwards, bend the wrist up towards your forearm

E With the palm facing upwards, bend the wrist up towards your forearm

29. A 22-year-old man has sustained a sports injury. He scuffs the top of his right shoe along the floor as he walks and cannot turn his foot outwards against resistance. Which is the *single* most likely distribution of sensory compromise? ★

A Dorsum of the foot

B Lateral calf

C Lateral calf + dorsum of the foot

D Medial calf

E Medial calf + dorsum of the foot

30. A 66-year-old man has been feeling 'slowed down' over a 6-month period. He is struggling to cope around the house and is becoming increasingly reliant on his wife. She has noticed him to be lower in mood and less expressive and effusive generally. He has a resting tremor and a slow gait of small steps. Which *single* further feature would be suggestive of Parkinson's disease, rather than parkinsonism? ★

A Asymmetrical symptoms

B Inability to look up

C Postural dizziness

D Short-term memory problems

E Urinary retention

31. A 74-year-old man visits his family doctor due to increasing difficulty walking over the past 6 months. He has a fixed facial expression and a unilateral tremor of his right hand. Which is the *single* most appropriate next step? ★

A Check serum dopamine levels

B Refer to a movement disorders specialist (neurologist or geriatrician)

C Request a computed tomography (CT) head scan

D Start a dopamine agonist

E Start levodopa

32. A 30-year-old woman has been reported to have had a seizure. It happened in the standing area at the end of a 2-hour concert. She remembers feeling nauseated and sweaty beforehand. Her partner describes her falling to the ground where she jerked her limbs for several seconds. She did not bite her tongue and was not incontinent of urine. Two hours later in the emergency department, she is lucid, although distressed. The junior doctor examines her, refers her for an electroencephalogram (EEG), and sends her home. The registrar feels it is unlikely to be a seizure. Which *single* detail from the history is most likely to have made the registrar reach this conclusion? ★

A Lack of tongue biting

B Lack of urinary incontinence

C Nausea beforehand

D Prolonged standing

E Sweating beforehand

33. A 42-year-old woman has been feeling more and more tired at the end of her days at work. When she gets home, she struggles to lift anything and is too weak to eat or even use the telephone. She has bilateral ptosis, and on counting down from 50, her voice becomes increasingly quiet. Which *single* pathological process most accurately explains all of this woman's symptoms? ★

A Demyelination

B Dysfunction of the neuromuscular junction

C Mononeuritis multiplex

D Neuronal degeneration

E Space-occupying lesion

34. A 30-year-old woman has had difficulty walking for the past 12 hours. She first noticed it when she left work the previous night—her walk to the station, which usually takes only a few minutes, on this occasion took over an hour. She has grade 3 power in all muscle groups in both lower limbs and an extensor plantar response bilaterally. Which is the *single* most likely cause of her symptoms? ★

A Amyotrophic lateral sclerosis

B Guillain–Barré syndrome

C Multiple sclerosis (MS)

D Syphilis

E Vitamin B12 deficiency

35. A 27-year-old woman has been having regular headaches over the last few months. She describes the presence of bright 'zigzag lines' across her field of vision before the onset of the headache. She is otherwise well and takes only the oral contraceptive pill. Which *single* additional patient narrative from the history would be consistent with the most likely diagnosis? ★

A 'I have intense shooting pain around my eye and across my cheek'

B 'It's one side of my head. I feel nauseated and the light hurts my eyes'

C 'My eye looks blood-shot, the eyelid swells, and I produce more tears'

D 'The pain has started to wake me up and is worse when I lie down'

E 'Work has been very busy recently and I rarely have a chance to relax'

36. A 25-year-old woman has had uncontrolled headaches over a period of 6 months. These are unilateral and associated with nausea and photosensitivity. She has tried a number of simple analgesics, with no effect. After seeing a neurologist, she unsuccessfully tried an oral triptan. She is having to take large amounts of time off work now and feels increasingly anxious. She asks if she can take anything to prevent the headaches. Which is the *single* most appropriate prophylaxis? ★

A Amitriptyline

B Codeine phosphate

C Propranolol

D Sodium valproate

E Valproic acid

37. A 53-year-old man has had recurrent headaches for 3 weeks. These are accompanied by feelings of nausea and aggravated by lifting heavy boxes at work. His mother suffered with migraines for many years. A neurological examination is normal. Fundoscopy reveals no evidence of papilloedema. Which is the *single* most appropriate initial management? ★

A Referral to a neurologist within 2 weeks

B Send off urine for 5-hydroxyindoleacetic acid (5-HIAA) levels

C start PRN ibuprofen

D Start high-dose prednisolone

E Trial of oral sumatriptan

38. A 24-year-old man has fallen off a 2 m-high wall onto grass. He thinks he landed on his head. He has not lost consciousness at any time. His story, however, is unclear as he has drunk over 20 units of alcohol. Aside from the effects of drinking, he seems well and reports no drowsiness or nausea. The junior doctor is keen to discharge the man home. Which *single* examination finding should prompt the junior doctor to arrange a computed tomography (CT) scan first? ★

A Bleeding from the scalp

B Bruising behind the ears

C Coarse tremor in the hands

D Past pointing

E Romberg's test positive

39. A 30-year-old man has suffered a head injury. He was hit by a blunt object about 2 hours prior to coming to the emergency department. He remembers the incident well and has not been nauseated or vomited and he has no real headache. He was keen to stay at home and sleep it off, but his wife was concerned as she felt he was falling in and out of sleep and was rather confused. Which is the *single* most appropriate management? ★

A Computed tomography (CT) head scan

B Discharge home

C Magnetic resonance imaging (MRI) head scan

D Observe for 12 hours

E Skull X-ray

40. A 26-year-old man has had successive seizures, without regaining consciousness between them. After arriving at the emergency department, he had lorazepam 4 mg intravenous (IV) twice and was started on an infusion of phenytoin 15 mg/kg. It is now 40 minutes since the first seizure began. Which is the *single* most appropriate next step? ★

A Arrange for electroencephalogram (EEG) monitoring

B Diazepam 10 mg IV

C Fast-bleep the anaesthetist

D Repeat dose of lorazepam 4 mg IV

E Thiamine 250 mg IV

41. A 28-year-old woman lost consciousness at home an hour ago and is brought in to the emergency department. She has no previous medical history, and this has never happened previously. Her mother is worried that she has had a 'fit'. Which *single* feature from the history is most likely to confirm her mother's concerns? ★

A Biting the end of her tongue

B Feeling tired and wanting to sleep

C Incontinence of urine

D Still being confused when the ambulance arrived

E Twitching after she fell to the ground

42. A 20-year-old woman has had one seizure at home. She and her partner, with whom she lives, attend an appointment with an epilepsy specialist 3 weeks later. The decision is made to postpone starting any treatment. The couple remain concerned about the prospect of having another seizure and, in particular, about when they should contact the emergency services. Which *single* feature should prompt her partner to call the emergency services? ★

A A second fit starts before she has regained consciousness

B She experiences an 'aura' prior to the seizure

C She is incontinent of urine

D The clonic phase lasts for >10 minutes

E There is evidence of tongue biting

43. A 38-year-old man has been shot in the back of his right thigh. He says that the sole of his right foot feels numb. The junior doctor thinks he has damaged a nerve and examines him to confirm the diagnosis. Which is the *single* most appropriate instruction to confirm the diagnosis? ★

A Lift your foot up towards your knee

B Point your toes and place the soles of your feet together

C Turn the sole of your foot out to the side

D With a straight leg, bury your heel into the couch

E With your leg bent at the knee, straighten your leg against resistance

44. A 36-year-old woman who is 34 weeks pregnant has a strange sensation in her right hand. She has weakness of her abductor pollicis brevis and sensory loss over her radial three-and-a-half fingers and palm. Which *single* anatomical site is most likely to be the source of her symptoms? ★

A Between the brachialis and brachioradialis

B Between the two heads of the flexor carpi ulnaris

C Deep to the flexor retinaculum

D Medial to the brachial artery in the forearm

E Posterior to the medial humeral epicondyle

45. A 25-year-old man has noticed that his arms and legs have become weak over 2–3 days. He has noticed that his urine looks like cola. His reflexes are difficult to elicit but are probably present. Within 24 hours of admission to hospital, he has developed type 2 respiratory failure, requiring ventilation in the intensive therapy unit (ITU). Troponin I levels are extremely high. What is the *single* most likely unifying diagnosis? ★

A Maple syrup urine disease

B Necrotizing myopathy

C Fascioscapulohumeral dystrophy

D Spinomuscular atrophy

E Glycogen storage disorder

46. A 45-year-old man has been living rough for the past 6 months. He has a history of injecting recreational drugs. He presents with headache and confusion. On examination, he is drowsy and disorientated. His temperature is 37.2°C. Blood tests are normal. Magnetic resonance imaging (MRI) shows enhancement of the leptomeninges. A lumbar puncture is performed, and the opening pressure is very high. Protein is 1.2 g/dL; there are 76 white cells (lymphocytes), and glucose in the cerebrospinal fluid is 2.4. Unfortunately, the junior doctor forgot to send a matched blood sample.

What is the *single* most likely diagnosis? ★

A Cerebral lymphoma

B Cerebral vasculitis

C Cryptococcal meningitis

D *Listeria* meningitis

E Tuberculosis meningitis

47. A 32-year-old man has been dribbling saliva from the right side of his mouth and having difficulty closing his right eye over the last 48 hours. His wife has noticed that his face is drooping on the same side. He has normal facial sensation but cannot raise his eyebrow on the right side. Which is the *single* most appropriate next step? ★ ★

A No treatment

B Start oral aciclovir

C Start oral aciclovir ± oral prednisolone

D Start oral prednisolone

E Urgent magnetic resonance imaging (MRI) head scan

48. A 22-year-old man has had a headache increasing in intensity over the past 48 hours. He has started to feel nauseated and rather drowsy.

T 37.8°C, HR 100 bpm, BP 125/70 mmHg.

When the junior doctor asks him to lift his head from the pillow, the man is seen to involuntarily lift both legs in the air. Which is the *single* most accurate explanation for this finding? ★★

A Limb–girdle weakness

B Meningeal irritation

C Muscle spasm

D Raised intracranial pressure

E Sciatic nerve inflammation

49. A 21-year-old lady attends your clinic, having had a generalized tonic–clonic seizure witnessed by her mother. There was no warning. She has recently started a new job that necessitates an early start. She has occasional sudden jerks of her limbs and trunk in early mornings. She is keen to avoid further events. What do you recommend? ★★

A Commence a ketogenic diet

B Commence treatment with carbamazepine

C Commence treatment with lamotrigine

D Commence treatment with phenytoin

E Commence treatment with sodium valproate

50. A 43-year-old woman has had an increasingly severe headache for the last 6 weeks. She has latterly become nauseated and confined to a darkened room. Three months previously, she completed chemotherapy- and radiotherapy for a recurrent breast carcinoma.

T 37.6°C, HR 100 bpm, BP 95/70 mmHg.

Which *single* pathological process is most likely to have caused these symptoms? ★★

A Haemorrhage

B Infection

C Inflammation

D Metastasis

E Thrombosis

51. A 66-year-old man has noticed that one of his eyelids will not open properly. He also complains of pain and tingling in the shoulder and arm on the same side. He has hypertension, gout, and a chronic cough, having quit smoking 5 years previously. The right pupil is constricted, and the right side of the face is dry from sweat. Which *single* pathological process most accurately explains all of this man's symptoms? ★★

A Autonomic neuropathy

B Infection

C Mononeuritis multiplex

D Neoplasia

E Venous sinus thrombosis

52. A 70-year-old woman has begun dragging her right foot along as she walks. Two weeks previously, her left wrist felt weak such that she could not straighten it. She has had rheumatoid arthritis for 35 years and is currently using methotrexate 12.5 mg once weekly. Which is the *single* most likely neuropathological process to explain her symptoms? ★★

A Autonomic neuropathy

B Demyelination

C Entrapment

D Inflammatory peripheral neuropathy

E Mononeuritis multiplex

53. A 59-year-old woman has been unable to speak for the last 24 hours. Her daughter has noticed her to be irritable and slightly confused for most of the past week. She has also fallen several times in this period and complained of a headache that is worse in the mornings. On examination, you notice bilateral papilloedema.

Which *single* management option would be most likely to improve this woman's symptoms? ★★

A Alteplase 0.9 mg/kg intravenous (IV)

B Aspirin 300 mg oral (PO) once a day

C Dexamethasone 8 mg PO twice a day

D Nimodipine 60 mg PO six times a day

E Therapeutic lumbar puncture

54. A 78-year-old woman has a sudden onset of weakness in her right leg. She also has some difficulty with spontaneous speech and been incontinent of urine. There is no discernible visual or sensory loss. Which *single* affected vascular territory is most likely to explain this woman's neurological deficits? ★ ★

A Anterior cerebral artery

B Deep perforators

C Middle cerebral artery

D Posterior cerebral artery

E Posterior inferior cerebellar artery

55. A 58-year-old man is confused. He has no recollection of the events that brought him into hospital but says he has never been unwell before. Records show that this is his fifth admission within a 6-month period.

T 35.6°C, HR 110 bpm, BP 90/55 mmHg.

His eyes flicker from side to side, and when asked to walk, he can only stagger. He scores 0/10 in an abbreviated mental test. Which is the *single* most appropriate course of action? ★ ★

A Aspirin 300 mg oral (PO) once daily

B Dexamethasone 8 mg PO twice daily

C Glucagon 1 mg intramuscular (IM) immediately (STAT)

D Donepezil 5 mg PO at night

E Thiamine intravenous (IV) three times a day

56. A 78-year-old woman has had increasingly regular diarrhoea for the last 2 weeks. She has also noticed some blood mixed in with the stool. She has mild microcytic anaemia, with raised eosinophils. As she is awaiting a colonoscopy, she develops sudden-onset weakness of her left foot with pain. She finds that she cannot pick her foot up properly but drags it behind her, her toes scraping along the floor. She is otherwise only treated for asthma, which she developed in her 50s. Which is the *single* most likely pathological process that would explain this woman's symptoms? ★ ★

A Immunosuppression

B Infection

C Inflammation

D Malignancy

E Vasculitis

57. A 52-year-old Jamaican lady has felt an odd sensation around her abdomen over the past month. This feeling has become more prominent over the past week, and her legs have started to feel weak on climbing the stairs. She was embarrassed to mention that she has been incontinent of urine. On examination, you notice that there is a relative afferent pupillary defect on the left and left optic disc pallor. Her serum calcium levels are slightly elevated. A magnetic resonance imaging (MRI) spinal cord shows a long, thin central spinal cord lesion, extending from the brainstem down to the thoracic cord.

What *single* test is most likely to be diagnostic? ★★

A 24-hour calcium

B Aquaporin-4 antibodies

C Central motor conduction testing

D Computed tomography (CT) positron emission tomography (PET) scan

E Serum ACE

58. A 61-year-old lady presents with a 5-year progressive history of apathy and reduced speech with word errors. She does not always understand commands. More recently, she has been stealing food from other people's plates at the dining table. Her mother developed behavioural changes aged 56 but died in a road traffic accident before a diagnosis could be made.

What is the *single* most likely diagnosis? ★★★

A Alzheimer's disease

B CADASIL (cerebral autosomal dominant arteriopathy with subcortical infarcts and leukoencephalopathy)

C Dementia with Lewy bodies

D Frontotemporal dementia

E Prion disease

59. You review a 66-year-old man in the neurology clinic. He has a 3-year history of slow walking, shuffling gait, and a left-sided resting arm tremor. He was given a diagnosis of idiopathic Parkinson's disease by your predecessor. Things have now progressed. Which *single* clinical sign might make you re-evaluate the diagnosis? ★★★

A Deterioration in handwriting

B Postural hypotension

C Restricted range of vertical eye movements and dry eyes

D Tremor of the right hand

E Visual hallucinations

60. A 24-year-old woman has had 4 months of right-sided parietal headaches, with intermittent blurred vision. The headaches are most severe in the morning and get better through the course of the day. Which is the *single* most likely diagnosis? ★★★

A Idiopathic intracranial hypertension

B Cluster headache

C Giant cell arteritis

D Migraine

E Tension headache

61. An 81-year-old man has collapsed. When he comes round, he says he felt dizzy immediately prior to falling but does not remember exactly what happened. He recovers quickly and feels back to his normal self. He has hypertension, asthma, type 2 diabetes, and osteoporosis, and had been started on a new medication the previous day.

Which *single* medication is the most likely cause of the episode? ★★★

A Alendronic acid

B Doxazosin

C Gliclazide

D Rosiglitazone

E Salbutamol

62. A 67-year-old woman had an extended right hemicolectomy with a primary anastomosis yesterday. She started eating a light diet today and was recovering well. At 1 a.m., the nursing staff call the junior doctor on call because she is confused and tremulous and has been trying to climb out of bed for 2 hours. The patient says that she wants to get out of bed 'to find her cat, which ran past the end of the bed earlier'.

T 37.4°C, HR 90 bpm, BP 105/88 mmHg, SaO$_2$ 95% on air.

Capillary blood glucose 5.5 mmol/L.

Sodium 131 mmol/L, potassium 4.1 mmol/L, creatinine 88 micromol/L, haemoglobin (Hb) 95 g/L, mean corpuscular volume (MCV) 104 fL.

Which is the *single* most appropriate next step in management? ★★★

A Administer 2 L of oxygen via nasal cannulae

B Cross-match for a 2 U blood transfusion

C Start haloperidol 2.5 mg oral (PO)

D Start a reducing regime of chlordiazepoxide

E Start trimethoprim for a presumed urinary tract infection

63. A 60-year-old woman has a sudden episode of weakness in her left arm. It lasts for no more than an hour but is associated with slurring of her speech. She has hypertension and takes bendroflumethiazide 2.5 mg oral (PO) once daily and simvastatin 20 mg PO once daily. A neurological examination reveals no residual deficit. An electrocardiogram (ECG) is carried out (Figure 8.3).

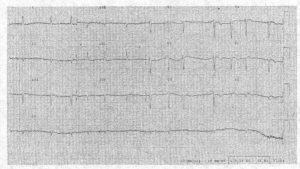

Figure 8.3

Which is the *single* most appropriate course of action? ★ ★ ★

A Computed tomography (CT) head scan, then start oral anticoagulation if appropriate

B Review in clinic in 3 months, and start oral anticoagulation if appropriate

C Start oral anticoagulant immediately

D Start oral anticoagulant only if there are further episodes of weakness

E Start oral anticoagulant only if the pulse rate is not adequately controlled

64. A 17-year-old woman has had a seizure at home, having felt sick for the preceding 2 hours. It was witnessed by her father who describes 1 minute of her stretching her arms and legs out, followed by 10 minutes of all four limbs shaking. She was incontinent of urine and was bleeding from the side of her tongue. This is her first such episode. No specific trigger can be detected. Twelve hours later, she has recovered well, apart from being unable to lift her left arm. The consultant suggests starting lamotrigine. Which *single* factor is most likely to have influenced the consultant's decision? ★ ★ ★

A Lack of a specific trigger

B Left arm weakness

C Pre-seizure sickness

D Tongue biting

E Urinary incontinence

65. A 67-year-old man has been brought into the emergency department in the early hours of the morning with a head injury following a fall at home 30 minutes ago. All he remembers is finding himself on the floor; he is not sure whether he lost consciousness. Which *single* feature should prompt a request for an urgent computed tomography (CT) head scan (within 1 hour)? ★ ★ ★

A He fell down five stairs

B He has vomited twice since the fall

C He is > 65 years old

D He suffers from epilepsy

E His Glasgow Coma Scale (GCS) score is currently 14

66. A 71-year-old man with rheumatoid arthritis went swimming in a lake. When he got out of the water, he was unsteady and his legs gave way. His symptoms then progressed over the next 3–4 weeks. He presented to hospital with worsening leg weakness and numbness. On examination, he has stiff legs, with extensor plantars and a positive Hoffman sign. Joint position sensation was abnormal in the upper and lower limbs, and there was a sensory level to pinprick at T4 level.

What is the most likely diagnosis? ★ ★ ★

A Compressive cervical myelopathy

B Guillain–Barré syndrome.

C Myasthenia gravis

D Myelitis

E Myopathy

67. A 33-year-old woman has had recurrent spells of tingling in her arms for the past 6 months. The tingling is noticeably worse when she is trying to use her arms and often seems to come on after she has had a hot bath. She has otherwise been well and does not smoke or drink alcohol. Which *single* investigation, or pair of investigations, would be the most likely to support the diagnosis? ★ ★ ★

A Anti-acetylcholine receptor antibodies

B Computed tomography (CT) thoracic outlet

C Magnetic resonance imaging (MRI) brain + spinal cord

D Nerve conduction studies

E Vitamin B12 + folate

68. A 78-year-old man has become acutely confused over the last few hours. He is recovering from a lower respiratory tract infection and is awaiting rehabilitation placement. He has hypertension, chronic obstructive pulmonary disease (COPD), Parkinson's disease, and type 2 diabetes. He is unsteady on his feet and has increased tone in all four limbs, more so than is usual for him. Which *single* medication is the most likely to have caused his deterioration? ★★★

A Amoxicillin

B Diazepam

C Metoclopramide

D Prednisolone

E Rosiglitazone

69. A 28-year-old woman has had a severe headache for the past 2 weeks. Her family doctor examines her eyes. The left eye constricts directly to light, with a consensual response in the right. However, as he swings the torch from the left to the right eye, he notes that both pupils appear to dilate. Which would be the *single* most accurate explanation of this finding? ★★★

A Argyll Robertson's pupil on the right

B Myotonic right pupil

C Normal variation

D Raised intracranial pressure

E Relative afferent pupillary defect on the right

70. A 72-year-old woman describes waking up 3 days ago, feeling like she is 'on a boat'. She has also noticed that after she rolls over in bed, especially to the right, the room spins around her for 15–20 s. She has also had to be careful when she has bent down to put on her shoes and getting things out of high cupboards.

No nystagmus seen. Romberg negative.

The doctor seeing her tries to explain why she is experiencing these symptoms. What is the *single* most likely explanation for why she is experiencing these symptoms? ★★★

A A benign growth on the acoustic nerve

B A blockage in the blood supply to the back of the brain

C Displaced crystals in the inner part of the ear

D Excessive fluid found in the inner ear

E Inflammation involving the inner ear

71. A 48-year-old man has had a painful neck for the last few months. The doctor examining him thinks he has symptoms consistent with a C8–T1 nerve root compression. Which *single* test result confirms this diagnosis? ★ ★ ★

A Numb fifth (little) and ring fingers

B Numb middle finger

C Reduced tricep jerks

D Weak biceps and deltoid

E Weak triceps and finger extension

72. An 84-year-old man is found unrousable in the bed of his nursing home. He has type 2 diabetes.

Sodium 156 mmol/L, potassium 5.5 mmol/L, urea 33 mmol/L, creatinine 288 micromol/L.

Random venous glucose: 55 mmol/L.

Which is the *single* most appropriate choice of infusion fluid? ★ ★ ★

A 0.45% saline

B 0.9% saline

C 5% glucose

D 5% glucose/0.9% saline

E Sodium bicarbonate

73. A 67-year-old man is brought to hospital by his family with a 3-week history of odd behaviour and poor recall memory. He was found on the bathroom floor that morning drowsy and confused, having been incontinent of urine. Routine bloods and computed tomography (CT) brain are reported to be normal.

A lumbar puncture reveals normal protein and two white cells. Viral cerebrospinal fluid (CSF) polymerase chain reaction (PCR) is negative.

What is the *single* most likely diagnosis? ★ ★ ★ ★

A Alzheimer's disease

B Dementia with Lewy bodies

C Herpes simplex encephalitis

D LGI-1 (leucine-rich glioma-inactivated 1) receptor limbic encephalitis

E NMDA (*N*-methyl-*D*-aspartate) receptor encephalitis

74. A 32-year-old man claims he has taken 30 temazepam 20-mg tablets 5 hours ago. He has a long history of depression and recurrent suicide attempts. He smells of alcohol; his speech is slurred, and he has an unsteady gait.

RR 12/min, SaO$_2$ 96% on air. Chest: scattered crepitations.

Which is the *single* most appropriate next step? ★ ★ ★ ★

A Activated charcoal

B Flumazenil intravenous (IV)

C Neurological observations until consciousness level improves

D Urgent referral to the intensive therapy unit for intubation and ventilation

E Urinary alkalinization

75. An 82-year-old woman has rapidly become unable to speak. Her family report that she has been increasingly tired over the last 3 weeks and latterly has been restricted to sitting in a chair. Prior to this, she walked with a stick and was independent with regard to all activities of daily living. She is awake, but not able to follow commands, and is therefore difficult to examine.

T 38.4°C, HR 105 bpm, BP 100/65 mmHg.

Tone and reflexes are globally increased, with equivocal plantars, but no focal neurology. Which *single* investigation is the most likely to produce a definitive diagnosis? ★ ★ ★ ★

A Blood culture

B Computed tomography (CT) scan of the brain

C Electroencephalogram (EEG)

D Lumbar puncture

E Magnetic resonance imaging (MRI) of the brain

76. An 18-year-old man has been brought to your clinic by his mother. She is worried about her son's behaviour. He has become withdrawn and is not sleeping. He sits in your office, with fidgeting movements of his arms and legs. His father has recently been admitted to a psychiatric institution. You find him to be withdrawn, with limb rigidity. Saccadic eye movements are slow.

What *single* action should you take next? ★ ★ ★ ★

A Arrange a sleep study

B Commence sertraline

C Draw a family tree and suggest genetic testing

D Measure very long-chain fatty acids

E Refer him to a psychiatrist

ANSWERS

1. A ★   OHCM 10th ed. → p. 452

The anterior interosseous nerve arises from the median nerve about 5 cm above the medial epicondyle, supplying the flexor digitorum profundus and the flexor pollicis longus muscles. It can be compromised by direct trauma or by compression by surrounding muscles (pronator teres), ligaments, or scar tissue. The result is the inability to pinch the thumb and forefinger together (in the way shown in Figure 8.1), and thus difficulty with fine motor pincer movements.

2. C ★   OHCM 10th ed. → p. 505

There are three symptoms described: postural falls, urinary retention, and constipation. Whilst they may occur in someone who is cognitively impaired, dementia itself does not cause them. They are all processes modulated by the autonomic system and likely to be affected by diabetes. Whilst they can coexist with Parkinson's disease in the 'Parkinson's plus' syndrome multi-system atrophy, there is no hint of parkinsonism in this patient.

3. A ★   OHCM 10th ed. → p. 500

All the other options can occur in any case of facial nerve palsy. Only A is seen in Bell's (idiopathic) palsy due to hyperacussis from stapedius palsy.

4. E ★   OHCM 10th ed. → p. 65

This is benign essential tremor, a rhythmic tremor (4–12 Hz) that is only present when the affected muscle groups are moved. It can be worsened by stress, demands to perform a task under pressure, cold, caffeine, and some drugs. It usually improves following small amounts of alcohol and beta-blockers.

Tremor can be a side effect of salbutamol but is more likely to occur intermittently after overuse of the drug, rather than progressively and constantly. Micrographia (small writing) and resting tremor are features of Parkinson's disease, which would be more likely to begin in just one hand. A tremor which disappears on movement is classic of Parkinson's disease, whilst the opposite is true in essential tremor.

5. E ★   OHCM 10th ed. → p. 498

The gradual presentation, together with a 'normal' magnetic resonance imaging (MRI) scan of the brain and raised intracranial pressure, suggests a diagnosis of idiopathic intracranial hypertension (IIH). This replaces the term 'benign intracranial hypertension', since this condition can cause visual loss due to compression of the optic nerves. It is associated with obesity in young women. Diagnosis requires the opening pressure to be measured during a supine lumbar puncture, and vision must be recorded and tracked (acuity, colour vision, and visual fields). Beware that IIH can cause secondary migraine.

6. B ★   OHCM 10th ed. → p. 498

It can be difficult to consider metastatic disease as a diagnosis if there is no knowledge of a primary cancer. However, the gradual onset of neurological symptoms over a 2-week period essentially rules out a vascular process, and thus all other options. They would all cause symptoms much more suddenly than in this case: in minutes for A, minutes to hours for C, seconds for D, and minutes (resolving in <24 hours) for E. The fact that symptoms continue to develop suggests that there is an ongoing process. In this case, it is likely due to the worsening oedema surrounding the mass. Given the discovery of an intracerebral mass, it would be essential to try to identify a primary (e.g. breast, bowel, skin), although the intracerebral mass may itself be the primary.

7. D ★   OHCM 10th ed. → p. 484

This man presents with acute confusion. This is delirium. He has a temperature and is tachycardic, tachypnoeic, and hypoxic, suggesting the most likely cause of his delirium is a lower respiratory tract infection.

A. These are used in the workup after a vascular event, which is unlikely to present with confusion.

B. These are part of a dementia screen; dementia is unlikely to present so suddenly and should not be suspected until sepsis has been excluded.

C. An acute coronary syndrome can present with delirium, but there is no suggestion of cardiac dysfunction in this case.

E. These are used to investigate diabetic ketoacidosis; hypoglycaemia is more likely to cause delirium.

8. D ★   OHCM 10th ed. → p. 503

This is often weakened in carpal tunnel syndrome and tests the abductor pollicis brevis innervated by the median nerve.

A. This tests the dorsal interossei (ulnar nerve).

B. This tests the extensor carpi radialis longus (radial nerve).

C. This is Finkelstein's test for de Quervain's tenosynovitis.

E. This tests the dorsal interossei/abductor digiti minimi (ulnar nerve).

9. A ★   OHCM 10th ed. → p. 502

This is 'cubital tunnel syndrome', which has been caused by intraoperative compromise and compression of the ulnar nerve at the elbow. The second most common entrapment neuropathy to carpal tunnel syndrome, the ulnar nerve is particularly vulnerable around the elbow.

B. This tests the opponens pollicis (median nerve).

C. This tests wrist extension (radial nerve).

D. This tests the pronator teres (median nerve).

E. This tests wrist flexion (median nerve).

10. D ★   OHCM 10th ed. → p. 470

The sudden-onset weakness, in combination with slurred speech, in a patient who has been admitted with atrial fibrillation should serve as an alert to a possible stroke.

A. This might explain some of the nocturnal delirium.

B and C. These are consistent with a fall.

E. This may be due to the infection.

11. D ★   OHCM 10th ed. → p. 72

This man's head tilt is characteristic of a trochlear nerve lesion—patients usually tilt away from the side of the lesion in order to reduce their diplopia. The trochlear nerve has three roles: intorsion, depression, and abduction of the globe. It is most commonly disturbed by head trauma but can be affected—as here—in microvasculopathies such as diabetes. Diplopia is worse on downward gaze and gaze away from the affected muscle.

A, B, and E. These occur together in palsies of the oculomotor nerve and result in an eye resting in the 'down and out' position.

C. Patients with left lateral rectus palsy cannot fully abduct the affected eye and so develop an esotropia (convergent squint) and resulting diplopia.

12. A ★   OHCM 10th ed. → p. 492

In someone with poorly controlled seizures the issue of drug compliance should be discussed. If there are still doubts, National Institute for Health and Care Excellence (NICE) guidance recommends monitoring drug levels. Ideally this should happen in the outpatient setting, with the aim of preventing admission to hospital. The other options may all lead to seizures and should be considered as a screen, particularly in someone with a first fit.

National Institute for Health and Care Excellence (2012). *Epilepsies: diagnosis and management*. Clinical guideline [CG137].

→ www.nice.org.uk/guidance/CG137

13. C ★   OHCM 10th ed. → p. 490

This man has had his second tonic–clonic seizure and has presented with a reduced Glasgow Coma Scale (GCS) score in the post-ictal phase.

A. This usually occurs against a background of daytime somnolence (narcolepsy).

B. This generally occurs in older people, usually women.

A non-epileptic attack disorder was known previously as 'pseudoseizures'. It is often difficult to tell apart from generalized epilepsy but would be less likely in a man with a low GCS score following the seizure; however, increasingly, video telemetry is required to disentangle non-epileptic attack disorders from epilepsy.

E. He would not be as drowsy following a simple faint.

14. B ★   OHCM 10th ed. → p. 788

This woman's Glasgow Coma Scale score is 9 (E2, V2, M5). Her airway has become partially obstructed, and this simple manoeuvre will help open it. A head tilt should not be attempted, to protect the cervical spine, which has not been cleared following a significant fall from height.

15. D ★★   OHCM 10th ed. → p. 71

It can be difficult to assess the severity of headaches, especially if there are no associated symptoms. In this case, however, the continued nausea and vomiting and the focal neurology suggest a serious cause. The features indicate a 3rd nerve palsy, which can be caused by compression from an aneurysm of the posterior communicating artery.

16. A ★   OHCM 10th ed. → p. 502

This is a common peroneal nerve injury, which runs a course around the neck of the fibula and has been damaged by the fracture. The other movements are all functions of the tibial nerve.

B. This tests the small muscles of the foot.

C. This tests the tibialis posterior (inverts the foot at the ankle).

D. This tests the gastrocnemius.

E. This tests the flexor digitorum longus.

17. E ★   OHCM 10th ed. → p. 457

This question clearly describes a new onset of cluster headaches in a middle-aged male smoker. His age, sex, and smoking status are all risk factors. Whilst imaging would be valuable to ensure that there is no underlying structural cause of these headaches, their frequent stereotyped nature and unilaterality with autonomic features make them unlikely to be anything else. Whilst waiting for imaging, it should be a priority to attempt symptomatic treatment. First-line treatment is usually abortive with high-flow oxygen and/or a triptan. A number of preventative medications, such as verapamil or lithium, can also be used if headaches are frequent or severe enough to justify this.

18. B ★   OHCM 10th ed. → p. 702

This man has a short history of problems affecting gait and hand strength. The presence of areflexia and autonomic dysfunction should quickly raise suspicion of a generalized acute demyelinating neuropathy (Guillain–Barré syndrome). This is a neurological emergency, since around 30% of patients develop respiratory weakness severe enough to require mechanical ventilation. This can occur rapidly and silently. Treating physicians should therefore be aware of the need to rapidly assess for respiratory weakness by measuring the forced vital capacity at the bedside. The presence of a resting tachycardia raises the possibility of dysautonomia, again raising concerns about the need for more intensive monitoring.

19. E ★   OHCM 10th ed. → p. 452

The image shows both wrist and finger drop, depicting a radial nerve injury. Up to 18% of humeral fractures are associated with radial nerve palsy, most commonly from mid-shaft fractures.

→ www.wheelessonline.com/ortho/radial_nerve_palsy_following_frx_ of_the_humerus

20. B ★   OHCM 10th ed. → p. 476

Patients with acute neurological symptoms that resolve completely within 24 hours [i.e. suspected transient ischaemic attack (TIA)] should be given aspirin 300 mg immediately and assessed urgently within 24 hours by a specialist physician in a neurovascular clinic or an acute stroke unit. Patients with a confirmed diagnosis of TIA should receive clopidogrel (300 mg loading dose and 75 mg daily thereafter). Patients who are in atrial fibrillation and suffer a TIA should be offered anticoagulation therapy. Dipyridamole has been superseded by the use of clopidogrel and will only be used in rare cases.

Royal College of Physicians Intercollegiate Stroke Working Party (2016). *National clinical guideline for stroke*. Royal College of Physicians: London.

21. E ★   OHCM 10th ed. → p. 476

Recurrent episodes of neurological disturbance in someone with hypertension are highly suggestive of transient ischaemic attacks (TIAs). The diagnosis would be clinched by the rapid resolution of symptoms (<24 hours). Given the high rates of stroke in those who suffer TIAs, this woman needs to have a workup for stroke, including an ultrasound scan of her carotids, with a view to urgent endarterectomy if carotid stenosis is confirmed.

22. A ★   OHCM 10th ed. → p. 512

This lady has generalized myasthenia gravis. Acetylcholine receptor antibody testing is the only diagnostic test listed, except for anti-MuSK antibodies which are much less commonly causative. Neurophysiology with repetitive stimulation demonstrating a decrement in neuromuscular transmission is also a valuable diagnostic test, but this option is not given. Patients should have imaging of the mediastinum to exclude a thymoma, which is sometimes the substrate for antibody production. A useful of review of myasthenia gravis is given in:

Gilhus NE. Myasthenia gravis. *N Engl J Med*. 2016;**375**:2570–81.

23. E ★   OHCM 10th ed. → p. 792

Patients with acute ischaemic stroke should only receive blood pressure-lowering treatment if there is an indication for emergency treatment, such as: systolic blood pressure above 185 mmHg or diastolic blood pressure above 110 mmHg when the patient is otherwise eligible for treatment with thrombolysis; hypertensive encephalopathy; hypertensive nephropathy; hypertensive cardiac failure or myocardial infarction; aortic dissection; and pre-eclampsia or eclampsia. Instead, concentrate on diagnosing and treating infections.

24. A ★   OHCM 10th ed. → p. 166

Aspiration signifies inhalation of gastric contents into the lower airways, which then causes an infective process. Most at risk are those who cannot protect their own airway, as in the early stages after a stroke. Whilst this patient is at risk of all options after a stroke, her chest signs and hypoxia are most suggestive of A The doctor who sees her in this condition should certainly investigate her with blood cultures and a chest X-ray, and treat her with intravenous antibiotics to include cover for anaerobes.

25. C ★   OHCM 10th ed. → p. 826

At 15 minutes, this woman is still in 'early' status. According to the National Institute for Health and Care Excellence (NICE) guidelines, she therefore needs a bolus of lorazepam, along with her usual antiepileptic drugs (if she is on any). A maximum of two doses of first-line treatment—per rectum (PR) diazepam/buccal midazolam/intravenous (IV) lorazepam or diazepam (including pre-hospital)—should be administered. If her seizures continue, then a phenytoin infusion may be started. If these initial measures do not help, anaesthetic support may be required.

National Institute for Health and Care Excellence (2012). *Epilepsies: diagnosis and management*. Clinical guideline [CG137].

→ www.nice.org.uk/guidance/CG137

26. A ★   OHCM 10th ed. → p. 510

When starting a statin, patients should be made aware of the risks of developing myopathy and advised to report any muscle weakness or pain as soon as it develops. In this event, it is important to measure the creatine kinase (CK) level promptly. If it is more than five times the upper limit or if myopathy is suspected on clinical grounds (as in this case), then treatment should be discontinued. If symptoms resolve and levels of CK return to normal, then the statin could be tentatively re-introduced or an alternative could be considered.

Wierzbicki AS. Statins: myalgia and myositis. *Br J Cardiol.* 2002;**9**:193–4.

→ bjcardio.co.uk/2002/04/statins-myalgia-and-myositis

27. C ★   OHCM 10th ed. → p. 453

Rupture of the supraspinatus is the most common rotator cuff injury. The supraspinatus muscle arises from the supraspinous fossa on the scapula and inserts into the greater tubercle of the humerus. The infraspinatus and teres minor insert here as well, with the subscapularis inserting into the lesser tubercle.

28. D ★   OHCM 10th ed. → p. 502

This is a radial nerve injury which runs a course in the groove around the mid-shaft of the humerus and has been damaged by the fracture.

A. This tests the opponens pollicis (median nerve).

B and C. These test the palmar interossei (ADductors) and dorsal interossei (ABductors) (both ulnar nerve).

E. This tests the forearm flexors (median nerve).

29. C ★   OHCM 10th ed. → p. 454

This man has a foot drop and weak eversion—symptoms of a common peroneal nerve lesion. The common peroneal nerve is commonly damaged by trauma to the lateral side of the knee. It is here that it winds around the head of the fibula, covered only by skin and subcutaneous tissue. After entering the peroneus longus muscle, it divides into deep and superficial branches. It is the superficial branch that provides sensory innervation to the skin of the lower lateral calf and dorsum of the foot. The deep branch is primarily a motor nerve.

→ emedicine.medscape.com/article/1141734-overview

30. A ★   OHCM 10th ed. → p. 494

C and E suggest the autonomic complications associated with multi-system atrophy, whilst B and D reflect two symptoms (defective vertical gaze and dementia) common in progressive supranuclear palsy. Parkinsonism is a syndrome of tremor, rigidity, bradykinesia, and loss of postural reflexes. Parkinson's disease is one cause of Parkinsonism.

31. B ★   OHCM 10th ed. → p. 494

The National Institute for Health and Care Excellence (NICE) recommends that if there is any suspicion of a patient having Parkinson's disease, they should be referred to a physician with an interest in Parkinson's disease, usually a geriatrician or a neurologist, before drug treatment is initiated. This is to reduce misdiagnosis, unnecessary treatment, and the use of increasingly complex drug regimes.

32. D ★ OHCM 10th ed. → p. 460

Both C and E could represent the aura prior to a partial seizure, whilst neither tongue biting (A) nor urinary incontinence (B) occurs in every case of an epileptic seizure. The history certainly suggests a case of vaso-vagal syncope and, although the brief jerks may have made the junior doctor think of epilepsy, the story as a whole is not concerning for this. In cases of probable syncope, the National Institute for Health and Care Excellence (NICE) guidelines state that an electroencephalogram (EEG) should not be performed (due to possible false positives). An EEG should only be used to support a diagnosis of epilepsy in those in whom the history is suggestive.

National Institute for Health and Care Excellence (2012). *Epilepsies: diagnosis and management.* Clinical guideline [CG137].

→ www.nice.org.uk/guidance/CG137

33. B ★ OHCM 10th ed. → p. 512

The scenario describes fatiguable weakness affecting several muscle groups: extraocular (ptosis), bulbar ('too tired to eat'), and limb–girdle ('struggles to lift anything'). This pattern is strongly suggestive of myasthenia gravis, which is a disease of the neuromuscular junction.

34. C ★ OHCM 10th ed. → p. 496

This woman has acute lower limb weakness which sounds like transverse myelitis. Although multiple sclerosis (MS) can present in a variety of ways, this is a common clinical syndrome. More commonly, patients present with one symptom that improves, only for another different problem to develop some time later. Anyone in this demographic who gives a history of unexplained, and seemingly unrelated, neurological symptoms lasting a few days or weeks that subsequently resolve should raise suspicion and prompt an in-depth history and careful examination.

A. Amyotrophic lateral sclerosis is the most common variant of motor neurone disease. It presents with wasting, weakness, and fasciculations. Sometimes, there are bulbar features. The sequence of symptoms varies from person to person, but it would be unlikely that a sufferer would deteriorate as rapidly as the woman in this case.

B. Guillain–Barré syndrome could cause such rapid weakness, but not with upgoing plantars. It often occurs following a viral illness.

D. Quaternary syphilis can cause an ataxic gait and numbness, but not such rapidly weak legs.

E. This can give rise to a cord syndrome and peripheral neuropathy, but these are likely to develop gradually and not cause weakness.

35. B ★   OHCM 10th ed. → p. 458

Migraine can be associated with an aura, which is often teichopsia (a transient visual sensation of flashing lights/colours), usually followed by the headache within the hour. Other migrainous features include photophobia, phonophobia, motion sensitivity, vertigo, and irritability.

36. C ★   OHCM 10th ed. → p. 458

This is an appropriate first-line treatment for migraine prophylaxis at a dose of 80–240 mg daily and will also help her anxiety. Topiramate is the other first line option recommended by NICE. Opioids (**B**) can cause medication overuse headache and dependence, and should not be used. The other options are useful second-line options: tricyclic antidepressants (**A**) and antiepileptics (**D** and **E**). Sodium valproate should be avoided in young women, as it causes a higher incidence of fetal malformations.

Duncan CW, Watson DPB, and Stein A. Diagnosis and management of headache in adults: summary of SIGN guidelines. *BMJ.* 2008;**337**:a2329.

37. A ★   OHCM 10th ed. → p. 456

This man has headaches of recent onset, with features of raised intracranial pressure. A 'normal' fundoscopy examination will not be able to definitively rule out papilloedema, and with this history, an urgent referral for investigations is warranted.

B. This is raised in carcinoid syndrome.

C and **E.** These are reasonable treatments for migraines.

D. This would be indicated if temporal arteritis were suspected.

38. B ★   OHCM 10th ed. → p. 828

It is difficult to assess for neurological deficits in those who have been drinking. Guidance is therefore that these people should be admitted. Furthermore, if there are any signs of a basal skull fracture, then a computed tomography (CT) head scan should be performed. **B** refers to Battle's sign (ecchymosis of the mastoid process) and, along with periorbital ecchymosis, cerebrospinal fluid rhino-/otorrhoea, and haemotympanum, should prompt urgent imaging.

A. This is not a significant finding in the assessment of a head injury.

C. This might suggest alcohol withdrawal but is unlikely in this situation.

D. This is a cerebellar sign.

E. This is positive in conditions causing sensory ataxia.

National Institute for Health and Care Excellence (2007). *Head injury: Triage, assessment, investigation and early management of head injury in infants, children and adults.* Clinical guideline [CG56].

→ www.nice.org.uk/Guidance/CG56#documents

39. A ★   OHCM 10th ed. → p. 828

It can be difficult to be clear about the management of head injuries, but, broadly summarized, computed tomography (CT) scans should be performed on those with normal consciousness but a skull fracture and all those with abnormal consciousness. (Note that it is not just skull fractures that demand imaging in those with a Glasgow Coma Scale score of 15/15; others are persisting severe headache, nausea and vomiting, irritability or altered behaviour, and seizure.)

By this rationale, the patient in this case deserves a CT head scan. This is because the chances of finding intracranial pathology in someone with disturbed consciousness is 20%, whilst in someone who is fully conscious and has no other features, the chances are <1%.

C. This is usually not used in the acute setting for head injuries.

D. In those who are drowsy or confused, it might be acceptable to observe them for at most 4 hours from the time of injury; if they still have failed to recover full consciousness, it would then be appropriate to request a CT head scan.

E. If a CT scan is planned, there is no need to carry out a skull X-ray. These are used in those situations where a CT scan is not planned but there is evidence of skull fracture.

National Institute for Health and Care Excellence (2007). *Head injury: Triage, assessment, investigation and early management of head injury in infants, children and adults*. Clinical guideline [CG56].

→ www.nice.org.uk/Guidance/CG56#documents

40. C ★   OHCM 10th ed. → p. 826

This man is now in established status epilepticus. He has received the necessary drug treatments (bolus + subsequent infusion of antiepileptic drugs) and is heading towards the general anaesthesia phase. Prior to this, an anaesthetist, and thus the intensive therapy unit (ITU), should be contacted. An anaesthetist will be needed to protect this man's airway and oversee the administration of a drug like propofol, whilst the ITU should be preparing itself to accept this man who will need close monitoring and possibly electroencephalogram (EEG) monitoring.

National Institute for Health and Care Excellence (2012). *Epilepsies: diagnosis and management*. Clinical guideline [CG137].

→ www.nice.org.uk/guidance/CG137

41. D ★   OHCM 10th ed. → p. 460

Although tiredness and fatigue can occur with syncope, confusion lasting >2 minutes after regaining consciousness should be regarded as a sign that this woman may well have had a seizure. Urinary incontinence can occur with syncope if the bladder were full at the time of the attack.

A deep bite of the lateral border of the tongue is suggestive of a seizure, but the tongue can also be bitten during a syncopal episode. Twitching and jerking can occur due to simple hypoxia, but tonic and then clonic movements for >1 minute should be regarded as suspicious of a seizure.

McCorry D and McCorry A. Collapse with loss of awareness. *BMJ.* 2007;**334**:153.

42. **A** ★ OHCM 10th ed. → p. 490

According to the National Institute for Health and Care Excellence (NICE) guidelines, there are four circumstances in which the emergency services should be contacted:

- If seizures develop into status epilepticus
- If there is a high risk of recurrence
- If it is a first fit
- If there is difficulty monitoring the individual's condition.

A second fit starting before the person has regained consciousness is one of the definitions of status epilepticus, the other being seizures lasting >30 minutes.

National Institute for Health and Care Excellence (2012). *Epilepsies: diagnosis and management.* Clinical guideline [CG137].

→ www.nice.org.uk/guidance/CG137

43. **B** ★ OHCM 10th ed. → p. 502

This man is unable to plantar flex or invert his foot due to an injury to the tibial nerve. The tibial nerve supplies a sensory branch to the sole of the foot and a motor branch to the hamstrings, tibialis posterior, gastrocnemius, flexor digitorum longus, and small muscles of the foot.

A and C. Both movements—dorsiflexion and eversion of the foot—are powered by the common peroneal nerve.

D. This tests the gluteus maximus (inferior gluteus nerve).

E. This tests the quadriceps femoris (femoral nerve).

44. **C** ★ OHCM 10th ed. → p. 452

This is carpal tunnel syndrome and can occur in pregnancy as a result of fluid retention causing compression of the median nerve in the carpal tunnel below the flexor retinaculum.

A. This is the radial nerve.

B. This is the ulnar nerve.

D. This is the anterior interosseus branch of the median nerve, but if the site of symptoms arose from here, there would be weakness of wrist flexion due to innervations of the forearm flexors.

E. This is the ulnar nerve.

45. B ★   OHCM 10th ed. → p. 510

This man has a dramatic acute myopathy affecting the skeletal muscles and cardiac muscle. The cola-like urine indicates myoglobin is being excreted by the kidneys, a by-product of muscle breakdown. The only differential that is likely to present with such an acute disseminated myopathy is inflammatory-mediated necrotizing myopathy.

46. E ★   OHCM 10th ed. → p. 393

All of these options might present with headache and confusion, and they might all cause a raised lymphocyte count (as opposed to neutrophil count) in the cerebrospinal fluid (CSF). A decreased CSF-to-serum glucose ratio is implied, which would be less likely in vasculitis and lymphoma. Both tuberculosis (TB) meningitis and cryptococcal meningitis can cause very high opening pressures; the others are less likely to do so. TB is suggested by his living circumstances.

47. D ★★   OHCM 10th ed. → p. 500

In the treatment of Bell's palsy, prednisolone and aciclovir used to be given in combination. However, a meta-analysis comparing prednisolone alone with prednisolone and aciclovir showed no significant benefit. Current practice is therefore to use prednisolone alone.

Quant EC, Jeste SS, Muni RH, *et al. BMJ.* 2009;**339**:b3354.

48. B ★★   OHCM 10th ed. → p. 822

The junior doctor has elicited Brudzinski's neck sign. As with Kernig's sign, this is a notoriously insensitive marker of meningeal irritation. Even though it is very specific, the fact that it has been absent in 95% of proven cases of meningitis in some studies has led people to question its value in the pre-treatment workup of meningitis. It is, however, quick to perform and non-invasive, and may be of use in borderline cases.

Thomas KE, Hasbun R, Jekel J, and Quagliarello VJ. The diagnostic accuracy of Kernig's sign, Brudzinski's sign, and nuchal rigidity in adults with suspected meningitis. *Clin Infect Dis.* 2002;**35**:46–52.

49. C ★★

This young lady probably has juvenile myoclonic epilepsy (JME). The early morning myoclonic jerks are the clue. The change in routine and early starts may be the precipitant for the seizures. Whilst this condition responds well to sodium valproate, this is one of the most teratogenic antiepileptic medications and should only be given to young women in exceptional cases. Lamotrigine would be a better first choice in generalized epilepsy.

National Institute for Health and Care Excellence (2012). *Epilepsies: diagnosis and management.* Clinical guideline [CG137].

→ www.nice.org.uk/guidance/CG137

50. D ★★

This is carcinomatous meningitis whereby metastasis has occurred from the primary to the meninges; imaging may show the suggestion of meningeal uptake—magnetic resonance imaging (MRI) is more likely to do so than a computed tomography (CT) scan—but the best way to detect malignant cells in the meninges is via a lumbar puncture.

Chamberlain MC. Neoplastic meningitis. *J Clin Oncol.* 2005;**23**:3605–13.

51. D ★★   OHCM 10th ed. → p. 50

The symptoms and signs (ptosis, miosis, and anhydrosis) described are those of Horner's syndrome and of nerve impingement (C8–T2). In an ex-smoker who continues to cough, this could be explained by an apical lung tumour (Pancoast's tumour) that is impacting on both brachial and cervical sympathetic plexuses.

52. E ★★   OHCM 10th ed. → p. 502

When two peripheral nerves are compromised, the term mononeuritis multiplex is used. It is rare but is associated with diabetes, some vasculitides, and rheumatoid arthritis.

A. This does not affect peripheral nerves, rather a range of functions, including postural blood pressure, sweating, and bladder and bowel function.

B. The main example of this is multiple sclerosis.

C. This would be the most likely cause of an isolated nerve lesion.

D. The classical inflammatory neuropathy is Guillain–Barré syndrome— an acute, mainly motor, demyelinating neuropathy.

53. C ★★   OHCM 10th ed. → p. 498

Evolving neurological signs against a background of headache and personality changes are highly suspicious of an intracranial space-occupying lesion. The papilloedema supports this suspicion, indicating raised intracranial pressure. Immediate management should consist of treating the associated cerebral oedema with steroids.

A. This is used for thrombolysis of those presenting within 4.5 hours with symptoms of an ischaemic stroke (see link at end of this answer).

B. This is used in the treatment of transient ischaemic attacks and stroke.

D. This is a calcium channel blocker used occasionally in the treatment of malignant hypertension. Headache and visual disturbances are possible with a blood pressure >200/140 mmHg, but it is unlikely to be associated with other gross neurological changes.

E. This can be used to relieve the symptoms of benign intracranial hypertension; this is a key differential diagnosis in these cases and may turn out to be the cause if brain imaging is normal. Whilst investigations are pending, however, cases of raised intracranial pressure, together with evolving neurology and personality changes, need to be treated as for a space-occupying lesion.

→ www.sign.ac.uk/assets/qrg108.pdf

54. A ★★   OHCM 10th ed. → p. 450

The clinical features of leg weakness (without arm weakness), impaired spontaneous speech, and urinary incontinence suggest a lesion of the parasagittal region served by the anterior cerebral artery.

55. E ★★   OHCM 10th ed. → p. 714

The acute onset of ophthalmoplegia (nystagmus as here, or lateral rectus or conjugate gaze palsies), an ataxic gait, and global confusion is known as Wernicke's encephalopathy; it results from thiamine deficiency (which is common in heavy alcohol users) and can proceed to the more serious Korsakoff's syndrome (characterized by retrograde amnesia resulting in confabulation). Untreated, mortality rates are 20% in Wernicke's encephalopathy and 85% in Korsakoff's syndrome. Apart from arresting the decline into Korsakoff's syndrome, thiamine has been shown variously to reverse all three clinical problems within hours. Therefore, in any patient with one or more of the three symptoms and no other more likely cause, give two pairs of thiamine ampoules intravenous (IV) in 50–100 mL of 0.9% saline over 30 minutes three times a day for 3–7 days before converting to oral thiamine.

A. Aspirin is started after a transient ischaemic attack or ischaemic stroke.

B. This is used to treat cerebral oedema in space-occupying lesions.

C. Glucagon can be used to treat hypoglycaemia, although it does not work as well in patients who have been drinking alcohol.

D. This can be used as symptomatic treatment in Alzheimer's dementia but would not be indicated in this context.

Day E, Bentham P, Callaghan R, Kuruvilla T, and George S. Thiamine for Wernicke–Korsakoff syndrome in people at risk from alcohol abuse. *Cochrane Database Syst Rev.* 2009;**2**:CD004033.

→ cochranelibrary-wiley.com/doi/10.1002/14651858.CD004033.pub2/abstract;jsessionid=79788930F4D1FFBA5923D0532606E11D.f03t01

56. E ★★   OHCM 10th ed. → p. 556

The scenario describes a case of Churg–Strauss syndrome. What is important is realizing that a vasculitic process should be considered as an explanation for any multi-system presentation. Churg–Strauss syndrome is a medium- and small-vessel autoimmune vasculitis that often affects the lungs, gastrointestinal system, and peripheral nerves.

57. B ★★   OHCM 10th ed. → p. 698

This lady has a spinal cord syndrome and optic neuropathy. Both sarcoid and neuromyelitis optica might present in this way. The clue to the diagnosis of neuromyelitis optica (Devic's disease) in this case is the long cord lesion which is reasonably specific to this condition. Aquaporin-4 antibodies are relatively specific to this.

58. D ★★★   OHCM 10th ed. → p. 486

This middle-aged lady is most likely to have frontotemporal dementia (FTD). She has both language problems and signs of a disorder of behaviour and social cognition, indicating degeneration of frontal and temporal brain structures. Around a third of cases of FTD are familial (autosomal dominant), and in this case, it is suspicious that her mother may have been affected. The history is too long for prion disease; the average survival is typically less than a year. A frontal variant of Alzheimer's disease is increasingly recognized, but rarely familial. A helpful overview of FTD is in:

Warren JD, Rohrer JD, and Rossor MN. Frontotemporal dementia. *BMJ*. 2013;**347**;f4827.

59. C ★★★   OHCM 10th ed. → p. 494

This question requires the candidates to identify the clinical feature(s) that would not be typical of idiopathic Parkinson's disease. Whilst postural hypotension is said to be an early and prominent feature of multisystem atrophy, it is also commonly seen in idiopathic Parkinson's disease, particularly later on in the disease course. A supranuclear gaze palsy is seen in progressive supranuclear palsy (previously known as Steele–Richardson syndrome) caused by an underlying neurodegenerative disease, characterized neuropathologically by the deposition of a specific form of the protein tau. Patients also have a staring expression, with reduced frequency of blinking. Consequently, they fail to lubricate their eyes and so they often complain of dry eyes.

60. A ★★★   OHCM 10th ed. → p. 498

Idiopathic intracranial hypertension presents as a mass might: headache and signs of raised intracranial pressure. Patients typically suffer most in the mornings. Symptoms of raised pressure include visual obscurations or tinnitus worse when bending or straining.

61. B ★★★   OHCM 10th ed. → p. 41

Doxazosin is an alpha-1 antagonist and is used in the treatment of benign prostatic hypertrophy and hypertension. The most likely cause of the collapse is a postural drop in blood pressure, which can occur after the first dose.

A. Alendronic acid is associated largely with gastrointestinal side effects.

C. Gliclazide can cause hypoglycaemic attacks, but these usually last longer, especially without treatment.

D. Rosiglitazone is associated with fluid retention and can precipitate heart failure, but is unlikely to cause loss of consciousness.

E. Salbutamol in high doses can cause tremor, tachycardia, and agitation but is unlikely to cause a collapse.

62. D ★★★   OHCM 10th ed. → p. 280

Delirium is common following surgery, especially in frail older patients. This woman, however, has a few features particular to a specific cause of delirium: alcohol withdrawal. This classically presents between 10 and 72 hours after admission with tremor, sweating, hypotension, tachycardia, and visual/tactile hallucinations. She should be given generous amounts of chlordiazepoxide (a benzodiazepine) for the first 3 days, which is then gradually reduced. Administration of intravenous thiamine is also important.

63. A ★★★   OHCM 10th ed. → p. 473

This woman has had a transient ischaemic attack (TIA) and is in atrial fibrillation (AF). According to the National Institute for Health and Care Excellence (NICE) guidelines, she needs to be anticoagulated, but before this can happen, a recent infarct and a haemorrhagic cerebral event need to be excluded, hence the computed tomography (CT) scan. The decision to anticoagulate is not based on the rate of AF (E) and should not be postponed (B and D). All those in AF should be risk-stratified for stroke, using the CHADS-VASc score. As this woman has just had a TIA, she immediately becomes high risk. Unless there are contraindications, all those in the high-risk group should be anticoagulated with warfarin to a target international normalized ratio (INR) of 2.5, or given a direct-acting oral anticoagulant (DOAC).

National Institute for Health and Care Excellence (2014). *Atrial fibrillation: management*. Clinical guideline [CG180].

→ www.nice.org.uk/cg180

64. B ★★★   OHCM 10th ed. → p. 492

In most cases, antiepileptic treatment does not start until after a second seizure. However, the National Institute for Health and Care Excellence (NICE) guidance highlights four situations in which it should be started after the first seizure:

- The individual has a neurological deficit
- The electroencephalogram (EEG) shows unequivocal epileptiform activity
- The individual considers the risk of further seizures unacceptable
- Imaging shows a structural abnormality.

Although this woman's deficit is likely to be temporary (Todd's paresis following a seizure involving the motor cortex), it is a sign that the seizure was likely to be epileptic in origin and that the risk of recurrence is high.

National Institute for Health and Care Excellence (2012). *Epilepsies: diagnosis and management*. Clinical guideline [CG137].

→ www.nice.org.uk/guidance/CG137

---

65. B ★★★   OHCM 10th ed. → p. 828

Vomiting more than once should prompt a request for an urgent computed tomography (CT) head scan, i.e. within 1 hour of arrival. Following a head injury, but no immediate triggers for an urgent scan, anyone >65 years with a dangerous mechanism of injury and amnesia of events >30 minutes can wait for up to 8 hours before the scan.

National Institute for Health and Care Excellence (2014). *Head injury: assessment and early management*. Clinical guideline [CG176].

→ www.nice.org.uk/CG176

---

66. A ★★★   OHCM 10th ed. → p. 466

The relatively acute onset of symptoms, the presence of upper motor neurone signs, and a sensory level in the high thoracic region localize this problem to the spinal cord, above the level of T4. The only plausible answers are myelitis or compressive cervical myelopathy. The pace and progression would be more consistent with compressive myelopathy, rather than myelitis. Furthermore, swimming might be more likely to trigger a mechanical compressive problem, rather than myelitis.

---

67. C ★★★   OHCM 10th ed. → p. 496

Multiple sclerosis (MS) remains a clinical diagnosis, in accordance with modified McDonald criteria (2017). Magnetic resonance imaging (MRI) will detect plaques in the central nervous system but is non-specific. Symptoms are often seen to worsen, or even present for the first time, when the body temperature rises (Uhthoff phenomenon), as it is thought that this slows conduction, especially through already demyelinated nerves.

A. This test is used if myasthenia gravis is suspected—this would be more likely to present with fatiguable weakness of muscle than paraesthesiae.

B. Thoracic outlet syndrome usually follows neck trauma and presents with paraesthesiae and weakness in an arm due to compression of neurovascular structures at the thoracic outlet. It would be unlikely to cause such a flitting picture that attacks both arms, as in this case.

D. Nerve conduction studies can be diagnostic for a radicular or peripheral nerve problem such as Guillain–Barré syndrome (GBS). GBS, however, is unlikely to run a course as long as this case—it has a progressive, rather than a fluctuant, pattern and is more likely to affect the lower, rather than the upper, limbs.

E. Subacute combined degeneration of the spinal cord is a reasonable differential diagnosis in cases of lower limb paraesthesiae, as it causes peripheral neuropathy. It is, however, progressive, rather than relapsing and remitting.

68. C ★★★ OHCM 10th ed. → p. 494

Metoclopramide will exacerbate the extra-pyramidal symptoms of Parkinson's disease due to its anti-dopaminergic effects. This manifests as confusion, difficulty walking, and an increase in tone. This can have very serious and prolonged consequences for the patient and should be avoided. Domperidone is the antiemetic of choice in Parkinson's disease patients.

69. E ★★★ OHCM 10th ed. → p. 72

The 'swinging flashlight test' reveals an abnormal response in the right pupil. The fact that the right eye produces less pupillary constriction suggests an afferent defect on that side. Although it may appear that both pupils are dilating, this is just relative—they are, in fact, both trying to constrict but failing to do so fully, due to the partial afferent nerve damage that distinguishes this condition. In this case—a young woman with concurrent headache—the damage may have occurred following optic neuritis and should make one think of the possibility of multiple sclerosis (subject to fulfilling other aspects of McDonald criteria, 2017). Full dilation and lack of a subsequent response would suggest a total optic nerve (cranial nerve II) lesion.

70. C ★★★ OHCM 10th ed. → p. 462

This is a classic history for benign paroxysmal positional vertigo (BPPV). Displaced otoconia can be relocated by the Epley manoeuvre or Brandt–Daroff exercises, and provide a cure in up to 80–90% of cases in some studies. The other descriptions correspond to these following diagnoses.

A. Acoustic neuroma.

B. Cerebellar stroke.

D. Ménière's disease.

E. Labyrinthitis.

71. A ★★★ OHCM 10th ed. → p. 452

This man has cervical spondylosis associated with radiculopathy—pain, reduced reflexes, dermatomal sensory disturbance, and lower motor neurone (LMN) weakness.

B, C, and E. These describe the involvement of the C7 nerve root.

D. This describes the involvement of the C5/6 nerve root.

72. B ★★★   OHCM 10th ed. → p. 834

Reduced consciousness level in a patient with type 2 diabetes is initially suggestive of a hyperosmolar state. This is clearly confirmed by the laboratory findings which show not only hyperglycaemia, but also hypernatraemia, considerable dehydration, and a raised serum osmolality [2 × (Na + K) + urea + glucose].

There are several important management steps at this time:

- Fixed-rate insulin infusion as per local protocol
- Consideration of prophylactic anticoagulation therapy, as these patients are at an increased risk of venous thrombosis
- Fluid replacement: most patients are fluid-depleted by 5 L or more. Normal-strength saline is effective at rapidly restoring the circulating volume and does so without dropping the serum osmolality too quickly, which is a risk for the development of cerebral oedema. If the sodium level remains high after 2–3 L of infusion fluids, then half-strength normal saline can be used. Clearly, it would be dangerous to use any glucose products. Given the amount of fluid that needs to be replaced, it is worth bearing in mind that these patients may need close monitoring in a high dependency unit.

73. D ★★★★   OHCM 10th ed. → p. 824

This middle-aged man presents with behavioural change and a history that is suspicious of seizures. The impairment of short-term recall memory implicates mesial temporal lobe structures. Whilst this history would be compatible with herpes simplex encephalitis, the normal white cell count and negative cerebrospinal (CSF) vital polymerase chain reaction (PCR) make this an unlikely diagnosis. Alzheimer's disease and Lewy body dementia can both cause recall memory problems and occasionally seizures, but the history is too short. Limbic encephalitis is caused by an antibody against the leucine-rich glioma-inactivated 1 (LGI-1) protein. It is twice as common in men and tends to present in late middle age. There is often a prodrome with behavioural change, a mood disorder, or drowsiness, as well as memory problems and seizures. A low serum sodium level is another clue.

74. C ★★★★   OHCM 10th ed. → p. 838

Treatment of benzodiazepine overdose is supportive with maintenance of the airway, regular assessment of consciousness level, and intravenous fluids.

A. This and gastric lavage are not used in pure benzodiazepine overdose.

B. Although flumazenil is a benzodiazepine antagonist, it is not used to reverse purposeful overdose because there is no way of being sure how much of the hypnotic has been taken. Flumazenil can trigger seizures via the benzodiazepine receptor as a result of a reduction in the seizure threshold. It is only used if the overdose has been caused during a procedure in the hospital environment.

D. There is no indication for this at the moment.

E. This uses sodium bicarbonate to produce urine with a pH of between 7.5 and 8. This can enhance elimination of weak acids such as cocaine, tricyclic antidepressants, and salicylates.

75. D ★★★★ OHCM 10th ed. → p. 824

This is suspicious for viral encephalitis. Cerebrospinal fluid examination obtained by a lumbar puncture is the most appropriate option. It usually shows a raised lymphocyte count, with a normal glucose concentration, but can be normal.

A. This is unlikely to help in the diagnosis.

B and E. The history is not suggestive of an abscess, space-occupying lesion, or stroke. Although imaging of the brain may aid in the diagnosis, it is not the choice that will 'produce the definitive diagnosis'.

C. Whilst an electroencephalogram (EEG) may show sharp wave activity in one or both temporal lobes of brains with viral encephalitis, it would be used diagnostically less often than a lumbar puncture.

76. C ★★★★ OHCM 10th ed. → pp. 27, 702

This young man has a reasonably non-specific presentation of behavioural change, with withdrawal and insomnia. This could be seen in primary psychiatric conditions; however, the increased limb tone and slow saccades indicate that there is an underlying central organic disorder. There is also a suggestion of a movement disorder. His father may also have a similar condition, but at a later stage of life. Huntington's disease is an autosomal dominant neurodegenerative disease that causes a movement disorder (chorea) and behavioural changes, and often eye movement abnormalities are seen. It is a trinucleotide repeat disorder and shows anticipation, i.e. the age of presentation may be earlier in later generations, as is the case here.

Chapter 9

Oncology and palliative care

Dan Furmedge

An ageing population, better prevention for ischaemic heart disease, and significant advances in treatment mean that cancer is becoming increasingly common, with patients living longer (sometimes decades) with it. This means living with the effects of cancer itself, as well as with the effects of the increasingly complex treatments used to treat it. It is important not only for doctors to be familiar with the presenting symptoms and signs of cancer, so it can be investigated and diagnosed, but also with the emergencies associated with it and the common side effects and complications related to the ever growing range of treatment options.

The importance of palliative and end-of-life care cannot be underestimated, and all doctors will come into contact with patients approaching the end of their lives. Increasing evidence suggests that early involvement of palliative care in patients with many terminal and chronic illnesses improves the quality of life and paradoxically can even improve the length of life. Importantly, palliative care is no longer associated just with cancer. It can help in almost any chronic illness, from chronic obstructive pulmonary disease (COPD) and heart failure to frailty and dementia.

All too often, particularly in hospitals, many patients receive active and aggressive treatments right up until their death when it has been evident they are approaching death for many days or weeks. All doctors should have a working understanding of the principles of palliative care, as well as how to recognize terminal illness and how to manage symptoms at the end of life.

QUESTIONS

1. A 49-year-old woman received her second cycle of chemotherapy for treatment of metastatic breast cancer 4 days ago. She reports feeling shivery all day but has no other symptoms.

T 38.5°C, HR 90 bpm, BP 106/74 mmHg, SaO_2 98% on air, RR 16/min. Physical examination is otherwise normal.

What is the *single* most important next step in her management? ★

A Arterial blood gas

B Intravenous antibiotics

C Intravenous paracetamol

D Intravenous fluids

E Intravenous steroids

2. A 37-year-old woman has a fever of 38.6°C. She completed her third cycle of chemotherapy 4 days ago for metastatic breast cancer.

Which is the *single* most important investigation? ★

A Arterial blood gas

B Blood cultures

C Chest X-ray

D Electrocardiogram

E Venous blood gas

3. A 76-year-old man undergoing treatment for multiple myeloma presents to hospital with acute hypoactive delirium. He is confused and drowsy.

Sodium 134 mmol/L.

Potassium 4.9 mmol/L.

Corrected calcium 3.62 mmol/L.

What is the next most appropriate step? ★

A Intravenous bisphosphonate

B Intravenous fluids

C Intravenous steroids

D Oral cinacalcet

E Subcutaneous calcitonin

4. A 51-year-old woman has completed treatment for ovarian cancer with a hysterectomy and bilateral salpingo-oophorectomy and adjuvant chemotherapy. She is radiologically disease-free after treatment.

Which is the *single* most appropriate blood marker which may be used to detect recurrence? ★

A CA125

B CA19-9

C CA15-3

D Carcinoembryonic antigen (CEA)

E Human chorionic gonadotrophin (hCG)

5. A 76-year-old man is diagnosed with carcinoma of the oesophagus. His staging is T4N3M0. He has locally advanced disease, with invasion of adjacent mediastinal structures and local lymph node involvement. There are no clear distant metastases.

He reports being increasingly unable to eat and drink and, in the last 4 days, has been unable to take more than very small sips of water.

What is the *single* most appropriate treatment at this stage? ★

A Antiemetics

B Chemotherapy

C Oesophageal stent

D Radical oesophagectomy

E Radiotherapy

6. A 70-year-old woman is seen in the emergency department, following a single self-terminating generalized tonic–clonic seizure lasting around 3 minutes. She has never had a fit before.

A computed tomography (CT) scan of the brain is performed, which is reported as: 'There is a 3 × 2 cm enhancing mass suspicious for cerebral metastasis, with significant surrounding oedema, but no significant mass effect. Infective causes should also be on the differential'.

What is the next *single* most appropriate course of action? ★★

A Cyclizine

B Dexamethasone

C Diazepam

D Levetiracetam

E Phenytoin

7. A 48-year-old woman is being treated for metastatic bowel cancer. She has significant pain from her bony metastases and requires analgesia. She has significant renal impairment with an estimated glomerular filtration rate (eGFR) of 13.

Given her renal impairment, which would be the least suitable agent to treat her pain? ★ ★

A Alfentanil

B Fentanyl

C Morphine

D Oxycodone

E Paracetamol

8. A 76-year-old man with advanced metastatic lung cancer is admitted with severe pneumonia. He is barely responsive and has a high volume of upper airways secretions. A decision is made with his wife that he is dying and will receive supportive palliative care. He is expected to die in the coming 24–48 hours.

Which is the *single* most appropriate method of managing his high-volume respiratory secretions? ★ ★

A Chest physiotherapy

B Nebulized sodium chloride

C Subcutaneous glycopyrronium

D Subcutaneous midazolam

E Subcutaneous morphine

9. A 53-year-old woman with a history of right-sided breast cancer treated 2 years ago with mastectomy, axillary node clearance, adjuvant chemotherapy, and hormonal therapy describes feeling increasingly unsteady on her feet over the past 6 weeks.

She has normal tone, reduced power 4/5 in the right lower limb and 3/5 in the left lower limb, normal reflexes, and normal sensation.

What is the next most appropriate step? ★ ★

A Computed tomography (CT) brain

B CT lumbar spine

C Magnetic resonance imaging (MRI) brain

D MRI lumbar spine

E MRI whole spine

10. A 69-year-old woman being treated for metastatic colon cancer takes 10 mg oral morphine immediate-release six times daily. She reports that this controls her pain fairly well and that she does not require any additional breakthrough doses, but that she is getting significant nausea and constipation related to this.

A decision is made to convert her to an alternative—oxycodone in a modified-release 12-hourly formulation—to try and reduce the side effect profile.

What is the equivalent dose of oxycodone modified-release? ★ ★

A Oxycodone modified-release 10 mg twice daily

B Oxycodone modified-release 15 mg twice daily

C Oxycodone modified-release 20 mg twice daily

D Oxycodone modified-release 30 mg twice daily

E Oxycodone modified-release 45 mg twice daily

11. A 57-year-old man with a large primary brain tumour has deteriorated at home and is admitted to a hospice for end-of-life care. He is now unresponsive. His main symptoms prior to admission were nausea and vomiting and seizures.

His oral medications are dexamethasone 4 mg twice daily (bd), sodium valproate 600 mg bd, metoclopramide 10 mg three times daily (tds), and ondansetron 8 mg tds.

What is the most appropriate drug to manage his risk of further seizures? ★ ★

A Intravenous levetiracetam

B Intravenous phenytoin

C Rectal diazepam

D Subcutaneous levomepromazine

E Subcutaneous midazolam

12. A 91-year-old woman is being treated for dehydration due to poor oral intake in hospital. She was admitted from her residential care home where she lives with advanced dementia. In the home, she requires constant supervision due to high risk of falls and a lack of safety awareness. She is frail.

Her admission chest X-ray shows right lung shadowing, and a computed tomography (CT) scan of her chest done in the acute medical unit is reported as: 'There is a large 6 × 4 cm mass in the right upper lobe, with surrounding local lymphadenopathy. This is highly suggestive of a primary malignancy of the lung. Urgent respiratory and oncology discussion recommended'.

What is the most appropriate investigation? ★★

A Bronchoscopy

B CT abdomen and pelvis

C CT-guided biopsy

D Endobronchial ultrasound

E No further investigation

13. A 47-year-old woman is diagnosed with breast cancer. She undergoes a total right mastectomy with axillary clearance and adjuvant chemoradiotherapy. After reviewing the histology, her oncologist recommends letrozole therapy.

What is the mechanism of action of letrozole? ★★

A Angiogenesis inhibitor

B Aromatase inhibitor

C Monoclonal antibody

D Oestrogen receptor antagonist

E Topoisomerase inhibitor

14. An 81-year-old man is lethargic, unsteady on his feet, and confused. His wife reports this started around 3 weeks ago and has progressively worsened. He has no medical history and does not take any regular medications. His initial investigations reveal:

Blood sodium 122 mmol/L.

Blood potassium 3.9 mmol/L.

Blood osmolality 255 mOsmol/kg.

Urine sodium 90 mmol/L.

Urine osmolality 110 mOsmol/kg.

Which is the *single* most likely option to have caused this presentation? ★★

A Adenocarcinoma of the lung

B Adenocarcinoma of the oesophagus

C Hepatocellular carcinoma

D Non-small cell lung carcinoma

E Small cell lung carcinoma

15. A 74-year-old woman has advanced chronic obstructive pulmonary disease (COPD). She is on maximal inhaler therapy and uses home nebulizers occasionally, as required.

She is cachectic and has a hyperexpanded chest which is clear, with reduced air entry throughout and no wheeze. Oxygen saturations are 94% on air.

Her main complaint is severe breathlessness on minimal exertion. She finds this very distressing.

What is the *single* most appropriate option for managing her breathlessness? ★★

A Long-term oxygen therapy

B Oral lorazepam 0.5 mg every 4 hours, as required

C Oral morphine 2.5 mg every 4 hours, as required

D Oral prednisolone 5 mg daily

E Salbutamol and ipratropium nebulizers every 4 hours

ANSWERS

1. B ★   OHCM 10th ed. → p. 528

This woman has chemotherapy-induced neutropenic sepsis until proven otherwise. Any patient presenting to the emergency department with a recent course of chemotherapy and fever is prioritized and must receive immediate broad-spectrum antibiotics. Neutropenic sepsis has a high mortality if not treated rapidly, and we should not wait for blood tests to confirm neutropenia. An arterial blood gas is probably not needed at this point with her normal observations. Intravenous (IV) fluids and paracetamol may be adjuncts to treatment with antibiotics. IV steroids do not currently have a place in the routine management of neutropenic sepsis.

National Institute for Health and Care Excellence (2012). *Neutropenic sepsis: prevention and management in people with cancer*. Clinical guideline [CG151].

→ www.nice.org.uk/guidance/cg151

2. B ★   OHCM 10th ed. → p. 528

A blood culture would be the most useful and vital investigation, and this may identify a bacteria and allow focused antibiotic therapy. A chest X-ray would be useful to look for a source of infection. A venous or arterial blood gas may be helpful in obtaining a lactate level if she is very unwell. An electrocardiogram makes up part of the routine investigation of acutely unwell patients admitted to hospital and may be useful if she is tachycardic or has other symptoms.

3. B ★   OHCM 10th ed. → p. 528

Hypercalcaemia is a common complication of many cancers, with multiple myeloma as a typical one. It causes a constellation of symptoms such as confusion, drowsiness, aches and pains, abdominal pain, polyuria, and polydipsia, and is commonly missed. Although all of the treatments listed can be used for hypercalcaemia, the priority is vigorous rehydration with intravenous (IV) fluids. As a general rule, if the calcium level remains significantly raised after this, then IV bisphosphonates would be the next choice. Cinacalcet is usually used in cases of hypercalcaemia caused by hyperparathyroidism where surgery is not an option.

4. A ★   OHCM 10th ed. → p. 531

Cancer antigen 125 (CA125) can be used as a tumour marker in post-treatment surveillance for some ovarian cancers. CA15-3 is mostly associated with breast cancers, CA19-9 with pancreatic malignancy, carcinoembryonic antigen (CEA) with bowel cancers, and human chorionic gonadotrophin (hCG) with germ cell testicular or gestational trophoblastic tumours.

5. C ★ OHCM 10th ed. → pp. 527, 618

This man has very locally advanced disease which is invading local structures. Although he has no distant metastases, from the limited information given, it is not likely that curative surgery would be an option. Antiemetics and chemo- and radiotherapy might form part of the management plan for this patient, but the most pressing issue is his inability to take fluid and food orally. Therefore, the only sensible option at this point is an oesophageal stent to partly relieve the obstruction. This is a palliative procedure but can often significantly improve symptoms in the short term and allow oral intake.

6. B ★★ OHCM 10th ed. → p. 529

This lady has had a seizure precipitated by her cerebral mass with significant cerebral oedema. Although it is likely she will need to be established on an anticonvulsant, such as levetiracetam, as she is at high risk of further seizures, dexamethasone is the most important intervention, given the significant surrounding oedema. Steroids will reduce inflammation and swelling around the mass and may therefore reduce the risk of further seizures. Cyclizine is an antiemetic and would not be appropriate. Diazepam might be used intravenously or rectally if this lady had a further fit which did not self-terminate, but it is not required at this point.

7. C ★★ OHCM 10th ed. → p. 533

Paracetamol is not affected by renal function, as this is cleared by the liver. Oxycodone and fentanyl can be used in patients with mild to moderate renal impairment, but with caution. Alfentanil is often used in patients with severe renal impairment. Morphine, however, should not be used in patients with impaired renal function, as it can build up and cause opiate toxicity, and therefore, of the options given, it is the least suitable agent to use.

8. C ★★ OHCM 10th ed. → p. 536

Morphine is used for pain or shortness of breath at the end of life and may be appropriate in this man. Midazolam is used to ease agitation and distress and may also be appropriate. Chest physiotherapy and nebulized sodium chloride are both active treatments which may be used in patients with pneumonia having active medical treatments, but they would be unsuccessful and possibly distressing in this man who is clearly at the end of his life. Glycopyrronium is a commonly used anticholinergic medication which effectively dries up secretions and can be used in a syringe driver for this indication. An alternative is hyoscine hydrobromide which acts in a similar way.

9. E ★★   OHCM 10th ed. → p. 528

In a patient with these features, with a history of a cancer which commonly metastasizes to the spine, urgent spinal imaging is needed to exclude metastatic spinal cord compression. This is often confused with cauda equina syndrome but is different, as the metastases and compression can occur at any level. In fact, the majority occur in the thoracic spine, hence the need for whole spine imaging. Imaging the lumbar spine alone could miss lesions. Magnetic resonance imaging (MRI) is the preferred image modality, but computed tomography (CT) imaging can be considered if there are contraindications to MRI scanning. Brain imaging may also be appropriate, depending on suspicion of intracerebral metastases, but again MRI would be preferred.

10. B ★★   OHCM 10th ed. → p. 533

Opioid dose conversions are not exact, but in general, oral oxycodone has double the potency of oral morphine. Therefore, 10 mg of oral morphine is roughly equivalent to 5 mg of oral oxycodone. For this lady, she takes 10 mg of oral morphine six times a day, which equates to a total dose of 60 mg of morphine daily, equivalent to 30 mg of oxycodone. As the oxycodone preparation will be a 12-hourly dose, the 30 mg equivalent dose is divided into two, giving a dose of 15 mg of oxycodone modified-release twice daily. Additional 'as required' immediate-release doses of around one-sixth of the total daily dose can be offered in addition, and if this is required, the regular doses can be increased accordingly.

Royal College of Anaesthetists. *Dose equivalent and changing opioids*.

→ www.rcoa.ac.uk/faculty-of-pain-medicine/opioids-aware/structured-approach-to-prescribing/dose-equivalents-and-changing-opioids

11. E ★★   OHCM 10th ed. → p. 536

In this situation, at the end of life, it is not usually appropriate to have intravenous devices which can be uncomfortable to insert and change (although in the hospital setting, if one is already in place, this might be appropriate). Rectal diazepam is used in the emergency management of seizures—in this case, the aim is to ensure the patient is comfortable and to prevent seizures in the first place. Subcutaneous midazolam is usually the preferred choice of seizure prophylaxis, but it needs to be given at reasonable doses which can cause sedation—but in this case, the patient is already unresponsive. Levomepromazine is used for nausea and agitation at the end of life and is not useful in the prophylaxis or management of seizures.

12. E ★★

This lady has advanced physical and cognitive frailty and clearly lacks mental capacity to make any decision about her healthcare. Any decision about further investigation or treatment of this cancer will need to be made in her best interests and probably with the input of her next of kin or with an advocate. However, the bottom line is that this lady is not going to be well enough for any major treatments like chemotherapy, radiotherapy, or surgery. She is far too frail to benefit from these, and her lifespan, even if she did not have cancer, is limited. Further investigation of the mass in terms of getting a tissue diagnosis is therefore academic and should only be pursued if the results will enact a change of use to the patient. Otherwise, we are putting a frail patient with dementia through potentially unpleasant and aggressive procedures, which she may not understand and may cause distress, and even harm. Therefore, the right thing for this lady is that no further investigation is attempted and her symptoms are managed appropriately with palliative care.

13. B ★★   OHCM 10th ed. → p. 524

Letrozole (and anastrozole) are aromatase inhibitors. Tamoxifen is an example of an oestrogen receptor antagonist. Both of these classes of drugs are classed as anti-oestrogens and are used in the treatment of breast cancer. Angiogenesis inhibitors include drugs like bevacizumab and sunitinib; monoclonal antibodies are emerging and increasingly popular drugs targeted to a specific tumour antigen. Topoisomerase inhibitors, such as etoposide, interrupt regulation of DNA winding.

14. E ★★   OHCM 10th ed. → pp. 529, 672

This man has the classic vague and non-specific symptoms of hyponatraemia (lethargy, dizziness, unsteadiness, confusion). His blood tests confirm significant hyponatraemia, and the supporting tests suggest the syndrome of inappropriate antidiuretic (ADH) secretion (SIADH) with a low serum osmolality and high urinary sodium excretion and urinary osmolality. There are many causes of SIADH, but one is a paraneoplastic phenomenon from a cancer. The cancer listed which most commonly causes this is small cell lung cancer. Pancreatic and prostate cancers and lymphoma are other cancers which more commonly cause SIADH.

15. C ★★   OHCM 10th ed. → p. 534

This lady is severely troubled by the symptom of breathlessness. She is on maximal therapy for her chronic obstructive pulmonary disease (COPD). The best evidence-based approach for symptomatic breathlessness is to try oral immediate-relief morphine at a very low dose. This helps to reduce the respiratory drive, and thus the sensation of breathlessness, and is very effective in some patients. Lorazepam is sometimes used due to the associated anxiolytic effects, but the evidence to support this as a useful adjunct in breathless patients is very limited. Her oxygen saturations are 94%, so she is unlikely to qualify for, or benefit from, long-term oxygen therapy. From the clinical examination, there are predominant signs of emphysema, rather than bronchitis, so regular steroids and increased nebulizers are unlikely to make any difference—and will not directly treat the symptom of breathlessness.

National Institute for Health and Care Excellence (2010). *Chronic obstructive pulmonary disease in over 16s: diagnosis and management.* Clinical guideline [CG101].

→ www.nice.org.uk/guidance/cg101

Chapter 10

Rheumatology

Rudy Sinharay

This specialty has been described by the British Society of Rheumatology as the 'branch of medicine that deals with the investigation, diagnosis, and management of patients with arthritis and other musculoskeletal conditions'. These include inflammatory arthritis, autoimmune disorders, vasculitides, soft tissue disorders, spinal problems, and metabolic bone disease.

Simplifying the assessment and approaching the patient in a logical manner, using history taking and examination, make it possible to narrow your differential:

- Is there any pain?
- How many joints are affected?
- Which joints?
- Is there swelling?
- Is there erythema?
- Is there loss of function?
- How is their gait?
- Is there any morning stiffness?
- Is there systemic upset?
- Are there extra-articular symptoms?
- Are there any related diseases?
- What is the patient's drug history?

Diseases that one comes across in the specialty of rheumatology vary between being ubiquitous (rheumatoid arthritis and osteoarthritis) to the vanishingly rare (scleroderma), and affect over 10 million adults and 12 000 children. As such, it is easy to feel out of one's comfort zone when discussing the possible causes of a patient's joint pain during a consultation. It is, however, a core skill for the budding physician to be able to assess and diagnose potential septic joints, flares of rheumatoid arthritis, and other autoimmune conditions. These conditions are often multi-system in nature, and it is crucial to recognize other organ involvement such as the kidneys or lungs, or indeed extra-articular signs in the generally unwell patient that may point one in the correct diagnostic direction.

There is significant morbidity from these conditions, with disability and loss of working days a problem, and it is important for the junior doctor to be aware of yellow and red flag symptoms. The impact on the ageing population also needs to be recognized, and involving the multidisciplinary team of physiotherapists and occupational therapists is essential. Although debilitating, joint problems are also often treatable. Treatment of rheumatological conditions invariably involves the use of systemic corticosteroids as first-line treatment, but this is now an exciting field itself with various biologic disease-modifying anti-rheumatic drugs

(DMARDs) in use and in development, owing to a better understanding of the mechanisms driving these conditions.

The aim of this chapter is then to provide and test knowledge gained in order to build up the confidence needed to suggest diagnoses and management plans. This will be done with a focus on the key bread-and-butter areas, as well as giving a flavour of the rarer conditions. After completing this chapter, you will be able to navigate overlapping presentations and symptoms, using the finer details of various requested investigations, and thus arrive at a unifying diagnosis.

QUESTIONS

1. A 29-year-old woman has been generally tired and lethargic for the past year. She has had intermittent crops of mouth ulcers that coincide with the flare-up of a skin rash over her cheeks.

Haemoglobin (Hb) 106 g/L, white cell count (WCC) 2.3 × 10⁹/L, platelets 87 × 10⁹/L.

Which *single* autoantibody is most consistent with the diagnosis? ★

A Anti-acetylcholine receptor

B Anti-double-stranded deoxyribonucleic acid (dsDNA)

C Anti-mitochondrial

D Anti-Scl-70

E Anti-smooth muscle

2. A 22-year-old man has been struggling to get out of bed in the morning for the past few months. As the day progresses, he feels his stiffness loosening, but by the evening, he has severe back pain. He has been otherwise fit and well, smokes ten cigarettes a day, and consumes 30 units of alcohol a week. Which *single* examination finding is most likely to support the diagnosis? ★

A Impaired sensation over L5–S1 dermatome

B Pain on straight leg raise

C Raised brown plaques on the soles

D Saddle anaesthesia

E Tender sacroiliac joints

3. A 68-year-old man has had progressively worsening lower back pain over the last month. He had previously been mobilizing with a frame, but this morning he felt too weak to get out of bed. He has not passed urine for over 12 hours. He receives a 3-monthly injection of goserelin for carcinoma of the prostate. Flexion at the hip is weak, especially on the right. Reflexes are brisk at the right knee and ankle, with an upgoing plantar. Sensation from the right mid thigh distally is dulled. Which is the *single* most appropriate course of action? ★

A Computed tomography (CT) head scan

B Magnetic resonance imaging (MRI) of the spine

C Ultrasound scan of the bladder

D X-ray of the lumbar spine

E X-ray of the pelvis

4. A 74-year-old woman has a large swelling in her left knee. It came on suddenly and grew rapidly in size over a 12-hour period. She is clammy and rather anxious. The knee is swollen and fluctuant. It is held in flexion at 20°. She is noted to have a urine output of <15 mL/hour.

Choose the *single* most likely diagnosis. ★

A Cellulitis

B Osteoarthritis

C Pseudogout

D Rheumatoid arthritis

E Septic arthritis

5. A 30-year-old woman has a painful and swollen right ankle. It has developed gradually over the last week or so. She has suffered flare-ups of the same joint at regular intervals over the last 18 months. The first attack occurred within a month of a urinary tract infection, but otherwise she has remained well.

Choose the *single* most likely diagnosis. ★

A Osteoarthritis

B Psoriatic arthritis

C Reactive arthritis

D Rheumatoid arthritis

E Septic arthritis

6. A 29-year-old woman has had painful fingers in cold weather for as long as she can remember. The tips change colour, turning from white to blue and then to red. Which is the *single* most appropriate explanation for this woman's symptoms? ★

A Aneurysms and thrombosis in medium-sized arteries

B Autoantibodies against platelet membranes

C Connective tissue weakness causing capillary dilatation

D Hyperactive sympathetic system causing vasoconstriction

E Inflammation of arteries and veins due to an unknown cause

7. A 66-year-old man has an acutely painful, swollen left knee. It started 3 days previously, and he has since been unable to fully bend the knee or weight-bear. He has had a high fever and felt off his food. He recalls no preceding trauma. There is no overlying cellulitis, but the joint is hot to touch and the patella tap test is positive. What is the most appropriate initial course of action? ★

A Aspirate the joint effusion

B Organize an ultrasound scan of the knee

C Organize an X-ray of the knee

D Request a review by an orthopaedic surgeon

E Start broad-spectrum intravenous antibiotics

8. A 38-year-old woman has had pain in her lower back for the past 2 weeks. She cannot relate it to any trauma and has noticed no pattern in how it affects her. It has forced her to miss 2 weeks of work, just after she had returned following 3 months off with wrist pain. She is using codeine 60 mg oral (PO) four times daily and citalopram 30 mg PO once at night. There is no evidence of soft tissue or skeletal injury, and there is a full range of lumbar flexion and extension both forward and laterally. Which is the *single* most important consideration when monitoring her symptoms? ★

A She is already on a high-dose analgesia regimen

B She is at risk of developing chronic pain

C She is at risk of missing significant time at work

D She is liable to suffer an acute depressive episode

E Her symptoms may be linked to a previous wrist injury

9. A 72-year-old woman has had a headache for the past week. It is mainly over her right temple where she has also been particularly tender. Her neck and shoulder had been stiff for the preceding few weeks, during which time she has felt tired and generally unwell. Which *single* further feature would necessitate urgent admission for high-dose steroid therapy? ★

A Flashing lights seen

B Night sweats

C One transient episode of loss of vision

D Pain in the left temple as well

E Weight loss

10. A 25-year-old woman has had a rash on her thighs and shins over the last week. She has no relevant past medical history and is recovering well 3 weeks after being diagnosed with glandular fever, which improved with symptomatic treatment only. The lesions are tender, smooth, shiny nodules. They are purple-coloured and between 1 and 3 cm in diameter.

Choose the *single* most likely diagnosis. ★

A Erythema chronicum migrans

B Erythema marginatum

C Erythema multiforme

D Erythema nodosum

E Pyoderma gangrenosum

11. A 60-year-old woman has a 3-week history of morning stiffness and pain in his shoulders and hips. He has had a poor appetite associated with a 2-kg weight loss. She has a normal serum creatine kinase (CK) level and a raised erythrocyte sedimentation rate (ESR).

What is the *single* most likely diagnosis? ★

A Dermatomyositis

B Fibromyalgia

C Giant cell arteritis

D Polymyalgia rheumatica

E Polymyositis

12. A 52-year-old woman has systemic sclerosis and has been told by her team of specialists that she has reached the end-stages of the disease. She is being treated palliatively but has intractable pain. She asks the on-call junior doctor to relieve her pain once and for all and suggests adding large amounts of potassium to her intravenous (IV) fluids. The palliative care registrar had earlier documented her full capacity for decisions around her medical treatment. Which is the *single* most appropriate next step? ★★

A Contact her next of kin before making a decision either way

B Give potassium as requested, as it would be in her best interests to die

C Give potassium as requested, as she has capacity

D Refuse, as active euthanasia is illegal

E Refuse, as it would be in her best medical interests to live

13. A 20-year-old man has suddenly developed a swollen right knee. He noticed it for the first time on waking this morning when he felt pain on attempting to weight-bear. He recalls no injury to the knee and has not experienced this before. He is otherwise well. The knee is warm, tender, and swollen, with an obvious effusion palpable. A diagnostic joint aspiration is carried out. Which *single* organism is most likely to be isolated on culturing the aspirate? ★★

A *Escherichia coli*

B *Neisseria gonorrhoeae*

C *Pseudomonas aeruginosa*

D *Staphylococcus aureus*

E *Streptococcus pneumoniae*

14. A 45-year-old man has had a painful, swollen great toe for the last 4 days. There is no history of trauma or previous joint problems. He has been self-medicating with anti-inflammatories, with good effect, but has developed some new troublesome symptoms and sees his doctor again. He has bipolar affective disorder and takes regular lithium therapy. What is the *single* most likely set of symptoms he has developed? ★★

A Ataxia and urinary frequency

B Headaches and vomiting

C Insomnia and diarrhoea

D Palpitations and sweating

E Paraesthesiae and fine tremor

15. A 28-year-old woman is seen in the ambulatory care unit with a swollen left leg. On examination, her left calf is tender and 3 cm larger than the right. She has a pink, mottling rash on both legs. Her past medical history includes well-controlled asthma and two previous miscarriages.

Which *single* autoantibody is most consistent with the diagnosis? ★★

A Anti-cyclic citrullinated peptide antibodies

B Anti-histone antibodies

C Anti-mitochondrial antibodies

D Anti-phospholipid antibodies

E Anti-smooth muscle antibody

16. A 68-year-old woman comes to the emergency department with pain in both legs and difficulty walking. She has felt generally weak for the last 2–3 weeks, associated with achy joints. On examination, she has a purple rash on her eyelids, as well as erythematous areas on her knuckles and elbows. She has 4/5 power on hip flexion bilaterally.

Which *single* autoantibody is most consistent with the diagnosis? ★★

A Anti-Jo-1

B Anti-La

C Anti-Scl-70

D Anti-Sm

E Anti-ribonucleoprotein (RNP)

17. A 72-year-old woman has had painful wrists and hands for the past 6 months. They are worse in the morning when she is stiff for at least 2 hours. She feels generally unwell. She is particularly tender over both ulnar styloids and all metacarpophalangeal joints which are swollen. Initial blood tests show that she is negative for rheumatoid factor. Which further blood test would be most useful to characterize her joint disease? ★★★

A Anti-cyclic citrullinated peptide (CCP) antibodies

B Anti-nuclear antibodies

C C-reactive protein (CRP)

D Erythrocyte sedimentation rate (ESR)

E Serum urate

18. A 51-year-old woman is having increasing difficulty swallowing and has noticed that the skin on her hands and feet is getting increasingly tight. Although she has previously enjoyed winter holidays, she now finds her hands get very cold, even on not particularly cold days. Which *single* autoantibody is most consistent with the diagnosis? ★★★

A Anti-centromere

B Anti-double-stranded deoxyribonucleic acid (dsDNA)

C Anti-Ro

D Anti-Scl-70

E Rheumatoid factor

19. A 44-year-old woman has felt lethargic, with generalized joint pain for the past 48 hours. She feels generally unwell. This is the third episode in the last year, despite continued treatment with azathioprine 150 mg oral (PO) once daily.

T 37.7°C, HR 85 bpm, BP 115/80 mmHg.

She has multiple mouth ulcers and non-tender cervical lymphadenopathy. Which would be the *single* most useful investigation to monitor disease activity? ★★★

A Complement

B Creatine kinase

C C-reactive protein (CRP)

D Joint aspiration

E Rheumatoid factor

20. A 55-year-old man has a swollen left foot. He does not remember any recent trauma or other provoking factors. He takes omeprazole 20 mg oral (PO) once daily for a previous duo-denal ulcer, smokes ten cigarettes a day, and drinks 40 units of alcohol a week.

T 37.1°C, HR 82 bpm, BP 142/75 mmHg.

The metatarsophalangeal joint of the big toe is hot, erythematous, and exquisitely tender. Which is the *single* most appropriate treatment for this man's symptoms? ★★★

A Allopurinol 100 mg oral (PO) once daily

B Colchicine 500 micrograms PO four times daily

C Indometacin 50 mg PO once daily

D Morphine sulfate 10 mg/5mL PO when required (PRN)

E Naproxen 500 mg PO twice daily

21. A 55-year-old woman has swollen, painful joints. The pain is present all the time but increases on movement and is worse by the end of the day. Her knees are swollen bilaterally, and crepitus can be felt on passive movement. Which *single* examination finding would be most likely to support the diagnosis? ★ ★ ★

A Hyperextension at the proximal interphalangeal joints

B Onycholysis

C Soft tissue swelling

D Squared thumb

E Thoracic kyphosis

22. A 75-year-old woman has felt lethargic for the month. She has noticed stiffness and pain in her neck and across her shoulders, particularly in the morning. She also feels she has lost weight in this time and reports low mood. Which *single* investigation is most likely to support the diagnosis? ★ ★ ★

A Calcium

B Erythrocyte sedimentation rate (ESR)

C Neck and shoulder X-rays

D Peripheral blood film

E Thyroid function tests

23. A 47-year-old man has had a painful right wrist for the past 3 months. It began gradually but is now so bad that he is finding it difficult to open bottle tops or turn on taps. His left wrist has also started to twinge. Both are particularly bad in the morning, remaining stiff for the first 3 or 4 hours of the day. He is otherwise well, except for a persistent itchy rash on the extensor surfaces of his arms and back. Which *single* further finding would most support the likely diagnosis? ★ ★ ★

A Early diastolic heart murmur

B Nodules on the elbows

C Onycholysis

D Squared thumbs

E Whitish nodule on the pinna of the ear

24. A 33-year-old man has excruciating pain in his lower back. It came on suddenly 2 days ago and is constant. It radiates into his buttock and, on movement, travels quickly down the back of his right leg and into his calf and foot. He can raise his right leg straight off the bed to an angle of 20° before the pain is reproduced. Which *single* examination finding will confirm the diagnosis? ★★★

A Dullness to percussion in the lower abdomen

B Hypertonia in the right leg

C Reduced perineal sensation

D Reduced sensation below both knees

E Reduced sensation in the plantar aspect of the right foot

ANSWERS

1. B ★   OHCM 10th ed. → p. 554

This woman has systemic lupus erythematosus (SLE) associated with a malar rash, leucopenia, and thrombocytopenia. There are a number of autoantibodies that are detected in this disease, including rheumatoid factor (RhF), anti-Ro, anti-ribonucleoprotein (RNP), and anti-Smith antibodies. Although anti-double-stranded deoxyribonucleic acid (dsDNA) antibodies are the most specific antibody in SLE, only about 60% of cases will be positive, whilst >95% of cases will be positive for anti-nuclear antibodies.

A. These antibodies are produced in myasthenia gravis.

C. Anti-mitochondrial antibodies are produced in primary biliary cirrhosis.

D. Anti-Scl-70 antibodies are produced in diffuse systemic sclerosis.

E. Autoimmune hepatitis involves anti-smooth muscle antibodies.

2. E ★   OHCM 10th ed. → p. 550

Non-traumatic back pain in a young person is always concerning, but persistent back stiffness in a young man is highly suspicious for ankylosing spondylitis which causes tender sacroiliac joints.

A. This describes a common peroneal nerve lesion—clearly unilateral and most likely after trauma to the lateral aspect of the knee.

B. This describes pain on hip flexion and extension that are suggestive of sciatic nerve root irritation.

C. The brown plaques are keratoderma blenorrhagica, which occurs with mouth ulcers in reactive arthritis, i.e. a sterile arthritis affecting the lower limbs within a month of urethritis.

D. These are worrying features that should raise the alarm for a potential cord compression, most commonly post-traumatic or due to metastatic disease.

3. B ★   OHCM 10th ed. → p. 543

This man is displaying the signs of acute cord compression—upper motor neurone signs below the lesion, with urinary retention. Whilst there are other causes of compression (e.g. myeloma, disc protrusion, spinal abscess), given this man's concurrent malignancy, it is most likely due to spinal metastasis. Once detected by magnetic resonance imaging (MRI), radiotherapy may be able to shrink any metastasis. A plain X-ray of the lumbar spine (**D**) may support clinical suspicions, but in an emergency such as this, there should be no delay in seeking the imaging most likely to seal the diagnosis—most trusts now have a specific pathway to support urgent MRI scanning.

4. E ★   OHCM 10th ed. → p. 544

This woman is in danger of becoming very unwell very quickly with septic arthritis. She is showing a systemic inflammatory response that has already started to affect her renal function. She needs an urgent knee aspiration, intravenous antibiotics, and a review by an orthopaedic surgeon for a possible knee washout.

5. C ★   OHCM 10th ed. → p. 550

Typically affecting the lower limbs, reactive arthritis occurs within a month of urethritis and can become chronic or relapsing, as in this case. The clue was the proximity to the 'urinary tract infection' and should prompt a sexual health screen.

6. D ★   OHCM 10th ed. → p. 708

This woman has been experiencing peripheral ischaemia that is characteristic of Raynaud's syndrome. Vasospasm is brought on by cold weather or stress and may be primary (idiopathic Raynaud's disease) or secondary (to connective tissue/haematological disorders—Raynaud's phenomenon).

A. This occurs in polyarteritis nodosum.

B. These are produced in idiopathic thrombocytopenic purpura.

C. This is hereditary haemorrhagic telangiectasia (Osler–Weber–Rendu syndrome).

E. This is Buerger's disease.

7. A ★   OHCM 10th ed. → p. 541

The management of the acutely hot, swollen joint is one of the few rheumatological emergencies. In all but a very few cases, the first step should be to aspirate the joint effusion (A). The appearance of the fluid can be instantly useful—if pus is withdrawn, an orthopaedic surgeon needs to be informed immediately to consider surgical washout of the infected joint. Otherwise, the fluid can be sent to the lab for analysis, whilst intravenous antibiotics can be started (E). If the joint is prosthetic, then joint aspiration should not be attempted and an orthopaedic surgeon notified (D). An X-ray (C) offers little to the diagnosis but will be useful in determining the health of the joint; however, in effusions that are difficult to aspirate, an ultrasound scan (B) can prove useful in locating the fluid.

Coakley G, Mathews C, Field M, et al. (2006). BSR & BHPR, BOA, RCGP and BSAC guidelines for management of the hot swollen joint in adults. *Rheumatology*. 2006;**45**:1039–41.

8. B ★ OHCM 10th ed. → p. 559

All options are reasonable to differing degrees. However, crucial to this case are the 'yellow flags' for the development of chronic pain: depression, time off work, and extended rest. These are some of the psychosocial factors that are known to put an individual at risk of developing long-term disability. It is therefore essential to see the bigger picture in such a case and to understand that the presence of this collection of problems is predictive of serious long-term impairment—whilst each immediate problem needs to be addressed, more important is holistic attention over time.

Bernstein IA, Malik Q, Carville S, and Ward S. Low back pain and sciatica: summary of NICE guidance. *BMJ*. 2017;**356**:i6748.

→ www.bmj.com/content/356/bmj.i6748

Samanta J, Kendall J, and Samanta A. Chronic low back pain. *BMJ*. 2003;**326**:535.

→ www.bmj.com/content/326/7388/535

9. C ★ OHCM 10th ed. → pp. 456, 556

This is a typical story for giant cell arteritis. Once the diagnosis is suspected, steroid therapy should be commenced and a temporal artery biopsy requested. In the absence of neuro-ophthalmic symptoms (jaw/tongue claudication or visual symptoms), the recommended steroid dose is >0.75 mg/kg (usually 40 mg). However, a dose of at least 60 mg or even intravenous methylprednisolone for 3 days is recommended in the presence of the following symptoms:

- Evolving visual loss
- History of amaurosis fugax (C)
- Established visual loss.

Weight loss (E) and night sweats (B) are both suggestive of systemic upset and support the diagnosis but are not worrying features. Bitemporal pain (D) is not either, whilst seeing flashing lights (A) may indicate a migraine.

Dasgupta B, Borg FA, Hassan N, et al. BSR and BHPR guidelines for the management of giant cell arteritis. *Rheumatology*. 2010;**49**:1594–7.

10. D ★ OHCM 10th ed. → p. 562

Erythema nodosum is associated in this case with Epstein–Barr virus, but in 30–50% of cases, no cause is identified. Common causes include sarcoidosis, drugs (sulfonamides, contraceptive pill, dapsone) and streptococcal infection. It occurs as a result of inflammation of subcutaneous fat.

11. D ★ OHCM 10th ed. → p. 557

Polymyalgia rheumatica (PMR) is a chronic inflammatory condition with an unknown pathogenesis. It usually occurs at age >50 years with a subacute onset and presents as symmetrical aching, tenderness, and morning stiffness in the shoulders, hips, and proximal limb muscles. Systemic symptoms include fatigue, fever, and weight loss. Investigations include increased C-reactive protein (CRP) and erythrocyte sedimentation rate (ESR) (>40), with normal creatine kinase (CK) levels. Management is with prednisolone 15 mg/day where a dramatic improvement should be observed within a week. An alternative diagnosis should be considered if there is no improvement with this.

A. As polymyositis, with skin signs, including rash and Gottron's papules.

B. Widespread pain that is chronic in nature (>3 months). Investigations are all normal, and it does not respond to steroids.

C. Symptoms include headache and temporal artery and scalp tenderness. Can result in amaurosis fugax and sudden-onset blindness. Treated with high-dose steroids, e.g. prednisolone 60 mg/day.

E. This presents with progressive symmetrical proximal weakness and is associated with raised muscle enzymes, including CK.

12. D ★★

As the Lillian Boyes case showed (in which her doctor was charged with attempted murder having injected her with two ampoules of potassium chloride—he remains the only doctor ever to have been convicted in the UK of 'mercy killing'), no matter how compassionate the action of the doctor, actively helping a patient to die remains illegal in the UK, regardless of whether the patient has capacity to ask for that help.

13. B ★★   OHCM 10th ed. → p. 544

In a young person (aged 19–25 years), this is the most common pathogen responsible for a septic joint. This may be related to the nascent sexual activity common to this group. In older adults, *Staphylococcus aureus* is the most common cause.

14. A ★★   OHCM 10th ed. → p. 756

Following a number of patients receiving lithium being harmed, the National Patient Safety Agency (NPSA) produced an 'alert'—*Safer lithium therapy*, in December 2009. It noted that regular blood levels (and renal/thyroid function) were not being checked to allow reciprocal changes in dosage, and patients seemed unaware of side effects and symptoms of toxicity, as well as many widely available interacting medications.

This patient has probably suffered an episode of gout and, although successfully self-medicating with an over-the-counter non-steroidal anti-inflammatory drug (NSAID), has consequently reduced the excretion of his lithium.

A therapeutic lithium level can cause fine tremor and gastrointestinal upset, but toxic levels can cause ataxia, blurred vision, a coarse tremor, dizziness, muscle twitching, tinnitus, and polyuria, and patients need to be made aware of these.

→ cks.nice.org.uk/nsaids-prescribing-issues#!scenariorecommendation:5

→ www.nrls.npsa.nhs.uk/resources/?entryid45=65426&char=S

15. D ★★   OHCM 10th ed. → p. 554

This woman has presented with a deep vein thrombosis (DVT) in her left leg and has livedo reticularis. Along with the history of miscarriages, this is consistent with a diagnosis of anti-phospholipid syndrome. Thrombocytopenia is often present.

A. Associated with rheumatoid arthritis.

B. Associated with drug-induced systemic lupus erythematosus (SLE).

C. Associated with primary biliary cholangitis.

E. Associated with autoimmune hepatitis.

16. A ★★   OHCM 10th ed. → p. 552

This patient has dermatomyositis. As well as progressive symmetrical proximal muscle weakness, she has a heliotrope rash on her eyelids and Gottron's papules. Dermatomyositis may be associated with lung, bowel, ovarian, or pancreatic malignancies.

B. Associated with Sjögren's syndrome.

C. Associated with diffuse systemic sclerosis.

D. Associated with systemic lupus erythematosus (SLE) (20–30%).

E. Associated with SLE and mixed connective tissue disease.

17. A ★★★   OHCM 10th ed. → p. 546

Anti-cyclic citrullinated peptide (CCP) antibodies (A) have a sensitivity comparable to that of rheumatoid factor, but with a higher specificity. They seem to be present before symptoms have developed (up to 10 years before) and are also often present even in the absence of rheumatoid factor. They are also a predictor of erosive disease, so they are vital in the classification of disease type at the onset of symptoms.

The presence of anti-nuclear antibodies (B) can imply a connective tissue disease. They should not be requested, unless there are suggestive symptoms, as a slightly positive test can be misleading. It is worth knowing at the onset of rheumatoid arthritis (RA), however, as overlap syndromes are common and symptoms may take time to declare themselves. Erythrocyte sedimentation rate (ESR) (D) and C-reactive protein (CRP) (C) are clearly both important, perhaps more in the monitoring of disease progression than in the diagnosis. Serum urate is used in the monitoring of treatment of gout.

American College of Rheumatology (2003). *The use of anti-cyclic citrullinated peptide (anti-CCP) antibodies in RA.* American College of Rheumatology: Atlanta, GA.

18. A ★★★   OHCM 10th ed. → p. 552

This woman has limited systemic sclerosis, which includes the diagnosis of CREST (calcinosis, Raynaud's syndrome, (o)esophageal dysmotility, sclerodactyly, and telangiectasia), with anti-centromere antibodies detected in up to 30% of cases. She has dysphagia, sclerodactyly, and secondary Raynaud's phenomenon. Skin involvement is limited to the face, hands, and feet. Other changes consistent with this diagnosis are telangiectasia and oesophageal dysmotility.

B. This occurs in 60–75% of cases of systemic lupus erythematosus (SLE).

C. This occurs in 30% of SLE cases and 75% of primary Sjögren's syndrome cases.

D. This occurs in 50% of diffuse systemic sclerosis.

E. This occurs in <100% of Sjögren's syndrome and Felty's syndrome cases and 70% of rheumatoid arthritis.

19. A ★★★ OHCM 10th ed. → p. 554

The scenario describes a flare-up of systemic lupus erythematosus (SLE); as well as monitoring urine for blood and protein, determining the C-reactive protein (CRP), erythrocyte sedimentation rate (ESR), and blood pressure, the best way to monitor disease activity is via antibody titres and complement levels (they would be low during a flare-up, as they are consumed).

B. This is used to support a diagnosis of dermatomyositis.

C. This is a key marker of any acute inflammation or infection and is therefore useful here, but not specific.

D. This is the critical step in the management of an acutely hot—and therefore potentially infected—joint.

E. Rheumatoid factor is positive in approximately 70% of rheumatoid arthritis sufferers; a high titre with a high ESR is found in severe disease.

20. B ★★★ OHCM 10th ed. → p. 548

An 'exquisitely tender' single joint should always raise the suspicion of gout, particularly in someone with a high alcohol intake. Treatment is with high-dose, fast-acting, strong non-steroidal anti-inflammatory drugs (NSAIDs) (such as indometacin) (C), unless contraindicated—as in this case where the patient has had peptic ulcer disease. Although it is slower-acting, colchicine is next in line (caution needs to be taken in those with renal impairment). Allopurinol (A) should not be started in an acute attack, although it should be continued in those already using it. The latest guidance (2017) suggests that urate-lowering therapy, such as allopurinol, should be offered to all patients after a first attack of gout, not just in those with recurrent exacerbations. Opioids (D) are useful as adjuncts in pain control.

Hui M, Carr A, Cameron S, *et al.* The British Society for Rheumatology guideline for the management of gout. *Rheumatology.* 2017;**56**:e1–20.

→ academic.oup.com/rheumatology/article-lookup/doi/10.1093/rheumatology/kex156

21. D ★★★ OHCM 10th ed. → p. 544

A story of background joint pain that worsens with activity is strongly suggestive of osteoarthritis. Post-menopausal women are prone to generalized disease, suffering damage to the distal interphalangeal joint of the hands and of the knees. It is also known as 'nodal osteoarthritis', as they are more likely to develop Heberden's nodes ('lumps' at the distal interphalangeal joint), as well as deformity of the thumbs.

A. This is found in rheumatoid arthritis, which normally causes pain and swelling of the small joints of the hands and feet and is worse in the morning.

B. This is seen in psoriatic arthritis; joint pain usually follows the onset of psoriasis, but not always. There are five patterns of psoriatic arthritis, but it would be unlikely for any of them to comprise the distribution of joints affected in this case.

C. This is a sign of crystal arthropathy, which is more likely to affect one single joint for a short time (acute monoarthropathy).

E. This is found in ankylosing spondylitis, which usually presents in younger men with gradual onset of lower back stiffness that is worse in the morning.

22. B ★★★ OHCM 10th ed. → p. 557

Despite being one of the most common reasons for long-term steroid use in the community, the diagnosis of polymyalgia rheumatica (PMR) has been an inexact science. This has been addressed by a working group who developed guidelines for the British Society of Rheumatology. They stipulate the following inclusion criteria:

- Age >50 years, duration >2 weeks
- Bilateral aching of the neck, shoulders, and/or pelvic girdle
- Morning stiffness >45 minutes
- Evidence of an acute phase response (**B**).

Importantly, the following exclusion criteria are also flagged up:

- Active infection
- Active cancer
- Active giant cell arteritis (GCA).

Having performed a full set of screening investigations, the crucial step is assessing response to a standard dose of prednisolone 15 mg daily. A dramatic improvement in patient-reported symptoms within a week, with return of inflammatory markers to baseline within a month, would be consistent with the diagnosis of PMR; any lesser response should prompt the search for an alternative cause.

A. A test for calcium would be carried out if either sarcoidosis or a malignancy were suspected. Both are unlikely here.

C. This would be important to exclude both cervical spondylosis and osteoporosis, and should therefore happen before the diagnosis of PMR can be pronounced.

D. This woman's symptoms could fit with a haematological malignancy, but these tests would only be indicated if basic blood tests showed abnormalities of the cell lineages.

E. Again, these would be essential at the start of the investigation process but are unlikely to prove diagnostic.

Dasgupta B, Borg FA, Hassan N, *et al*. BSR and BHPR guidelines for the management of polymyalgia rheumatica. *Rheumatology*. 2009;**49**:186–90.

23. C ★★★　　OHCM 10th ed. → p. 551

An important skill to develop is the ability to classify joint pain and to begin to suggest a diagnosis. This man has an asymmetrical oligoarthritis (suggestive of either a crystal, reactive, or psoriatic arthritis), with morning stiffness and loss of function (typical of an inflammatory process). As with any joint complaint, it is important to perform a full extra-articular examination. Nail changes would be strongly supportive of the diagnosis in this case, as they occur in 80% of psoriatic arthritides. Varying patterns of arthritis occur in 10–40% of psoriasis sufferers.

A. This is a potential extra-articular finding in ankylosing spondylitis, indicative of aortic regurgitation.

B. This is seen in rheumatoid arthritis, which is more likely to cause polyarthritis.

D. This is a feature of osteoarthritis, due to bony enlargement and remodelling of the carpometacarpal joint.

E. This is a description of the tophi that usually only appear in chronic sufferers of gout.

24. E ★★★　　OHCM 10th ed. → p. 502

This is classic sciatica, involving impingement of the sciatic nerve at the level of S1. Pain is felt in the distribution of the sciatic nerve in the thigh and below the knee. The history and positive straight leg raise confirm this diagnosis.

A. Urinary retention (along with loss of the cremasteric reflex, elicited by stroking the superomedial part of the thigh) would suggest compression of the L1–L2 nerve root.

B. Together with hyperreflexia, this is a feature of a right-sided upper motor neurone lesion.

C. This is a feature of cauda equina syndrome, caused by compression of the cauda equina below L2.

D. Together with absent ankle reflexes, this is a feature of subacute combined degeneration of the cord, due to vitamin B12 deficiency.

Koes BW, van Tulder MW, and Peul WC. Diagnosis and treatment of sciatica. *BMJ*. 2007;**334**:1313–17.

→ www.bmj.com/cgi/content/extract/334/7607/1313

Chapter 11

Surgery

Shelly Griffiths

Starting a surgical job can feel like learning a completely new language. It may be the first time seeing patients in acute severe pain with a variety of lumps and bumps and a past history of previously unheard of complex operations. It can be easy to get hung up on whether the distended large bowel loop on the X-ray is a caecal or sigmoid volvulus or whether the strangulated hernia is femoral or inguinal.

Ultimately, however, the most important point is that, as a junior doctor, it is being able to recognize that the patient is acutely unwell and may require an operation that will save lives.

Ironically, a surgical rotation involves little time in the operating theatre—mostly, it will be spent dealing with problems during the perioperative period. This may start a week or two before the patient is even admitted, in the shape of a pre-assessment clinic, though these are increasingly nurse-led clinics with minimal input from junior doctors. Such clinics are, however, a good opportunity to see stable patients with interesting pathology and good clinical signs and to establish how well they look before the majority of their large bowel or their stomach is removed.

The preoperative preparation of the patient goes beyond bloods and a cursory chat, and will require one to be on the lookout for previously undiagnosed cardiorespiratory or rheumatological conditions, among others, that might affect the patient getting to sleep or staying safely asleep under anaesthesia. Liaising with the anaesthetist about possible sources of difficulty well in advance of the planned procedure will ensure that operations do not get cancelled.

The acute abdomen will take centre stage during general surgical takes. A thorough history and sound anatomical knowledge will help create a list of differential diagnoses. Accurate and careful palpation of the abdomen will reveal peritonism and the presence of any masses, and simple bedside observations and tests can greatly aid the diagnosis.

Surgical specialties have a heavy reliance on imaging—erect chest X-ray, ultrasound, computed tomography (CT)/magnetic resonance imaging (MRI) scan—each providing different information for the symptoms displayed. The theory behind selecting the right medium can be easily learnt, but the ability to interpret it may take a good deal longer. It is essential too to become accustomed to a multitude of surgical tubes—two- and three-way urinary catheters, central venous pressure (CVP) lines, naogastric and nasojejunal tubes, intravenous (IV) lines, and post-operative drains—each one giving different information on how the patient (and the doctor) is coping with the stresses of surgery.

Post-operatively, analgesia and a stepwise approach to progression using the World Health Organization analgesic ladder enable us to offer the patient the most comfortable and speedy recovery.

Patient-controlled analgesia and epidurals are becoming more common-place, and pain teams will often review patients daily, providing good learning opportunities and points of reference if difficulties arise.

This chapter emphasizes the fact that the time between the knife breaking the skin and the wound being closed is a tiny fraction of the whole process of 'surgery'. Preoperative preparation, consent, know-ledge of anaesthesia, and post-operative management of pain, fluids, and complications will be where our skills are employed—and tested.

QUESTIONS

1. A 58-year-old man is found to have an expansile mass in his abdomen. He undergoes an ultrasound examination and is found to have an abdominal aortic aneurysm (AAA), which is 4.5 cm in diameter. He is told that the aneurysm can enlarge and asks for advice about reducing his risk of rupture. He is currently taking metformin for type 2 diabetes. His body mass index (BMI) is 31 kg/m².

T 36.6°C, HR 85 bpm, BP 150/90 mmHg.

Which is the *single* most appropriate management? ★

A Close blood glucose monitoring

B Computed tomography (CT) scan every 6 months

C Lose weight

D Reduce blood pressure

E Ultrasound scan every 3 months

2. A 23-year-old man has had 24 hours of central abdominal pain. He has passed urine on eight occasions already today and is complaining of pain each time he goes. He opened his bowels today and has not had any diarrhoea, although he vomited earlier in the day. He has taken analgesia at home, without much effect.

T 37.4°C, HR 88 bpm, BP 130/75 mmHg.

He is maximally tender in the right iliac fossa.

C-reactive protein (CRP) 30 mg/L, white cell count (WCC) 15 × 10⁹ / L, bilirubin 28 micromol/L.

Which is the *single* most likely explanation for the blood results? ★

A Appendicitis

B Gallstones

C Pancreatitis

D Paracetamol overdose

E Urinary tract infection

3. A 31-year-old woman has pain in her upper abdomen. It has been constant for 4 hours and radiates to her back. She feels nauseated but has not vomited. She recalls a similar episode 3 months previously, but she did not see a doctor at that time. She drinks 20 units of alcohol a week. She cannot get comfortable, and her abdomen is tender to deep palpation in the right upper quadrant.

T 36.9°C, HR 95 bpm, BP 130/90 mmHg.

Which is the *single* most likely diagnosis? ★

A Biliary colic

B Chronic pancreatitis

C Hepatitis C

D Peptic ulcer disease

E Renal colic

4. A 44-year-old woman has generalized abdominal pain. It has been intermittent but is getting progressively more intense. She is feeling shivery and nauseated. She recalls a similar episode 3 months ago, but that passed after a few days. She has recently been advised to amend her diet, as her cholesterol levels are raised.

T 38.2°C, HR 110 bpm, BP 95/65 mmHg.

Which is the *single* most likely examination finding to confirm the diagnosis? ★

A Epigastric pain, even on light palpation

B Pain and discoloration around the umbilicus and in the flanks

C Pain more in the right iliac fossa than in the left iliac fossa when the left is pressed

D Pain on palpation of the loins

E Pain on palpation of the right upper quadrant (RUQ) that interrupts deep inspiration

5. A 72-year-old woman has cramps in her buttocks after walking for 20 m. The pain eases once she rests but comes on again at that fixed distance. She has ischaemic heart disease and type 2 diabetes. The junior doctor performs an examination of her lower limb arterial system, including peripheral pulses. Which is the *single* most important additional examination to perform? ★

A Auscultation of the carotid arteries

B Auscultation of the heart

C Lower limb venous system

D Musculoskeletal examination of the lower limbs

E Palpation of the abdomen

6. A 75-year-old woman has had a painful left leg for 24 hours. The entire leg is swollen and red. She has 24-hour care and requires help to transfer from bed to chair, following a stroke 3 years ago. She has chronic obstructive pulmonary disease (COPD) and uses home oxygen.

T 36.2°C, HR 88 bpm, BP 155/90 mmHg, SaO$_2$ 92% on air.

Which is the *single* most likely diagnosis? ★

A Cellulitis

B Deep vein thrombosis (DVT)

C Lymphoedema

D Ruptured Baker's cyst

E Superficial thrombophlebitis

7. A 55-year-old woman has had a scaly, itchy rash on her right nipple for 3 weeks. She has been using a moisturizer but has not seen any improvement. She has not felt a lump in her breasts or had any discharge from the nipples. There is no family history of breast cancer, and a mammogram last year was normal. Which is the *single* most appropriate next step? ★

A Hydrocortisone cream 1% twice daily

B Patch allergy testing

C Reassure and ask her to come back in 6 weeks if it is still present

D Routine referral to a dermatologist

E Two-week wait referral to the breast unit

8. A 45-year-old woman has had severe abdominal pain for the past 48 hours. It radiates through to her back and can only partially be relieved by bending forwards. She has vomited several times. She is otherwise well and does not drink alcohol.

T 37.6°C, HR 120 bpm, BP 95/45 mmHg.

Her abdomen is tense and generally tender, especially at the epigastrium.

Which *single* further factor would most support the likely diagnosis? ★

A 10-kg weight loss in past month

B Familial hyperlipidaemia

C On oral contraceptive pill

D Previous total abdominal hysterectomy

E Recent foreign travel

9. A 75-year-old lady has had 3 days of intermittent abdominal pain with vomiting. She had an abdominal hysterectomy 15 years previously. Her abdomen is distended, with tinkling bowel sounds. There is a tender lump palpable in the right groin.

T 37.5°C, HR 110 bpm, BP 110/80 mmHg.

Which is the *single* most likely diagnosis? ★

A Band adhesions

B Lymphoma

C Obstructed femoral hernia

D Pancreatic cancer

E Ulcerative colitis

10. A 19-year-old woman has a 2 cm × 2 cm mobile, non-tender, soft lump with smooth edges in her right breast. She takes the combined oral contraceptive pill. Her mother had breast cancer aged 48. She is referred and undergoes standard quadruple assessment at the local breast unit.

Which is the *single* most likely management? ★

A Aspirate the lump and send the contents for cytology

B Core biopsy of the lump

C Leave the lump and no need for follow-up

D Leave the lump, but if it is still there in 2 months' time, remove it surgically

E Surgical excision of the lump

11. A 62-year-old man is sweating and shivering 5 days after he had a lump in his groin resected. The on-call junior doctor is bleeped to the ward to review the observations chart (Figure 11.1).

Which *single* process is most likely to explain the pattern seen on the chart? ★

A Abscess

B Fistula

C Haematoma

D Haemorrhage

E Sinus

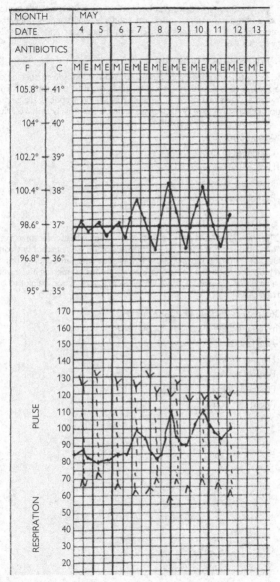

Figure 11.1

12. An 88-year-old woman has had severe pain in her left leg for the past week. It came on suddenly whilst at rest. She has carcinoma of the bronchus with cerebral metastases and smokes 20 cigarettes a day.

HR 90 bpm, BP 165/90 mmHg.

The leg is dark blue and mottled up to mid calf, with fixed staining of the toes. It is cold, with no pulses palpable distal to the popliteal. The surgeon explains that the only possible management options are amputation or palliative care. Which *single* factor is most likely to have influenced the surgeon's opinion? ★

A Age >80 years

B Continues to smoke

C Limb is non-viable

D Metastatic disease

E Patient does not have capacity

13. A 32-year-old man has had severe pain, whilst defecating, over the last 2 months. The pain starts as he passes stool but continues long after he has finished. He has seen small amounts of bright red blood on the tissue paper and is now nervous of opening his bowels as a result of the pain. A digital rectal examination is too painful to be carried out.

T 36.2°C, HR 70 bpm, BP 128/75 mmHg.

Which is the *single* most likely diagnosis? ★

A Anal fissure

B Haemorrhoids

C Perianal abscess

D Proctalgia fugax

E Rectal carcinoma

14. A 29-year-old woman has had abdominal pain for 3 days. It began around the umbilicus but is now worse on the right side of her abdomen. She has a poor appetite and intermittent nausea. Her periods are regular but heavy, and she is currently mid cycle. Her abdomen is tender to light palpation and percussion in the right iliac fossa.

T 37.4°C, HR 105 bpm, BP 95/65 mmHg.

Urinary beta-human chorionic gonadotrophin (β-hCG): negative.

Which is the *single* most likely diagnosis? ★

A Acute appendicitis

B Ectopic pregnancy

C Endometriosis

D Ovulation pain

E Pelvic inflammatory disease

15. A 42-year-old man has developed acute pain over an inguinal hernia. He is vomiting and unable to tolerate oral analgesia. He is prescribed intramuscular (IM) morphine. Which is the *single* safest area of the gluteal muscle in which to administer the injection? ★

A Central

B Inferolateral

C Inferomedial

D Superolateral

E Superomedial

16. A 53-year-old woman has had a swelling and an aching sensation in her left groin for the past 6 months. She had some varicose veins removed from her right leg 5 years ago. The swelling is below and lateral to the pubic tubercle and does not disappear on lying down. There is no cough impulse detected. Which is the *single* most likely cause of the groin swelling? ★

A Femoral hernia

B Inguinal hernia

C Lipoma

D Lymph node

E Saphena varix

17. A 72-year-old man collapses at home. He has had 4 hours of back pain. Prior to this episode, he has been fit and well. He is now alert, but in pain.

HR 120 bpm, BP 90/70 mmHg.

There is an expansile mass palpable in his abdomen. Which is the *single* most appropriate course of action? ★

A Arrange consent for an immediate laparotomy

B Ask the surgical registrar to assess immediately

C Computed tomography (CT) scan of the abdomen

D Insert a urinary catheter

E Ultrasound scan of the abdomen

18. A 68-year-old woman has had central abdominal pain for the last 12 hours. She feels more bloated than usual, and although she has vomited on four occasions, this has made her feel better. She opened her bowels today, with normal soft stool. There is a Kocher scar on her abdomen, which is soft but slightly distended, and there are only occasional bowel sounds heard. Blood tests are normal. Which is the *single* most likely diagnosis? ★

A Gallstone ileus

B Large bowel obstruction

C Paralytic ileus

D Pseudo-obstruction

E Small bowel obstruction

19. A 55-year-old man has a painful right calf. It has come on suddenly and is making it difficult for him to walk. He is in such pain that he has come to the emergency department out of hours. The entire right leg is swollen, with the calf >5 cm larger than the left. There is pitting oedema to the knee, with tenderness locally over the mid calf. Which is the *single* most appropriate management? ★

A Defer treatment until after a Doppler ultrasound scan

B Measure D-dimer

C Start low-molecular-weight heparin

D Start unfractionated heparin

E Start warfarin

20. A 76-year-old man is given intravenous (IV) fluids and catheterized during conservative treatment of an attack of acute pancreatitis. On the second day, he feels much better and the catheter is removed at 8 a.m. That evening, the on-call junior doctor is called because the man has lower abdominal pain and distension. He has not passed significant amounts of urine since the catheter was removed.

T 36.6°C, HR 100 bpm, BP 140/80 mmHg.

Which is the *single* most appropriate next step in management? ★

A Abdominal ultrasound scan

B Abdominal X-ray

C Catheterize the patient

D Insert a nasogastric tube

E Urgent amylase

21. A 25-year-old man has worsening scrotal pain over a 4-hour period. It started as a dull ache but is now excruciating. His pain is partially relieved by elevation of the testes. The cremasteric reflex is absent. Which is the *single* most likely diagnosis? ★

A Acute epididymo-orchitis

B Indirect inguinal hernia

C Strangulated inguinal hernia

D Testicular torsion

E Testicular tumour

22. A 55-year-old man with severe abdominal pain undergoes a laparotomy. He is found to have a badly devascularized transverse colon. Which *single* arterial supply is most likely to have been compromised? ★

A Ascending colic artery

B Ileocolic artery

C Middle colic artery

D Right colic artery

E Superior rectal artery

23. An 18-year-old man is brought to the emergency department, having fallen off his bicycle. He was clipped on his right side, with his left side landing on the kerb. He has bruising to his left chest, flank, and thigh. His abdomen is tender in the left hypochondrium.

HR 120 bpm, BP 105/80 mmHg, RR 22/min, SaO$_2$ 97% on air.

Which is the *single* most likely diagnosis? ★

A Colonic perforation

B Haemothorax

C Liver capsule rupture

D Renal haematoma

E Splenic rupture

24. A 72-year-old man has had severe pain in his lower abdomen for the past 12 hours. He is nauseated and unable to walk.

T 37.2°C, HR 100 bpm, BP 90/60 mmHg.

There is a lump in his right groin that neither the patient nor the doctor can reduce. Which is the *single* additional feature that should prompt the most urgent attention? ★

A Bowels not opened for the past 4 days

B Lump has previously always been irreducible but only became acutely painful when his lower abdominal pain started

C Lump is warm and tender to touch

D The patient has had three previous laparotomies

E Pain radiates down into the scrotum

25. A 30-year-old man has had a swelling in his scrotum for several weeks. He says it disappears when lying down and that occasionally he has an aching feeling in his groin. There is a soft, irregular lump palpable in the left testicle. It is non-tender and does not transilluminate. It is possible to get above it, and there is no cough impulse present.

Which is the *single* most likely diagnosis? ★

A Hydrocele

B Inguinal hernia

C Spermatocele

D Testicular tumour

E Varicocele

26. An 82-year-old woman has become increasingly drowsy through the course of an evening. Two days previously, she underwent emergency repair of an incarcerated femoral hernia. The on-call junior doctor is contacted by the ward staff who relays the woman's latest observations over the phone:

T 38.2°C, HR 110 bpm, BP 90/70 mmHg, SaO$_2$ 94% on air, urine output 25 mL/hour.

Which is the *single* feature that is most of concern? ★

A Increasing drowsiness

B Low oxygen saturation and no oxygen therapy

C Low urine output

D Pulse rate higher than systolic blood pressure

E Raised temperature 48 hours after surgery

27. A 75-year-old man has had sudden-onset central abdominal pain for 30 minutes. He is confused, and a collateral history is taken from his wife. He smokes 20 cigarettes per day and drinks 30 units of alcohol per week. He opens his bowels every 3 days and takes bendroflumethiazide once daily for hypertension.

T 36.8°C, HR 110 bpm, BP 90/50 mmHg, BM 7.5 mmol/L.

Which is the *single* most likely diagnosis? ★

A Acute pancreatitis

B Perforated diverticula

C Perforated duodenal ulcer

D Ruptured abdominal aortic aneurysm (AAA)

E Ureteric colic

28. A 62-year-old man has had epigastric and central abdominal pain over the last 4 days. He feels bloated and has been vomiting for the last 12 hours. His bowels have not opened for 3 days. Which *single* further feature in the history would be most supportive of the likely diagnosis? ★

A Drinks 40 units of alcohol per week

B Eats a lot of takeaway foods

C Previous open cholecystectomy

D Recent foreign travel

E Regularly takes naproxen for back pain

29. A 74-year-old man has been troubled by pain in his calves for many years. The walking distance at which it comes on has dropped from 50 to 10 m, despite him giving up smoking, losing weight, and lowering his blood pressure. The patient declines surgical intervention, and his surgeon is considering starting a new medication. Which is the *single* most appropriate class of medication? ★

A Beta-blocker

B Calcium channel inhibitor

C Diuretic

D Inotropic sympathomimetic

E Peripheral vasodilator

30. A 33-year-old man is undergoing an elective hernia repair. The anaesthetist uses the same agent for induction and maintenance.

As he injects it, he tells the patient that it will sting a little around the injection site. Which *single* agent has the anaesthetist most likely used? ★

A Desflurane

B Midazolam

C Propofol

D Suxamethonium

E Thiopental

31. A 53-year-old man is attending a preoperative assessment before an elective cholecystectomy. He had an inferior myocardial infarction 3 years ago but otherwise has had no health problems. He is taking aspirin 75 mg oral (PO) once daily, simvastatin 40 mg PO once at night, perindopril 4 mg PO once daily, and atenolol 50 mg PO once daily. Which is the *single* most appropriate piece of advice regarding his medications during the perioperative period? ★

A All his medications need to be stopped the week before the planned operation

B All his medications should be continued, including on the morning of the operation

C Subcutaneous heparin injections should replace aspirin for 5 days before the operation; the other medications can be continued

D Aspirin should be changed for clopidogrel a week before the planned operation

E Aspirin should be stopped 7 days before the operation, but all his other medications continued as normal

32. A 36-year-old man has had pain around his anus and fresh rectal bleeding for 24 hours. He opens his bowels every 3 days and passes hard, pellet-like stools. He has had small amounts of rectal bleeding previously and, over recent weeks, felt 'something come down' as his bowels opened, which he then pushes back inside. He has a thrombosed external haemorrhoid, but no necrotic tissue. Which is the *single* most appropriate management? ★

A Banding of the haemorrhoid

B Emergency open haemorrhoidectomy

C Emergency stapled haemorrhoidectomy

D High-fibre diet

E Ice pack therapy with analgesia

33. A 55-year-old man has severe central abdominal pain that radiates into his back. It started 2 hours ago, and although it initially settled, it returned after his lunch and he has vomited twice. His pain is reduced, but not eliminated, by intravenous (IV) morphine. He has mild exercise-induced asthma and has had an epigastric hernia for years.

T 36.3°C, HR 85 bpm, BP 140/70 mmHg.

Abdomen: soft, central tenderness, scanty bowel sounds.

An abdominal X-ray shows a few small bowel loops on the right side of the abdomen.

Which *single* additional history supports the diagnosis? ★

A His bowels have not opened for 3 days

B The epigastric hernia has not got bigger recently

C The pain is better sitting forward

D There has been no haematemesis

E There is a family history of colorectal cancer

34. A 36-year-old woman has an infected insect bite and has been feverish for a week. The emergency department doctor refers the patient to the surgical on-call team. The surgical registrar is on the way to the operating theatre but tells the surgical junior doctor that the patient does not have a surgical problem and that he should discharge her with antibiotics and no follow-up. The area of cellulitis covers an area about 8 × 8 cm and has surrounding induration. The junior doctor is unsure whether there is an abscess present. Which is the *single* most appropriate next step? ★

A Arrange an outpatient ultrasound scan and give her a week of oral antibiotics

B Call your registrar to see the patient when she is out of the theatre

C Discharge her with a course of antibiotics and no outpatient follow-up

D Give her oral antibiotics and ask her to return if things do not improve

E Use a needle and syringe, and try to aspirate pus from the inflamed area

35. A 24-year-old woman has had abdominal pain for the last 48 hours. It has been associated with nausea, but no vomiting. Her last menstrual period was normal and finished 3 days ago. She has had no vaginal discharge and is not sexually active. She has had a recent persistent coryzal illness.

T 36.6°C, HR 63 bpm, BP 125/75 mmHg.

Urine dipstick: trace blood.

Her abdomen is soft, but tender in the right iliac fossa, with no guarding or rebound tenderness. Which *single* additional finding is most likely to support the diagnosis? ★

A Cervical excitation

B Pause in inspiration on palpation of the right upper quadrant

C Right renal angle tenderness

D Soft stool on digital rectal examination

E Tender lymph nodes palpable in the neck

36. A 40-year-old woman has had a small sebaceous cyst on her back removed. The doctor wants to use 1% lidocaine as a local anaesthetic before closing the wound (maximum dose is 3 mg/kg). The patient weighs 50 kg. Which is the *single* maximum amount of 1% lidocaine that can be administered? ★

A 1.5 mL

B 3 mL

C 5 mL

D 15 mL

E 30 mL

37. A 66-year-old woman has pain in her right hip 24 hours after having varicose veins stripped. The junior doctor is called to the ward. As he is reviewing the history, he realizes that he failed to make an entry in the notes during the morning ward round. It is now mid afternoon.

Which is the *single* most appropriate action? ★

A Find whoever led the morning round and ask them to make an entry

B Ignore the omission and move on to the next consultation

C Write the notes in now, but mark the entry 'in retrospect'

D Write the notes in now with the current time

E Write: 'patient not seen on morning ward round'

38. A 28-year-old woman has had pain under her right ribs for the last 12 hours since eating a lunch of chicken and chips. It radiates to her back and is associated with three or four bouts of vomiting. Although she has had this type of pain before, it has never been as bad as on this occasion. She had a Caesarean section 3 years ago and takes the progestogen-only pill each day.

T 36.2°C, HR 80 bpm, BP 130/66 mmHg.

Her abdomen is soft, but tender in the right upper quadrant in the mid-clavicular line on inspiration. Which is the *single* most appropriate initial imaging? ★

A Abdominal computed tomography (CT) scan

B Endoscopic retrograde cholangiopancreatography (ERCP)

C Hepatobiliary iminodiacetic acid (HIDA) scan

D Magnetic resonance cholangiopancreatography (MRCP)

E Ultrasound scan of the gall bladder

39. An 82-year-old man is seen in the emergency department with an incarcerated inguinal hernia. The surgical team deems him to have the capacity to decide the course of treatment, and he consents to an urgent laparotomy. Whilst he is awaiting a theatre slot, his pain increases and he becomes more unwell. He tells nursing staff that he no longer wants the operation and would like to withdraw his consent.

Which is the *single* most appropriate course of action? ★

A Ask his next of kin to persuade him to have the operation

B Proceed to theatre, as consent cannot be revoked

C Proceed to theatre under a section of the Mental Health Act 2007

D Reassess his capacity, given the change in his condition

E Respect his wishes, as he has already been shown to have capacity

40. A 77-year-old man has had loose bloody bowel motions for the last 3 months. He has mixed Alzheimer's and vascular dementia, with a mini-mental state examination (MMSE) score of 14/30. The surgical team plan to investigate his symptoms with a colonoscopy. When seeking his consent, it is clear that he does not understand the explanations, cannot retain information, and cannot weigh up the risks and benefits. Which would constitute appropriate consent in this case? ★

A Verbal consent from the man

B Verbal consent from the man's next of kin

C Written consent by a doctor as proxy

D Written consent from the man

E Written consent from the man's next of kin

41. A 67-year-old man has a sudden onset of epigastric pain that woke him up 4 hours ago. He has never had pain as severe as this before—it moves into both flanks, although it seems to improve if he sits forward. He has vomited four times but just feels nauseated now. He takes perindopril 4 mg once daily for hypertension. He drinks 6 units of alcohol per week.

T 36.6°C, HR 86 bpm, BP 135/75 mmHg.

His abdomen is soft, but tender, particularly over the upper and central abdomen. Which is the *single* most likely diagnosis? ★

A Acute appendicitis

B Acute pancreatitis

C Mesenteric ischaemia

D Perforated duodenal ulcer

E Upper small bowel obstruction

42. A 57-year-old man has needed to pass urine with little warning for the last 6 months and now struggles to go out, unless he knows where toilets are going to be. He has a good urinary flow, but his symptoms have persisted despite reducing his caffeine intake.

Urine dipstick test: unremarkable.

The doctor wants to start him on some medication to see whether he can reduce the urinary frequency. Which is the *single* most appropriate choice of medication? ★

A Desmopressin

B Finasteride

C Solifenacin

D Tamsulosin

E Trimethoprim

43. A 73-year-old woman has had central abdominal pain and vomiting for the last 12 hours. She has a painful lump in the groin, which she thinks appeared at the same time as the symptoms started. She is thought to have an incarcerated femoral hernia.

Where would the lump be found? ★

A At the lateral border of the rectus abdominis

B Between the anterior superior iliac spine and the pubic tubercle

C Just inferior and lateral to the pubic tubercle

D Just superior and medial to the pubic tubercle

E Just superior to the mid-point of a line between the anterior superior iliac spine and the pubis

44. A 55-year-old man has noticed bright red blood in the toilet each time he passes a stool for the last couple of months. It seems to coat the stool and, on occasion, drips into the pan. He has an intermittent perianal itch. His weight is stable, and he is otherwise well.

What is the most likely diagnosis? ★

A Anal fissure

B Angiodysplasia

C Caecal cancer

D Haemorrhoids

E Ulcerative colitis

45. A 78-year-old male smoker presents with an 8-week history of progressive difficulty swallowing. He is now unable to swallow solids, though he can drink liquids. He has lost 6 kg in weight. Abdominal, chest, and neck examinations are unremarkable.

What is the most likely diagnosis? ★

A Achalasia

B Gastric cancer

C Globus

D Oesophageal cancer

E Scleroderma

46. A 66-year-old woman has had diarrhoea associated with pain in the left side of her abdomen over the last 3 days. Normally, she opens her bowels once or twice a week, but over the last 12 hours, she has passed very loose stools with a large amount of mucus and bright red blood.

T 37.7°C, HR 86 bpm, BP 138/76 mmHg.

Her abdomen is soft, but distended and tender in the left iliac fossa. She is admitted and treated with antibiotics and returns 6 weeks later for a colonoscopy. Which is the *single* most likely finding on colonoscopy? ★★

A Friable sigmoid colon mucosa that bleeds on contact

B Large ulcerated lesion in the ascending colon

C Mucosal projections through the circular muscle of the colon

D Multiple pedunculated polyps in the distal colon

E Patchy ulcerated fissures throughout the colon

47. A 28-year-old man undergoes an emergency laparotomy, following a gunshot wound to his abdomen. The anaesthetist requires a rapidly acting paralysing agent in order to be able to intubate the non-starved patient safely. Which is the *single* most appropriate choice? ★★

A Bupivacaine

B Dantrolene

C Lidocaine

D Propofol

E Rocuronium

48. A 20-year-old man has extreme pain in his right calf after walking only short distances over the past few weeks. It eases quickly with rest and came on suddenly. He is a non-smoker and a keen athlete. His family doctor refers him for a magnetic resonance imaging (MRI) scan of his calf. Which *single* process is most likely to be responsible for his symptoms? ★★

A Autoimmune inflammation of vascular walls

B Entrapment of vessel

C Inflammation of artery

D Impingement of nerve

E Stenosis of artery

49. A 38-year-old woman is undergoing a mastectomy and latissimus dorsi reconstruction. She has been given a non-depolarizing neuromuscular-blocking agent intraoperatively. Following completion of the operation, the anaesthetist needs to reverse this block and is going to use neostigmine. Which drug must be given in conjunction with neostigmine? ★★

A Atracurium

B Glycopyrronium

C Sevoflurane

D Suxamethonium

E Thiopental

50. A 70-year-old man had right iliac fossa pain for 10 days and underwent an open appendicectomy of a gangrenous appendix. Two days post-operatively, he is taking sips of fluids but feels bloated, has vomited twice, and is sweaty. His abdomen is distended, with mild generalized tenderness.

T 36.2°C, HR 90 bpm, BP 140/80 mmHg, RR 30/min.

Which is the *single* most appropriate next step? ★★

A Abdominal ultrasound + urine microscopy, culture, and sensitivity (MC&S)

B Computed tomography (CT) pulmonary angiogram + low-molecular-weight heparin

C Electrocardiogram (ECG) + cardiac enzymes

D Nasogastric tube + intravenous (IV) fluids

E Urinary catheter + furosemide 40 mg IV

51. A 62-year-old man has developed pain in his upper abdomen, which radiates into his back and loin. He returned from the high-dependency unit to a general surgical ward 3 days after a complex bowel resection. He is on a sliding-scale insulin infusion for type 1 diabetes.

T 38.4°C, HR 110 bpm, BP 110/60 mmHg, SaO₂ 96% on air.

Urinalysis: nothing abnormal detected.

He is tender in the right upper quadrant. Which is the *single* most likely explanation for these new symptoms? ★★

A Basal pneumonia

B Cholecystitis

C Intra-abdominal collection

D Pyelonephritis

E Renal stone

52. A 21-year-old woman has had right iliac fossa pain, which started during the previous evening following her dinner. She vomited twice, but now she just feels nauseated and is not hungry. She has passed three loose stools over the last 12 hours and has also found that she needs to pass urine more often than usual.

T 37.6°C, HR 100 bpm, BP 130/75 mmHg.

Urine dipstick: blood 1+, leucocytes 1+.

Which is the *single* most likely diagnosis? ★ ★

A Appendicitis

B Gastroenteritis

C Mesenteric adenitis

D Pelvic inflammatory disease

E Urinary tract infection

53. A surgical ward round is in progress. The next patient has had a femoral–popliteal bypass but is in a side room because he is positive for *Clostridium difficile* toxin. In the side room, the doctor handles the patient's observation chart and then his drug chart. He does not have any physical contact with the patient before he moves on to the next patient. Which is the *single* most appropriate step before seeing the next patient? ★ ★

A Nothing—he did not touch the patient

B Nothing, unless he examines the next patient

C Put on a pair of gloves before examining the next patient

D Wash his hands with alcohol gel

E Wash his hands with soap and water

54. A 66-year-old man has passed blood with his stools for the last 6 weeks. Which is the *single* clinical feature that would be most suggestive of a carcinoma, rather than haemorrhoids? ★ ★

A Anaemia

B Change in bowel habit

C Fresh rectal bleeding

D Itching around the anus

E Rectal mucus discharge

55. A 76-year-old woman is to undergo an elective hemicolectomy for a caecal carcinoma. She has type 2 diabetes and has had previous arterial ulcers in the left leg [most recent ankle–brachial pressure index (ABPI) 0.4]. The junior doctor is asked to prescribe compression stockings as prophylaxis for venous thromboembolic disease (VTE).

Which is the *single* most appropriate course of action? ★★

A Elevate the legs, with no compression

B High-pressure compression

C Keep the legs dependent, with no compression

D Low-pressure compression

E Low- or high-pressure compression at night only

56. A 33-year-old woman is a front-seat passenger in a head-on collision with another car. She sustains multiple long bone fractures and a splenic tear. During a laparotomy, she undergoes a splenectomy and fixation of her fractures. She is transferred to the intensive therapy unit for initial post-operative management. Which is the *single* most appropriate step to take before discharge? ★★

A No specific prophylaxis or treatment is recommended once she has left the hospital

B The patient should be booked in for an influenza vaccination at the start of the winter months

C The patient should receive *Haemophilus influenzae* type B (HiB), pneumococcal, and meningitis C vaccines and take regular penicillin on discharge

D The patient should have a 2-week course of penicillin at home to take, should she become unwell

E Vaccines are not indicated, but the patient may require immunoglobulin treatment if she becomes unwell in the future

57. A 65-year-old woman has had left-sided abdominal pain, been off her food, and felt tired for the last 3 days. She has passed three or four loose stools each day and urine frequently. Her bowels usually open twice weekly, often followed by a few days of loose stools. Any pain that she has previously had settles after spending a few days in bed.

T 37.8°C, HR 92 bpm, BP 155/82 mmHg.

Her abdomen is soft, but slightly distended and tender in the left iliac fossa.

Which is the *single* most likely diagnosis? ★★

A Coeliac disease

B Colonic carcinoma

C Diverticulitis

D Irritable bowel syndrome

E Viral gastroenteritis

58. A 58-year-old man has felt feverish and has had a distended upper abdomen for the last 2 days. He has only recently left hospital, prior to which he recalls severe abdominal pain and vomiting.

He drinks 40 units of alcohol per week.

T 38.2°C, HR 90 bpm, BP 156/90 mmHg.

His abdomen is soft, but there is a 10 cm × 8 cm mass in the upper abdomen.

Which is the *single* most likely cause for the abdominal mass? ★★

A Ascites

B Gastric volvulus

C Hepatomegaly

D Liver abscess

E Pancreatic pseudocyst

59. A 64-year-old man has had pain in his left lower leg for the last 4 days. He says he has lost feeling in the lower part of it over the last day or two. He has hypertension, type 2 diabetes, and schizophrenia. The limb is very pale, and no pulses are palpable. The on-call surgical team explain to the man that, at this stage, the best option would be a below-knee amputation of the limb. The man refuses. Which is the *single* most appropriate next step? ★★

A Assess the man's capacity to make such a decision

B As the man has a mental illness, operate in his best interests

C Operate, having detained the man under a section of the Mental Health Act 2007

D Respect the man's wishes and do as he wants

E Seek consent for surgery from his next of kin

60. A 44-year-old man has severe right-sided abdominal pain, which moves down into his groin. The pain started suddenly and comes and goes in waves. He vomited twice when the pain started, and his bowels have not opened today. He admits to eating a poor diet with regular takeaway meals and drinks 20 units of alcohol per week, usually all at the weekend. He is taking oral non-steroidal anti-inflammatory drugs (NSAIDs) for a soft tissue injury. Which is the *single* most useful piece of advice for this man to prevent further presentations? ★★

A Cut down on alcohol binges

B Drink 2–3 L of fluid per day

C Follow a low-fat diet

D Only take NSAIDs after meals

E Use regular laxatives and aim for two soft stools per day

61. A 46-year-old lady underwent a day-case laparoscopic chole-cystectomy 5 days ago. She re-presents with worsening right upper quadrant pain and feeling generally unwell.

T 38.2°C, HR 105 bpm, BP 145/70 mmHg, SaO₂ 98% on air.

White cell count (WCC) 16.2, alkaline phosphatase 206, alanine aminotransferase (ALT) 207, bilirubin 19.

What will be the most useful investigation? ★★

A Abdominal ultrasound

B Abdominal X-ray

C Computed tomography pulmonary angiogram (CTPA)

D Endoscopic retrograde cholangiopancreatography (ERCP)

E Magnetic resonance cholangiopancreatography (MRCP)

62. A 58-year-old woman has had left-sided abdominal pain, been off her food for the last week, and now requires morphine for analgesia. Initially, she passed loose stools with mucus and small amounts of blood, but her bowels have not opened for the last 48 hours. Since a teenager, she has always had a tendency to be constipated but can also be affected by episodes of loose stools over a number of days and abdominal pain relieved by passing flatus.

T 37.9°C, HR 90 bpm, BP 142/82 mmHg.

Haemoglobin (Hb) 118 g/L, white cell count (WCC) 14.2 × 10⁹/L, platelets 340 × 10⁹/L.

Her abdomen is soft, but tender in the left iliac fossa.

Which is the *single* most appropriate management? ★★

A Blood transfusion + laparotomy

B Colonoscopy + water-soluble enema contrast

C High-fibre diet + laxatives

D Intravenous (IV) antibiotics + analgesia

E Nasogastric tube + IV fluids

63. A 66-year-old man presents with painless visible haematuria. He is systemically well. He has a background of hypertension and gastro-oesophageal reflux disease.

What is the most appropriate course of action? ★★

A Make a routine urology referral

B Make an urgent (2-week wait) urology referral

C Organize a computed tomography (CT) kidney, ureters, and bladder (KUB)

D Treat with a prolonged course of levofloxacin

E Treat with a short course of trimethoprim

64. A 62-year-old man has been passing small amounts of blood with his bowel movements for 2 months. He is not sure whether it is mixed with the stool, but the blood is bright red in colour, and he thinks it is getting less. He has always been troubled by constipation, but he has not noticed any change in his bowels recently. He has osteoarthritis and takes regular diclofenac for symptomatic relief. He has no family history of bowel cancer. Which is the *single* most appropriate management? ★★★

A Add omeprazole 40 mg oral (PO) once daily

B Commence regular lactulose 20 mL PO twice daily

C Routine referral to the surgical outpatients clinic

D Send a full blood count, and review if he is anaemic

E Urgent 2-week referral to the surgical outpatients clinic

65. A 42-year-old man has started passing small amounts of fresh blood with his bowel motions over the last 4 weeks. He is opening his bowels three times daily, whereas before he opened them only once daily, but this is not associated with any other change in his stools. He has not noticed any tiredness, weight loss, or change in his appetite. His abdomen is soft and non-tender. A digital rectal examination reveals soft stool with no blood or mucus. Which is the *single* most appropriate next step? ★★★

A Arrange to review in 2 months

B Arrange to review in 2 weeks

C Reassure and ask to return if things do not improve

D Routine referral to surgical outpatients clinic

E Urgent referral to surgical outpatients clinic

66. A 44-year-old woman is having a laparotomy for adhesional small bowel obstruction. She had an open cholecystectomy 18 years ago but otherwise has been in good health and has no other medical problems. The operation goes well, and the abdomen is closed in layers. The skin in the midline is closed with metal clips. Which is the *single* earliest day after her operation that the clips could start to be taken out? ★★★

A 2 days

B 4 days

C 6 days

D 8 days

E 10 days

67. An 85-year-old woman has had lower abdominal pain for 1 week. She has been vomiting and not had her bowels open for 10 days. She lives alone and has vascular dementia. Her abdomen is distended and diffusely tender, with tinkling bowel sounds. The surgical registrar explains to the woman that she needs emergency surgery—she flatly refuses to give her consent. The surgeon notes that she is unable to comprehend and retain information about her clinical situation or to weigh up the risks and benefits of the proposed treatment. Which would be the *single* most appropriate course of action? ★★★

A Ask a member of the woman's family to persuade her that surgery would be in her best interests

B Ask a psychiatrist to admit the woman under the Mental Health Act 2007, so that he can legally proceed to surgery

C Proceed to surgery if the surgeon feels it would be in the woman's best interests

D Respect the woman's wishes

E Seek consent from the woman's next of kin

68. An 81-year-old man has metastatic prostatic carcinoma. He is taking 30 mg of modified-release morphine orally twice daily for pain, with three 10-mg doses of morphine liquid for breakthrough pain over a 24-hour period. He is rapidly deteriorating, and the on-call registrar feels that the best strategy now would be to commence a diamorphine syringe driver. The junior doctor has been asked to write the prescription. Which is the *single* most appropriate 24-hour dose of subcutaneous diamorphine? ★★★

A 30 mg

B 45 mg

C 90 mg

D 135 mg

E 180 mg

69. A 32-year-old man is knocked off his bicycle at 35 mph, landing heavily on his left side, and has pain in his left shoulder. He was wearing a helmet and did not lose consciousness. His Glasgow Coma Scale (GCS) score is 15/15. He has some bruising and marked tenderness over the left eight and ninth ribs posteriorly and tenderness over the left clavicle. The trauma series of X-rays show no abnormalities. A left shoulder X-ray shows an undisplaced fracture of the clavicle. Which is the *single* most appropriate next step? ★ ★ ★

A Admit and observe for 24 hours before discharge

B Computed tomography (CT) scan of the abdomen

C Discharge home with analgesia and a sling

D Facial X-rays

E Magnetic resonance imaging (MRI) of the left shoulder

70. A 58-year-old man has had rapidly worsening pain near his rectum for 4 days. He has had normal bowel movements and has passed no blood.

T 37.8°C, HR 90 bpm, BP 125/80 mmHg.

His abdomen is soft and non-tender. The medial side of his right buttock is erythematous, indurated, and warm and tender, but with no obvious focus. A digital rectal examination reveals no external sites of bleeding and an empty rectum with no blood, but a thickened right lateral wall. Which *single* additional feature in the history would be most concerning? ★ ★ ★

A He has a family history of colorectal cancer

B He has previously had haemorrhoids

C He has recently completed a course of antibiotics

D He has type 2 diabetes

E He is nauseated and has vomited

71. A 74-year-old woman has undergone a femoral hernia repair. She takes metformin for type 2 diabetes and stopped her aspirin a week ago. She is commenced on enoxaparin 40 mg subcutaneous (SC) and has three doses of antibiotic prophylaxis perioperatively. She makes a slow post-operative recovery and on day 8, despite regularly receiving low-molecular-weight heparin (LMWH), develops a tender right calf. An ultrasound scan shows the presence of a deep vein thrombosis (DVT). Which *single* pair of investigations should be performed? ★ ★ ★

A Activated partial thromboplastin time (aPTT) + international normalized ratio (INR)

B Factor V Leiden + factor VII

C Fibrinogen + haemoglobin

D Platelets + potassium

E Protein S + protein C

72. A 77-year-old woman has had severe pain in her left hand for 3 hours. It came on suddenly and is associated with numbness and tingling. She has had two previous myocardial infarctions and takes digoxin 62.5 micrograms oral (PO) once daily for an irregular heart rhythm. Her left hand is cold and white, with a capillary refill time of >2 s. Sensation is decreased from the wrist distally, but power is unaffected. Which would be the *single* most appropriate treatment? ★ ★ ★

A Amputation

B Angioplasty

C Bypass

D Embolectomy

E Heparinization

73. An 82-year-old man has had central abdominal discomfort for the past 3 months. It radiates through to his back and is associated with nausea. He has lost his appetite and has lost 11 kg over this period.

Bilirubin 146 micromol/L, alkaline phosphatase (ALP) 766 IU/L, aspartate aminotransferase (AST) 32 IU/L, gamma-glutamyl transpeptidase (GGT) 480 IU/L.

Which is the *single* most appropriate next step? ★ ★ ★

A Computed tomography (CT) scan of the abdomen

B Endoscopic retrograde cholangiopancreatography (ERCP)

C Hepatobiliary iminodiacetic acid (HIDA) scan

D Magnetic resonance cholangiopancreatography (MRCP)

E Ultrasound scan of the liver

74. A 64-year-old woman has had loose stools, rectal bleeding, and weight loss for the last 6 months. The day after a colonoscopy, she has an episode of chest pain whilst getting washed and dressed.

T 36.6°C, HR 105 bpm, BP 125/80 mmHg, SaO$_2$ 93% on 6 L O$_2$.

Which is the *single* most appropriate immediate management? ★★★

A Computed tomography pulmonary angiogram (CTPA)

B D-dimer

C Erect chest X-ray

D Therapeutic dose of low-molecular-weight heparin (LMWH)

E Ventilation/perfusion (V/Q) scan

75. A 28-year-old man has had a painful swelling for 2 weeks. He was started on a course of flucloxacillin 1 week ago but feels things have worsened since then. The swelling is in the midline of the upper part of the gluteal region. It is fluctuant, 2 cm × 2 cm in size, and the surrounding skin is erythematous. Which is the *single* most appropriate explanation for the cause of this lump? ★★★

A An in-growing hair characteristically is the cause

B Chronic constipation is recognized to increase the incidence

C High alcohol consumption typically is linked with these lumps

D Poor anal hygiene is characteristically to blame

E Poor diabetic control is recognized to increase the incidence

76. A 60-year-old woman has come to the pre-assessment clinic to discuss the surgical repair of her para-umbilical hernia. She is accompanied by her husband. He is very keen that the operation goes ahead and does most of the talking. The patient herself appears rather anxious and does not say much. The surgeon running the clinic explains the risks and benefits of the surgery, with a view to gaining the patient's written consent to proceed to theatre. Which is the *single* most appropriate way for the surgeon to gain consent for the operation? ★★★

A Ask the husband to give written consent, as he has been the main point of contact

B Ask the patient to give written consent, as she has been given a full explanation

C Ask to talk to the patient on her own before addressing consent

D Postpone gaining written consent until the morning of surgery

E Verbal consent is sufficient if a full explanation has been given

77. A 77-year-old man has a rectal adenocarcinoma and has had his consent taken for an anterior resection. The surgeon has left instructions in the medical notes for the patient to be given bowel preparation the day before the operation. The nursing staff call the junior doctor to prescribe the medication for the patient. Which is the *single* most appropriate preparation to prescribe? ★★★

A Sodium docusate

B Lactulose

C Macrogol (polyethylene glycol 3350)

D Senna

E Sodium picosulfate

78. A 25-year-old woman has noticed a lump in her neck. She is worried about it, as she also thinks she has lost some weight recently. The mass is fluctuant and moves superiorly when she swallows and protrudes her tongue. Which is the *single* most likely anatomical site of the lump? ★★★

A Arising from the jugular lymph sac

B Inferior to the angle of the mandible

C Midline below the hyoid bone

D Superior to the carotid bifurcation

E Upper third of the sternocleidomastoid

79. A 47-year-old man has a sudden onset of upper abdominal pain that radiates into his back. He has vomited six or seven times but now just feels nauseated. His bowels opened normally today, and he has no urinary symptoms. He drinks 30 units of alcohol a week.

T 36.6°C, HR 86 bpm, BP 165/75 mmHg.

His abdomen is soft, but tender, particularly in the epigastric region.

The junior doctor is asked to assess the severity of this man's condition. Which *single* result will be most useful? ★★★

A Amylase

B Creatinine

C Early warning score

D Lipase

E Urea

80. A 22-year-old woman has an emergency bowel resection for a superior mesenteric artery thrombosis. Which *single* diagnostic test is most likely to identify the cause? ★★★★

A Anti-phospholipid antibodies

B Anti-thrombin

C Factor V Leiden

D Protein C

E Protein S

81. A 55-year-old man undergoes a laparoscopic anterior resection. His operation is uneventful, and he has a fentanyl/bupivacaine epidural post-operatively for pain relief, with good effect. He is given low-molecular-weight heparin (LMWH) subcutaneously as thromboprophylaxis. On day 2 post-operatively, he is starting to tolerate oral fluids and eat. The decision is taken to stop the epidural. Which is the *single* earliest time at which the epidural can be safely removed after the dose of LMWH? ★★★★

A Immediately

B 2 hours

C 6 hours

D 10 hours

E 24 hours

82. A 44-year-old woman has chronic pain due to an intra-abdominal malignancy. She currently takes morphine modified-release (MR) 30 mg twice daily and morphine liquid 10 mg, as required, for breakthrough pain (max. every 4 hours). Over the last month, the pain has gradually worsened, such that she now needs to take 10 mg of the morphine liquid regularly every 4 hours. Which is the *single* most appropriate change to her morphine regime? ★★★★

A MR 30 mg twice daily; liquid 20 mg every 4 hours as required

B MR 30 mg twice daily; liquid 20 mg every 1 hour as required

C MR 30 mg twice daily; liquid 40 mg every 4 hours as required

D MR 60 mg twice daily; liquid 10 mg every 4 hours as required

E MR 60 mg twice daily; liquid 20 mg every 4 hours as required

83. A 43-year-old man has abdominal pain, following an endoscopic retrograde cholangiopancreatography (ERCP) and sphincterotomy 2 days ago for a gallstone obstructing his common bile duct. He now has severe pain, which is worse in his right upper quadrant and radiates down into his flank, associated with nausea and vomiting twice this morning.

T 37.5°C, HR 90 bpm, BP 115/75 mmHg.

Sodium 135 mmol/L, potassium 3.5 mmol/L, creatinine 90 micromol/L, amylase 180 U/L.

His abdomen is tender, with guarding throughout the right side.

Which *single* investigation is most likely to confirm the diagnosis? ★ ★ ★ ★

A Abdominal ultrasound scan

B Abdominal X-ray

C Computed tomography (CT) scan of the abdomen

D Intravenous urogram (IVU)

E Magnetic resonance cholangiopancreatography (MRCP)

84. A 38-year-old man attends the preoperative assessment clinic a week before his inguinal hernia repair. He has no past medical history and takes no medications. He smokes ten cigarettes a day and drinks 25 units of alcohol a week.

T 37°C, HR 75 bpm, BP 130/70 mmHg.

The nursing staff asks the junior doctor which preoperative tests need to be done. Which *single* test is recommended preoperatively? ★ ★ ★ ★

A Chest X-ray

B Clotting screen

C Electrocardiogram (ECG)

D Full blood count

E No tests required

85. A 34-year-old woman has had a laparoscopic appendicectomy. The surgeon has resected a moderately inflamed, but not gangrenous, appendix. The abdominal wounds are closed layer by layer. The junior doctor has assisted on a number of laparoscopic operations, and the consultant asks him to close the skin using absorbable sutures.

Which is the *single* most appropriate choice? ★ ★ ★ ★

A Ethilon®

B Monocryl®

C PDS®

D Silk

E Vicryl®

86. A 69-year-old woman underwent a femoral artery aneurysm repair 4 days ago. She has become unwell over the last 48 hours with a cough productive of green sputum.

T 38.5°C, HR 88 bpm, BP 145/86 mmHg.

Sodium 139 mmol/L, potassium 4.1 mmol/L, creatinine 88 micromol/L.

Blood cultures grow multiresistant *Staphylococcus aureus* in both bottles. She is started on vancomycin 1 g intravenous (IV) twice daily. A trough level is taken before the third dose and is found to be 20.4 mg/L (trough level range <15 mg/L). Which is the *single* most appropriate next step? ★★★★

A It is on the borderline of normal limits, so give the 4th dose of 1 g

B No need to repeat the level; give the 4th dose at 750 mg

C Omit the 4th dose, and change the dosing regime to 1 g once daily

D Repeat the level in 12 hours, and change the dosing regime to 1 g every 18 hours

E Repeat the level in 12 hours, and give the 4th dose at 750 mg when in range

ANSWERS

1. D ★ 　　　OHCM 10th ed. → p. 654

The risk of rupture of an abdominal aortic aneurysm (AAA) of <5.5 cm in diameter is <1% per year. Aneurysms obey the Law of Laplace, namely that as a vessel increases in radius, the inward force on the vessel decreases and the aneurysm continues to expand until it ruptures. However, stopping smoking and controlling hypertension is the best way to reduce the rate at which this occurs.

The NHS abdominal aortic aneurysm (AAA) screening programme invites all men at the age of 65 to have an ultrasonograpic assessment of their abdominal aorta. Its introduction stemmed from evidence showing that deaths from ruptured AAAs could be reduced through early detection, appropriate monitoring, and treatment.

→ www.gov.uk/topic/population-screening-programmes/abdominal-aortic-aneurysm

2. A ★ 　　　OHCM 10th ed. → pp. 608, 700

This young man later underwent a laparoscopic appendicectomy for acute appendicitis. The mildly raised bilirubin is a result of Gilbert's syndrome, which has a prevalence of 1–2%. Urinary tract infections are rare in young men, and urinary symptoms can be seen in association with acute appendicitis due to irritation of the bladder.

3. A ★ 　　　OHCM 10th ed. → p. 634

The clues here are: this is a recurrent problem; constant pain, with nausea lasting <6 hours, radiation to the back; and correct demographic. Pain from intermittent obstruction of the biliary tree by gallstones can present with a variety of clinical signs but tends to include an inability to keep still, tachycardia, and tenderness in the upper abdomen with no guarding.

Sufferers of chronic pancreatitis normally live with a degree of pain, which occasionally flares up; they would be unlikely to present for the first time with two separate episodes of very short-lived pain. Hepatitis C is unlikely; if acute, it is often asymptomatic, and if chronic, it is likely to present with a range of associated chronic symptoms. Whilst peptic ulcer disease is a good differential diagnosis, it is more likely to present with ongoing pain that occasionally flares up, rather than two distinct episodes of pain, as in this case.

Renal colic is less likely.

4. E ★ 　　　OHCM 10th ed. → p. 634

The history is suggestive of biliary disease—a woman in her 40s with high cholesterol who has had similar previous episodes. She also has fever, rigors, and mild hypotension, so this is an attack of acute chole-cystitis. Examination of her abdomen would reveal epigastric or right upper quadrant (RUQ) pain. On palpation of the RUQ, she is likely to pause whilst trying to take a deep breath in. This is known as Murphy's sign, which is said to be 97% sensitive for cholecystitis.

Epigastric pain alone can be suggestive of acute pancreatitis. Periumbilical discoloration (Cullen's sign) and flank discoloration (Grey Turner's sign) are seen with retroperitoneal haemorrhage. They can rarely be seen in acute pancreatitis. Rovsing's sign, with pain more in the right iliac fossa than the left when the left is pressed, would support a diagnosis of appendicitis. Loin pain is found in renal or ureteric inflammation (pyelo-nephritis or calculus disease).

5. E ★   OHCM 10th ed. → p. 656

This woman has intermittent claudication caused by arterial disease. The most serious association of this would be an abdominal aortic aneurysm, hence the need to palpate the abdomen. All other options would be helpful in completing the picture, but it is **E** that is the one that simply cannot be missed.

→ guidance.nice.org.uk/CG147/NICEGuidance/pdf/English

6. B ★   OHCM 10th ed. → p. 578

Lower limb paralysis and her severe lung disease put her at a moderate to high risk of deep vein thrombosis (DVT) and make this the most likely diagnosis. Cellulitis is unlikely, as she is afebrile and systemically well. There is no history of malignancy or lymph node biopsies to suggest a risk of lymphoedema, and this would not present acutely. Neither rup-tured Baker's cysts nor thrombophlebitis would cause such widespread oedema.

7. E ★   OHCM 10th ed. → p. 708

An urgent 2-week wait referral should be made in the case of unilateral eczematous skin or nipple change that does not respond to topical treat-ment. In this case, Paget's disease of the breast needs to be ruled out.

→ www.nice.org.uk/guidance/ng12

→ www.nice.org.uk/CG80

8. B ★   OHCM 10th ed. → p. 636

The first thing to note is that this woman is hypotensive and tachycardic—with these vital signs, acute epigastric pain that radiates through to the back is relieved by sitting forward and, if associated with nausea, is highly suggestive of pancreatitis, even in those who do not drink alcohol. In someone presenting like this, it is vital to screen for other possible trig-gers: are they known to have gallstones? Has anyone in their family had them? Do they have high cholesterol/triglycerides (hyperlipidaemia may be responsible for 1–7% of all cases of acute pancreatitis)? If pancreatitis is suspected, then amylase should be sent and an ultrasound scan of the upper abdomen requested.

Weight loss is suggestive of a malignant process; if pancreatic, it would present with painless jaundice. Whilst cholestasis, which increases the risk of developing gallstones, is known to occur in pregnancy, there is no such association with the oral contraceptive pill. Recent foreign travel may cause gastroenteritis, which would be likely to cause diarrhoea, as well as vomiting, and a less serious clinical picture than the one depicted here (though marked dehydration can be a potential consequence of severe gastroenteritis, which may cause a similar physiological picture). Previous surgery raises the possibility of adhesional bowel obstruction, which would present with abdominal distension and pain, vomiting, and reduced bowel movements.

9. C ★   OHCM 10th ed. → p. 612

This woman has features of bowel obstruction. The key to the cause is tenderness of the groin lump. If it were non-tender, this would be less likely to be the cause of her symptoms. Femoral hernias are most common in older women, but inguinal hernias are still more common than femoral hernias in this group.

If there were no lump, then, given the surgical history, adhesions would be the most likely cause of obstruction. Lymphomas can present with enlarged 'rubbery' inguinal lymph nodes, but these are more likely to be painless and non-tender and associated with a range of other symptoms (e.g. malaise, night sweats, low-grade fever). Pancreatic cancer is unlikely to present in this way (it is usually either painless jaundice, epigastric pain, or anorexia and weight loss, depending on the part of the pancreas affected) or to spread to inguinal lymph nodes. Attacks of ulcerative colitis usually present with bloody diarrhoea and abdominal pain, rather than bowel obstruction, and are not typical for this age group.

10. C ★   OHCM 10th ed. → p. 603

This is a fibroadenoma—commonly found in teenagers, with an increased incidence in those on the oral contraceptive pill. It should only be removed if it causes pain or discomfort. It 'never' becomes malignant, but occasionally a lobular carcinoma can involve a fibroadenoma.

11. A ★   OHCM 10th ed. → p. 576

The chart shows a temperature that varies from normal or below normal to well above normal. The fact that this variation happens in a 'swinging' pattern is classically suggestive of a collection of pus. If such a finding leads to the suspicion of an abscess, then the normal course of events is to try to find its location; in this case, this is likely to be fairly straightforward, given the recent surgery. Imaging may be required, along with a course of antibiotics, but the most important step in management is drainage of the pus.

12. C ★   OHCM 10th ed. → p. 657

The length of symptoms and the clinical findings suggest that this woman's leg has suffered irreversible ischaemia. In cases such as this, where blood has stagnated in the arterial tree and clotted (hence the fixed dark blue staining), any attempt to revascularize the limb could be dangerous, as it risks a 'reperfusion injury'.

All other options are inappropriate. Neither the patient's age nor smoking habits should influence management, whilst the fact that she has cancer is a risk for the development of ischaemia in the first place but should not drive how it is treated. In scenarios where patients are said to have cerebral disease, it is tempting to assume they do not have capacity—this is clearly a mistake. In some cases, such as this one, however, palliation may be more appropriate than such aggressive surgical intervention. With a limb ischaemia like this, death will likely occur within days.

13. A ★   OHCM 10th ed. → p. 632

This is a typical description of an anal fissure and can initiate a cycle of: pain—fear to pass stool—constipation—pain. It is often too painful to perform a digital rectal examination, but a visual inspection of the perianal area will exclude other pathologies such as a perianal abscess. A trial of topical treatment, such as glyceryl trinitrate (GTN) or diltiazem ointment, should be considered.

Haemorrhoids do cause the passage of bright red blood, but they are not painful, unless they thrombose and become enclosed by the anal sphincter, causing distal venous engorgement. Proctalgia fugax is an idiopathic cause of an intense stabbing pain deep in the rectum, due to cramping of either the pubococcygeus or levator ani muscles. Pain can be brought on by defecation, but this can also relieve it and there is no associated blood loss. Rectal malignancy may uncommonly present in a young man with bleeding, but also with a range of other symptoms. It is not impossible, given this scenario, but certainly is not the most likely cause here.

14. A ★   OHCM 10th ed. → p. 608

This is as classical a presentation of appendicitis as you could wish for: the migratory nature of the pain (as visceral pain becomes local peritonism), nausea, low-grade fever, and tachycardia (Alvarado score >7, though this scoring system is little used in clinical practice). In female patients, the chief differential diagnosis is an ectopic pregnancy, but this is virtually excluded by a negative pregnancy test. Neither endometriosis nor pelvic inflammatory disease (PID) are likely to cause such rapidly developing clinical pictures, but PID at least would remain an important differential if laparoscopy revealed a macroscopically normal appendix. Other supporting evidence for an acute appendicitis would be a raised white cell count (WCC) and C-reactive protein (CRP).

→ www.biomedcentral.com/1741-7015/9/139

15. D ★

The 'upper outer quadrant' is the 'safe area', avoiding the sciatic nerve and the surrounding vasculature.

16. A ★   OHCM 10th ed. → p. 612

This woman has an incarcerated femoral hernia, and a cough impulse is not always present due to the small size of the femoral canal. The anatomy of the femoral canal is that the anterior border is the inguinal ligament, the posterior border is the pectineal ligament, the medial border is the lacunar ligament, and the lateral border is the femoral vein.

Classically, an inguinal hernia would be superior and medial to the pubic tubercle. A lipoma would be more firm and situated just below the surface of the skin. An enlarged inguinal lymph node would not be fluctuant. A saphena varix is a dilatation of the saphenous vein at its junction with the femoral vein but would disappear on lying down.

17. B ★   OHCM 10th ed. → p. 612

It is likely that this man has ruptured an abdominal aortic aneurysm (AAA). The priority has to be informing a senior member of the appropriate team. The key to management of a ruptured AAA is speed, and a person with decision-making ability needs to be present. This is because the detail of the situation will determine exactly what is necessary for that patient. Surgical assessment therefore must be the priority, and when referring these patients, the immediacy of the situation must be communicated clearly.

There are some situations where an immediate laparotomy may be appropriate, e.g. if a patient is becoming increasingly cardiovascularly unstable. However, the centralization of vascular services has meant that most vascular units have the ability to perform emergency endovascular aneurysm repair (EVAR). The recovery after EVAR is quicker, and the mortality and morbidity risks are lower than with open repairs in the planned setting, though evidence supporting this in the emergency situation is lacking. Computed tomography (CT) will also be able to demonstrate the anatomy of the aneurysm in a clear way to aid operative planning for an open approach. A senior decision-maker needs to ascertain whether performing a CT scan would be safe.

A urinary catheter is required but can be sited at a convenient time, rather than taking precedence over other more important management steps. Other such steps include securing good intravenous (IV) access, sending bloods and cross-matching, fluid resuscitation (often allowing for a degree of hypotension to avoid the risk of dislodging any clot which may have formed), and performing an electrocardiogram (ECG). An ultrasound scan is unhelpful in the emergency situation, as the information required from imaging is rarely obtainable from this modality.

Badger S, Forster R, Blair PH, Ellis P, Kee F, and Harkin DW. Endovascular treatment for ruptured abdominal aortic aneurysm. *Cochrane Database Syst Rev.* 2017;**5**:CD005261.

18. **E** ★ OHCM 10th ed. → p. 581

This is a small bowel obstruction secondary to adhesions from the previous open cholecystectomy procedure (which left the Kocher scar). This means a gallstone (**A**) cannot be the cause of the obstruction. Paralytic ileus (**C**) is more likely to occur in the acute recovery phase following surgery, and pseudo-obstruction (**D**) is like mechanical bowel obstruction with no cause found and usually involves the large bowel (**B**).

19. **C** ★ OHCM 10th ed. → p. 578

This is a common dilemma in the emergency department and requires the doctor to be able to use the Wells score for deep vein thrombosis (DVT) probability accurately. This man scores 4 and is thus in the 'likely' DVT group; as such, it is advised that he is started on a low-molecular-weight heparin, as long as it not contraindicated, whilst waiting for a Doppler ultrasound scan.

If the probability is high enough to warrant a scan, then, in this patient, treatment should be instigated in the interim. There are, of course, some more complex scenarios, particularly in post-operative patients, where the risk of bleeding needs to be weighed up more carefully against the risks of not anticoagulating.

If the Wells score is low, D-dimer should be measured. If normal, DVT can be excluded, and if raised, a Doppler ultrasound scan can be organized. Unfractionated heparin needs to be given continuously intravenously so is not used these days, as most of these patients can be managed on an outpatient basis. Warfarin should not be prescribed alone, as it is initially pro-thrombotic.

→ www.nice.org.uk/guidance/cg144

20. **C** ★ OHCM 10th ed. → p. 763

This man is in acute urinary retention and needs a catheter resited. This is one of the few genuine indications for an acute urinary catheter (the others being severe illness with significant haemodynamic instability, or severe skin breakdown and pressure sores in patients with urinary incontinence). Giving an alpha-receptor blocker at the same time would be useful, as it helps increase the chances of his bladder functioning normally the next time the catheter is removed. With the invention of the 'bladder scanner', patients can be left waiting in severe pain whilst a bladder scanner is found to confirm retention. If the patient is in pain and there is a palpable suprapubic mass with tenderness, do not wait for a bladder scan—just catheterize the patient.

21. **D** ★ OHCM 10th ed. → p. 652

The rapid progression of symptoms is concerning. The time course of the history associated with such severe pain that can be partially alleviated by positioning of the scrotum (Prehn's sign) should always raise the suspicion of torsion and prompt an urgent surgical review.

A tumour is unlikely to present this acutely, nor is a hernia—a strangulated hernia is more likely to present with symptoms of groin pain, with possible symptoms of bowel obstruction. The main differential in these circumstances is usually acute epididymo-orchitis (indeed they can occur together)—this is the most common cause of acute scrotal pain and presents with severe pain and a red, warm, and oedematous testicle. It is said that the most sensitive physical finding for separating the two is the cremasteric reflex (stroking the superior medial thigh causes elevation of the ipsilateral testicle)—in patients with torsion, it is absent; in those with epididymo-orchitis, it is present. However, such a subjective finding should not be relied upon. Torsion is a diagnosis not to be missed, and it is far better to err on the side of caution and explore what turns out to be a normal testis rather than risk missing this key diagnosis.

David JE, Yale SH, and Goldman IL. Urology: scrotal pain. *Clin Med Res.* 2003;**1**:159–60.

22. C ★ OHCM 10th ed. → p. 621

The middle colic artery (and the left colic artery, a branch of the inferior mesenteric artery) supplies the transverse colon.

23. E ★ OHCM 10th ed. → p. 606

Rupture of the spleen is the most common intra-abdominal injury following blunt trauma. It should be suspected in all those who present after such an event with tachycardia and abdominal pain.

Colonic perforation is more common following penetrating trauma of the abdomen but can happen with blunt trauma. Patients with inflammatory bowel disease are more at risk. A haemothorax is possible in such a scenario but unlikely, given his oxygen saturations and respiratory rate, so it is not the primary concern here. Liver injuries must be considered if the right side of the abdomen is more symptomatic. Renal injury can occur in blunt trauma, as the 12th rib compresses against the lumbar spine but would be more likely to present with frank haematuria.

24. B ★ OHCM 10th ed. → p. 612

Something has happened to this man's groin lump. The sudden onset of severe pain is concerning in itself, but the worst-case scenario would be strangulation (i.e. ischaemia of the bowel within the hernial sac). If a hernia that has always been irreducible suddenly becomes the source of severe pain, then strangulation has to be suspected, with an urgent trip to theatre essential. Whilst his bowels not opening suggest the hernia may be causing obstruction, the remaining answers are non-specific. Skin changes over the lump are also a concerning feature.

25. E ★ OHCM 10th ed. → p. 650

A varicocele is a largely asymptomatic and slowly developing testicular lump. It occurs via the same mechanism that leads to varicose veins in the legs. On examination, it can be revealed by asking the patient to stand or strain (anything to increase intra-abdominal pressure). It does not trans-illuminate and, on palpation, feels like a twisted mass (classically a 'bag of worms'). If idiopathic, 98% occur in the left testicle due to the venous drainage system (the left testicle drains via the renal vein, and the right drains directly into the inferior vena cava). If a right varicocele is diagnosed, then there may be concern for a pelvic or intra-abdominal malignancy.

Hydroceles are normally painless, although they can become uncomfort-able if large. They are said to transilluminate, i.e. light shone through one will be visible from the other side. A hernia will normally have a cough impulse, and it will not be possible to get above it when examining the testicles. Spermatoceles are small cystic masses that are separate from the testicle and they often transilluminate. A tumour would feel hard to palpation and may be associated with lymph node enlargement.

26. D ★   OHCM 10th ed. → p. 790

The figures relayed to the doctor are represented by the image shown in Figure 11.2 and are known colloquially as showing the 'Portsmouth sign'. The fact that the systolic blood pressure is falling below the heart rate is a poor prognostic sign and suggestive of shock. It suggests a deteriorating output, and thus end-organ instability, and is demanding of urgent atten-tion. Whilst all options should be of some concern, it is D that would be the hardest to reverse.

27. D ★   OHCM 10th ed. → p. 654

In an older man >55 years presenting with sudden abdominal pain, shock, and confusion, the most important diagnosis that must be ex-cluded is an abdominal aortic aneurysm (AAA).

28. C ★   OHCM 10th ed. → p. 610

This is adhesional small bowel obstruction following previous surgery. Treatment would initially be conservative with 'drip [intravenous (IV) fluids] and suck [nasogastric (NG) tube]'. If this fails, surgical adhesiolysis may be necessary. This is normally done via a laparotomy, but in some cases a laparoscopic approach may be used. A computed tomography (CT) scan may be useful to determine the level of the obstruction, which can aid planning a surgical approach, as well as exclude any other pathology.

High alcohol intake is linked to peptic ulcer disease [as are non-steroidal anti-inflammatory drugs (NSAIDs)] and pancreatitis. Obesity and poor diet increase the risk of gallstones. Foreign travel is associated with gastroenteritis. None of these conditions would present with features of obstruction.

29. E ★   OHCM 10th ed. → p. 656

The peripheral vasodilator licensed for use in intermittent claudication is naftidrofuryl oxalate, a selective antagonist of 5-HT$_2$ receptors. It is only

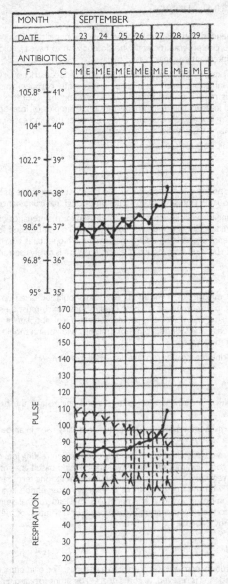

Figure 11.2 Patient observation chart demonstrating 'Portsmouth' sign (pulse higher then systolic blood pressure)
Courtesy of Dr Abhijit Datir.

recommended in those people who have not benefitted from a supervised exercise programme and who do not wish to have radiological or surgical intervention (angioplasty/bypass).

Beta-blockers would increase peripheral vasoconstriction. Calcium channel inhibitors, such as nifedipine, promote coronary vasodilatation, thus reducing myocardial oxygen consumption. Diuretics may be indicated in heart failure and hypertension. Examples of inotropic sympathomimetics are dobutamine and dopamine; they increase contractility of the heart, with little effect on the rate.

→ www.nice.org.uk/Guidance/TA223

30. C ★   OHCM 10th ed. → p. 572

Of the options listed, propofol would be most likely to be used as an intravenous (IV) infusion, from induction through to maintenance.

Desflurane is a volatile anaesthetic agent used for maintenance of anaesthesia. Midazolam is a sedative. Suxamethonium can be used for rapid sequence induction in an emergency setting. Thiopental is a barbiturate which can be used as an induction agent, though it is rarely used anymore.

31. B ★

The vast majority of medications can, and should, be taken up to, and including, the morning of surgery. Medications which must be stopped are warfarin and novel oral anticoagulants. Dual antiplatelet therapy often needs to be stopped, but monotherapy with aspirin should be continued in most cases.

→ emedicine.medscape.com/article/284801-overview

32. E ★   OHCM 10th ed. → p. 632

Conservative treatment with ice packs and analgesia is the treatment of choice.

Banding of haemorrhoids is a procedure regularly used in an outpatient setting.

General measures directed at avoiding constipation (eating lots of fibre, drinking good volumes of water, avoiding codeine-based analgesics, and toileting regularly) are important in the medium to long term but would not help with this acute situation. Emergency intervention in a patient with thrombosed external haemorrhoids can lead to anal stenosis or damage to the sphincter complex as a result of disruption of the normal anatomy by oedema.

33. C ★   OHCM 10th ed. → p. 606

This is acute pancreatitis secondary to gallstones. The pain often radiates to the back and is relieved, to some degree, by sitting forward. His bowel frequency does not add to this diagnosis. The history is not suggestive of bowel obstruction, and it is important not to be thrown by the sentinel loops on the abdominal X-ray. Although it may be nice to know that his hernia is no bigger, epigastric hernias rarely strangulate and pain from such a hernia would be unlikely to radiate to the back. Again, it is useful to know that there has been no haematemesis, but this history is more typical of acute pancreatitis than a gastric ulcer. Malignancy is not a likely cause in such an acute presentation, and therefore knowledge of a family history does not add to the diagnosis.

34. B ★

Recognizing and working within the limits of your competence is hugely important and ultimately protects not only the patient, but also the junior doctor. When the emergency department is busy, it would be tempting to try to aspirate the area (E) or just give her antibiotics and ask her to come back if things worsen (D). However, if you are not sure about the diagnosis, you must ask the patient to wait for a senior doctor review.

→ www.gmc-uk.org/guidance/good_medical_practice.asp

35. E ★   OHCM 10th ed. → p. 607

The causes of abdominal pain in a young woman are numerous. Although pain that localizes to the right iliac fossa should raise the alarm for a potential appendicitis, this woman has not vomited, is afebrile, and has no guarding or rebound tenderness (and none of the examination findings listed is specific to appendicitis). Mesenteric adenitis should be considered if other causes have been excluded (or deemed very unlikely) in the setting of a recent coryzal illness and palpable lymph nodes.

Cervical excitation is suggestive of a gynaecological pathology. Murphy's sign suggests acute cholecystitis. Renal angle tenderness suggests pyelonephritis. The presence of soft stool in the rectum is most likely to be a normal finding consistent with many diagnoses!

36. D ★

Lidocaine 1% means there is 1 g of lidocaine in 100 mL, or 10 mg/mL. The maximum dose the woman can have is 150 mg, which equates to 15 mL.

37. C ★

In busy jobs, this can happen. If the notes are not readily available, as the post-take surgical team are motoring from ward to ward, then even the speediest junior doctor is going to have trouble keeping up. Often the best approach in the absence of notes is to have a clear sheet of paper to hand and to record the consultation ready to go into the notes when they surface. If, however, as in this case where a record of the consultation simply was not made anywhere, then common practice is to admit as much by marking the entry relating to the consultation as 'retrospect', including the time to which it refers and the time at which it is eventually being written.

38. E ★ OHCM 10th ed. → p. 634

A simple ultrasound scan will detect gallstones. Biliary colic is the most likely cause of this woman's discomfort. Few patients with symptomatic gallstones are able to adequately control their symptoms with dietary changes alone. There is an increasing drive to perform cholecystectomy during the index admission to prevent further and frequent readmissions, though the availability of such a service is variable.

Hepatobiliary iminodiacetic acid (HIDA) scans are rarely used now but can aid the diagnosis of functional gall bladder problems, whilst endoscopic retrograde cholangiopancreatography (ERCP) and magnetic resonance cholangiopancreatography (MRCP) are used for diagnostic evaluation and therapeutic interventions in the pancreaticobiliary duct systems.

→ www.augis.org/wp-content/uploads/2014/05/Gallstone-disease-commissioning-guide-for-REPUBLICATION-1.pdf

39. D ★ OHCM 10th ed. → p. 568

An individual's capacity to make a decision may fluctuate or be temporarily affected by factors such as pain, fear, confusion, or the effects of medication. To respond to this, the surgical team in this case need to understand that assessment of capacity must be time- and decision-specific.

→ www.gmc-uk.org/guidance/ethical_guidance/consent_guidance_ac-cessing_capacity.asp

40. C ★ OHCM 10th ed. → p. 568

The man is shown to not have capacity for this decision and therefore cannot consent. If a patient lacks capacity, a decision must be made in their best interests. His next of kin cannot give informed consent, unless they have Power of Attorney for health and welfare or have been awarded Court of Protection deputyship for health matters. The team need to sign a form stating this, with one of them acting as proxy consent giver explaining why the procedure is necessary, but it is good practice to involve the next of kin in the decision-making. Most hospitals now have a range of different types of consent forms available and include forms which the doctor will sign as proxy when a patient does not have capacity to make decisions (typically called consent form 4). The guidance applies to emergency and elective situations.

→ www.gmc-uk.org/guidance/ethical_guidance/consent_guidance_making_decisions_patient_lacks_capacity.asp

41. B ★ OHCM 10th ed. → p. 636

This is most likely to be acute pancreatitis, probably due to gallstones. The sudden onset of the pain, which can radiate into the flanks and/or back, is a very different presentation to that experienced with appendicitis or small bowel obstruction. The fact that the pain is relieved by sitting forward points towards pancreatitis over mesenteric ischaemia or a perforated duodenal ulcer, all of which can present with sudden-onset epigastric pain.

42. C ★   OHCM 10th ed. → p. 648

The symptoms of an overactive bladder include urinary urgency with or without urge incontinence, frequency (>8 times in 24 hours), and nocturia (>2/night). There are many causes and contributing factors, but it is usually due to involuntary contractions of the bladder's detrusor muscle. The main class of drug therapy is anticholinergics (Ach), which cause bladder contraction, although their use is limited by significant side effects, which may be less prominent with the newer ones but nevertheless cause problems, particularly in frail older adults. Solifenacin is one example. Older agents like oxybutynin should be avoided now.

Desmopressin is used to treat children with primary nocturnal enuresis. Finasteride and tamsulosin are used in treating benign prostatic hypertrophy. Trimethoprim would be inappropriate, as there is no suggestion that the symptoms are infective in origin.

43. C ★   OHCM 10th ed. → p. 612

Femoral hernias are more common in middle-aged and elderly women. Because of the rigidity of the canal borders, femoral hernias are at high risk of strangulation. Emergency surgical repair is indicated.

Spigelian hernias occur through the linea semilunaris at the lateral edge of the rectus abdominis. They are often hard to detect clinically. Inguinal hernias are found superior and medial to the pubic tubercle. They are the most commonly occurring abdominal wall hernia. The femoral artery is found at the mid-inguinal point, which is the mid-point of a line between the anterior superior iliac spine and the pubis. It is important to differentiate between this and the mid-point of the inguinal ligament, halfway between the anterior superior iliac spine and the pubic tubercle, which indicates the deep inguinal ring.

44. D ★   OHCM 10th ed. → p. 632

The most likely cause of this man's symptoms is haemorrhoids. When assessing causes of rectal bleeding, it is important to distinguish between anorectal-type bleeding (bright red, fresh blood, separate from the stool) and colonic bleeding (dark or altered blood, mixed in with the stool). However, a flexible sigmoidoscopy is indicated to exclude other more serious pathology, before embarking on treatment of the haemorrhoids.

The predominant symptom from anal fissures is normally pain. Angiodysplasia is the most common vascular abnormality of the gastrointestinal tract but is found most commonly on the right, meaning a presentation with fresh bleeding is unlikely. They become increasingly common with age. A caecal cancer will be more likely to present as a change in bowel habit or iron deficiency anaemia. Ulcerative colitis would be unlikely to present in a man of this age but would normally be associated with a significant change in bowel habit.

45. D ★   OHCM 10th ed. → pp. 250, 618

This man most likely has oesophageal adenocarcinoma and should be referred for an oesophagogastroduodenoscopy (OGD) under the 2-week wait referral pathway for suspected cancer. Smoking is a significant risk factor.

Achalasia is an oesophageal motility disorder characterized by failure of the lower oesophageal sphincter to relax. Symptoms can be intermittent. It affects men and women equally and typically presents in middle age. Diagnosis can be confirmed through barium swallows or oesophageal manometry studies. Gastric tumours often present non-specifically with symptoms, including increasing dyspepsia, weight loss, vomiting, and iron deficiency anaemia. Dysphagia may be a prominent symptom, but less commonly than with oesophageal tumours. Globus, the sensation of a lump in the throat, can be differentiated from dysphagia by careful history taking. Scleroderma or systemic sclerosis is an autoimmune connective tissue disorder, affecting women more commonly than men. It can cause oesophageal dysmotility, though it is unlikely to present with this before other manifestations of the condition.

→ www.nice.org.uk/guidance/ng12/chapter/1-Recommendations-organised-by-site-of-cancer#upper-gastrointestinal-tract-cancers

46. C ★★   OHCM 10th ed. → p. 578

This woman had an acute attack of diverticulitis. This was treated with intravenous (IV) antibiotics and analgesia. A colonoscopy is not carried out during the acute phase, due to the risk of perforation, but when settled would demonstrate diverticulae—mucosa herniating through the colonic wall where the anterior and posterior branches of the marginal artery enter. These are very common with increasing age. Friable mucosa bleeding on contact is seen in ulcerative colitis. A large ulcerated lesion is most likely to be a carcinoma, whereas multiple pedunculated polyps are seen in polyposis syndromes. Patchy ulcerated fissures are characteristics of Crohn's disease.

47. E ★★   OHCM 10th ed. → p. 572

As this man is having emergency surgery, he has not been able to empty his stomach, unlike elective patients who have been prepared by remaining 'nil by mouth'. To prevent aspiration of gastric contents into his respiratory tract, 'rapid sequence induction' must be carried out using a fast-acting depolarizing neuromuscular-blocking agent such as rocuronium.

Bupivacaine and lidocaine are agents used for local or regional anaesthesia. Dantrolene is a treatment for malignant hyperpyrexia. Propofol can be used for induction of anaesthesia in both elective and emergency cases or for maintenance of anaesthesia in elective cases.

48. B ★★ OHCM 10th ed. → p. 656

The symptoms described sound like the pain of intermittent claudication that is caused by atherosclerotic limb ischaemia. However, in a young person with no risk factors, there is likely to be another pathology at play. The most likely of these is something relatively benign such as popliteal artery entrapment syndrome in which malformation of the gastrocnemius muscles leads to vascular compromise (either congenital or acquired—as can happen due to overgrowth in some athletes). This in itself is rare and not important—what is important is the lateral thinking that is required when dealing with common symptoms occurring in uncommon patient groups. It would be all too easy to tell this man to lose weight, improve his diet, and lower his blood pressure, whilst missing what may be a very treatable cause of his problems.

Vasculitis rarely causes limb ischaemia. Buerger's disease (thrombophlebitis obliterans), due to inflammation and thrombosis of the arteries, typically afflicts young heavy smokers. Nerve impingement would cause compromise only in the distribution of the affected nerve. A healthy non-smoker is unlikely to suffer from atherosclerosis, particularly at such a young age, which makes this option unlikely.

49. B ★★ OHCM 10th ed. → p. 572

In order to reverse the block, the anaesthetist has to select an agent that will increase the amount of acetylcysteine at the neuromuscular junction. The anticholinesterase neostigmine will do just this but has to be given with glycopyrronium to minimize its muscarinic side effects (such as build-up of secretions and bradycardia).

Atracurium and suxamethonium are both agents that block the neuromuscular junction. Sevoflurane is a volatile agent used for maintenance of anaesthesia, whilst thiopental can be used in induction.

50. D ★★ OHCM 10th ed. → p. 611

This man has post-operative ileus and needs to be treated by the 'drip and suck' regimen with intravenous (IV) fluids to rest the bowel and a nasogastric tube to decompress the stomach (which, in this case, is splinting his diaphragm and making it difficult for him to breathe).

51. C ★★ OHCM 10th ed. → p. 756

In any patient who becomes unwell after a procedure, it must always be initially assumed that the deterioration is a result of a complication of the procedure. In any patient who has had a bowel resection, an anastomotic leak, with a resulting intra-abdominal collection, must be the primary concern.

There is a high risk of basal pneumonia in such a scenario, but it is not the most likely cause, particularly with the normal oxygen saturations. Cholecystitis is a potential cause, but again not the most likely. However, it must be remembered that there is a risk of acalculous cholecystitis in any patient who has been acutely unwell or who has suffered a significant physiological insult, such as occurs during major surgery. The normal urinalysis makes any renal pathology unlikely.

52. A ★★   OHCM 10th ed. → p. 608

Appendicitis is the most common surgical emergency. However, it does not always present with typical migratory periumbilical-to-right iliac fossa pain. The position of the appendix determines the symptoms and signs produced, and this can mimic other diagnoses. This woman has right iliac fossa pain, nausea, vomiting, and tachycardia—although the history does not sound 'classical' (indeed, it is a reasonable history for gastroenteritis), in patients with right iliac fossa tenderness, it is always important to think of appendicitis.

53. E ★★   OHCM 10th ed. → p. 259

Despite not touching the patient, the doctor must clean his hands with soap and water because *Clostridium difficile* is spread by spores and cannot be 'washed' off with alcohol gel.

54. B ★★   OHCM 10th ed. → p. 616

Although many of these can be associated with both conditions, including severe anaemia as a result of haemorrhoids, a change of bowel habit should alert you to other pathologies and warrants further investigation.

55. A ★★   OHCM 10th ed. → p. 656

There are very few contraindications to compression stockings, but it is important to think before prescribing them to everyone. The two categories to be wary of are unstable cardiac failure and peripheral arterial disease. Those with no evidence of acute heart failure and an ankle–brachial pressure index (ABPI) >0.8 are safe to use high-pressure compression [indicated as therapy for ulcers of vascular aetiology, rather than venous thromboembolism (VTE) prophylaxis]. Those with an ABPI >0.5 but <0.8 should use low-pressure compression (into which category come most anti-VTE disease stockings or bandages), whilst those with an ABPI <0.5 or evidence of acute heart failure should be managed with leg elevation and no compression.

56. C ★★   OHCM 10th ed. → p. 373

The patient should have the *Haemophilus influenzae* type B (HiB), pneumococcal, and meningococcal C vaccines, before leaving hospital (this should ideally happen 14 days before surgery but is obviously not possible in emergency cases such as this). The pneumococcal vaccine should be repeated every 3–5 years. In addition to this, she should be commenced on penicillin V 500 mg twice daily as continual prophylaxis against encapsulated bacteria.

Davies JM, Lewis MP, Wimperis J, Rafi I, Ladhani S, and Bolton-Maggs PH. Review of guidelines for the prevention and treatment of infection in patients with an absent or dysfunctional spleen: prepared on behalf of the British Committee for Standards in Haematology by a working party of the Haemato-Oncology task force. *Br J Haematol.* 2011;**155**:308–17.

57. C ★★   OHCM 10th ed. → p. 628

This is an acute attack of diverticulitis affecting the sigmoid colon. The patient describes previous episodes with alternating constipation and diarrhoea, and pain in the left iliac fossa. Such a chronic history may be common to both coeliac disease and irritable bowel syndrome (but clearly not gastroenteritis), but the acute presentation is not typical for either. If this altered bowel habit were to continue for 6 weeks, this woman would warrant an urgent referral to surgical outpatients for suspected cancer.

58. E ★★   OHCM 10th ed. → p. 636

This man has an excessive alcohol intake and a likely recent admission for pancreatitis. This all points towards the diagnosis as being a pseudocyst where fluid pools in the lesser sac, the cavity posterior to the stomach and adjoining omentum.

Ascites causes generalized abdominal fullness, rather than a localized mass, whilst a liver abscess is unlikely to be felt as a mass at all. This man may indeed have hepatomegaly, but this is likely to be chronic and would not explain his acute medical problems. Gastric volvulus is more likely to present with vomiting and upper abdominal pain.

59. A ★★   OHCM 10th ed. → p. 568

The fact that a person has a mental illness does not mean they automatically lack capacity. A capacity assessment is vital. Those who are shown to have capacity can make decisions to refuse treatment, even if those decisions appear irrational to the doctor or may place the patient's health or their life at risk. Detention under the Mental Health Act can only be done if he is deemed not to have capacity. The next of kin cannot give consent on behalf of a patient, though it is very important to involve them in the decision-making process.

→   www.gmc-uk.org/guidance/ethical_guidance/consent_guidance_contents.asp

60. B ★★   OHCM 10th ed. → p. 638

This is a classical presentation of a renal stone. Good preventative advice would be to drink plenty of fluids and avoid certain foods, depending on the stone's biochemical make-up, e.g. oxalate levels are increased by chocolate, spinach, tea, and rhubarb. Whilst cutting down on alcohol binges is generally good lifestyle advice, in this particular situation, the main benefit is through remaining hydrated. Following a low-fat diet should be recommended for people with symptomatic gallstones.

61. A ★★   OHCM 10th ed. → p. 576

This patient most likely has a post-operative collection. This would explain her fever and high white cell count. Liver function tests are often slightly deranged after cholecystectomy, due to hepatocyte damage intraoperatively. An ultrasound scan would be able to identify a collection and also assess the biliary tree to ensure there is no intra- or extra-hepatic duct dilatation suggesting a bile duct injury, without subjecting her to the radiation from a computed tomography (CT) scan.

An abdominal X-ray would add little to the diagnosis, as there is no suggestion of obstruction. A CT pulmonary angiogram (CTPA) would be useful, should a post-operative pulmonary embolus (PE) be possible, though again this is not suggested by the history. The interventional nature of an endoscopic retrograde cholangiopancreatography (ERCP) means it carries far higher risks than the other investigations here and should not be used first line. It is most useful post-cholecystectomy for treatment of a confirmed bile leak. Magnetic resonance cholangiopancreatography (MRCP) is useful when a retained stone is suspected.

62. D ★★   OHCM 10th ed. → p. 628

This woman has had an acute attack of diverticulitis. This should be initially treated 'conservatively' with analgesia and intravenous (IV) antibiotics. A computed tomography (CT) scan would be useful and would most likely show fat stranding and the diverticulae in the colon and rule out perforation and abscess. A colonoscopy should not be carried out acutely, due to the risk of perforation. There is no evidence that patients with uncomplicated diverticulitis should be kept nil by mouth, and increasingly ambulatory management pathways with no dietary restrictions are being employed.

Jackson JD and Hammond T. Systematic review: outpatient management of acute uncomplicated diverticulitis. *Int J Colorectal Dis* 2014;**29**:775–81.

63. B ★★   OHCM 10th ed. → p. 644

This patient has a urinary tract malignancy, until proven otherwise, and requires an urgent referral to the urologists. Macroscopic haematuria can be associated with renal, bladder, and prostate tumours. Whilst imaging will be required, further investigations, such as cystoscopy, will also be indicated. It is more appropriate to refer to a specialist who can organize all the required investigations simultaneously.

A prolonged course of levofloxacin is the treatment for acute prostatitis, the presentation of which is characterized by pain. Trimethoprim is often the first-line treatment for uncomplicated urinary tract infections (UTIs), which again would not typically present with painless macroscopic haematuria.

→ www.baus.org.uk/_userfiles/pages/files/Publications/BAUS%20Cancer%20Guidelines%20Summary.pdf

64. E ★★★   OHCM 10th ed. → p. 616

In those over the age of 60 years, a history of fresh rectal bleeding of >6 weeks' duration should not be attributed to diclofenac (which would not cause fresh bleeding anyway) or haemorrhoids. Regardless of whether there is any change in bowel habit, an urgent referral should be made for the patient to be seen within 2 weeks in a surgical outpatients clinic. Guidance states that, when referring, all that is required is an abdominal and a rectal examination and a full blood count, so as not to delay specialist assessment.

National Institute for Health and Care Excellence (2017). *Suspected cancer: recognition and referral*. NICE guideline [NG12].

→ www.nice.org.uk/guidance/ng12

65. B ★★★   OHCM 10th ed. → p. 616

Anyone aged 40 years and older who reports rectal bleeding with a change of bowel habit towards looser stools and/or increased stool frequency persisting for 6 weeks or more should be urgently referred. The history in this case—although suspicious of a sinister cause—is only of 4 weeks' duration. Pending a review at 6 weeks, a full blood count should be taken to detect any anaemia present, ready for an urgent referral to surgical outpatients if things do not settle.

National Institute for Health and Care Excellence (2017). *Suspected cancer: recognition and referral*. NICE guideline [NG12].

→ www.nice.org.uk/guidance/ng12

66. E ★★★   OHCM 10th ed. → p. 571

Metal clips can start to come out between 10 and 14 days after the operation. Earlier removal risks wound breakdown. Patient factors which have an impact on wound healing, such as age, malignancy, smoking, and steroid use, should be considered. Metal clips are useful for skin closure when there is a high risk of wound infection, as it is possible to remove clips beforehand, if necessary, to allow any infection to drain.

67. C ★★★　OHCM 10th ed. → p. 568

As displayed by the surgeon's notes, this lady lacks capacity to make an informed decision. In other words, she cannot understand information relevant to that decision, she cannot retain it, she cannot weigh it up as part of the process to make a decision, and she is unable to communicate any decision.

Any act done to this woman or decision made on her behalf must be done or made in her best interests. If, after considered discussion with the patient and/or relatives/carers/attorneys, the surgeon feels that to proceed to theatre would be in her best interests (and this decision is not based on her age, appearance, or behaviour), then there can be said to be 'sufficient compliance' with the Mental Capacity Act 2005.

It may be reasonable for the woman's family to talk through the options with her, but they cannot be asked to persuade her (indeed, as she is lacking capacity, even should they persuade her, the consent would be invalid). Equally, the next of kin cannot make decisions on her behalf, unless they have been granted a Lasting Power of Attorney covering medical issues specifically. Psychiatric opinion is unlikely to be useful in such a situation where capacity is clearly lacking. It would be wrong for the surgeon to accept a decision from a patient whom it has been demonstrated is unable to make decisions—however, if the surgeon were to decide that conservative management, rather than surgery, was in her best interests, that is another matter. Palliation may, in fact, be the most appropriate course of action in this situation. It can also be useful to engage a geriatrician in the decision-making process, if possible.

→ www.gmc-uk.org/guidance/ethical_guidance/consent_guidance_making_decisions_patient_lacks_capacity.asp

68. A ★★★　OHCM 10th ed. → p. 533

In the palliative care setting, syringe drivers are given subcutaneously. The total daily dose of oral morphine is converted into a dose of subcutaneous diamorphine by dividing this by 3. Diamorphine is used in preference to morphine because of its greater solubility, when compared with morphine. This means that larger doses can be put into the syringe driver, should they be required.

69. B ★★★

The pain in the left shoulder could be attributed to the fractured clavicle. However, taking into account the mechanism of injury and bruising to the left posterior ribs, a splenic injury must be considered. Management of trauma is very important, and a rational approach must be consistently used. The most appropriate way to assess this patient is with a whole-body or trauma computed tomography (CT) scan, which includes the vertex to mid thigh. This is always indicated in adult patients with blunt major trauma and suspected or potential multiple injuries.

→ www.nice.org.uk/guidance/ng39

70. D ★★★ OHCM 10th ed. → p. 660

The scenario describes what sounds like a perianal infection. Whilst nausea and vomiting suggest systemic upset and the need for treatment, it is the association of diabetes and perianal infection that would be most concerning. This is because of the strong link between diabetes and the very serious necrotizing infections that can arise as complications of peri-anal abscesses. Fournier's gangrene is a polymicrobial necrotizing fasciitis of the genital, perianal, or perineal areas. The classical symptoms are severe pain, swelling, and fever. It most often affects those with systemic disease—20–70% of those who get Fournier's gangrene have diabetes. It is a surgical emergency, requiring prompt treatment in the form of anti-biotics and appropriate drainage, as well as wide debridement.

Whilst a family history of colorectal cancer or previous haemorrhoids would be red herrings in this scenario, non-resolution after a course of antibiotics would be concerning, as it suggests that this may be more than just a standard case of cellulitis.

Thwaini A, Khan A, Malik A, et al. Fournier's gangrene and its emergency management. *Postgraduate Med J*. 2006;**82**:516–19.

71. D ★★★ OHCM 10th ed. → p. 350

Development of a deep vein thrombosis (DVT) whilst on heparin should prompt investigation of heparin-induced thrombocytopenia (HIT). This is more common with unfractionated heparin, but it can develop, although much less commonly, with prolonged low-molecular-weight heparin (LMWH) therapy. Most commonly, this is after 5–10 days. Although the platelet count drops, this disorder is pro-thrombotic, with venous thromboembolism being about four times as common as arterial.

Heparin can also inhibit aldosterone secretion, and hence cause hyperkalaemia. Patients with diabetes mellitus, chronic renal failure, acid-osis, and raised potassium or who are taking potassium-sparing drugs seem to be more susceptible. The Committee on Safety of Medicines (CSM) recommends that baseline and regular measurements of potas-sium should be made in those at risk or those receiving therapy for >7 days.

→ emedicine.medscape.com/article/1357846-treatment

72. D ★★★ OHCM 10th ed. → p. 657

This woman has suffered an acute vascular event, causing ischaemia of her left hand. The two main causes of limb ischaemia are embolic (30%) and thrombotic (60%). This woman has three features that make an embolus the likely cause: sudden onset of symptoms (hours), upper limb affected (thromboses rarely occur in the upper limbs), and a fibrillating heart. Examination reveals a white hand, which suggests that the occlu-sion is recent, as there has not been time for the arterial tree to come out of spasm and allow deoxygenated blood into the tissues, turning them purple. Sensory deficit means the limb is in danger and in need of emergency surgery.

All other options are used to treat thrombotic ischaemia. Heparin is used, pending investigations prior to reperfusion therapies such as bypass or angioplasty, with amputation clearly a last resort for an irreversibly ischaemic limb.

73. A ★★★   OHCM 10th ed. → p. 270

All options would provide useful information regarding this man's diagnosis, which is almost certainly a pancreatic tumour. Whilst endoscopic retrograde cholangiopancreatography (ERCP) is likely to be necessary to treat his obstructive jaundice, it is important to perform a staging computed tomography (CT) scan prior to instrumentation of the biliary tree. This is because inflammatory change around the inserted stent can make assessment of the resectability of the tumour less accurate.

→ www.bsg.org.uk/resource/bsg-guidelines-for-the-management-of-patients-with-pancreatic-cancer-periampullary-and-ampullary-carcinomas.html

74. D ★★★   OHCM 10th ed. → pp. 190, 576

The history is suspicious of bowel cancer. Further to this, the woman has had an episode of chest pain associated with low oxygen saturations and tachycardia. A pulmonary embolism (PE) is top of the differentials. She should be given therapeutic low-molecular-weight heparin (LMWH), whilst investigations are organized to confirm the diagnosis. It is reasonable to start with a chest X-ray to exclude other pathologies, though a computed tomography pulmonary angiogram (CTPA) will be needed to confirm the diagnosis. D-dimer is sensitive, but not specific, and a negative result cannot be relied upon to exclude a PE in a high-risk patient. Ventilation/perfusion (V/Q) scans have largely been replaced by CTPA, though they are sometimes still used in pregnancy.

75. A ★★★   OHCM 10th ed. → p. 630

Although not proven, the most common cause for pilonidal abscesses is thought to be an ingrowing hair. Appropriate initial management is incision and drainage. A course of antibiotics is normally required.

76. C ★★★   OHCM 10th ed. → p. 568

A patient's consent to a particular treatment may not be valid if it is given under pressure or duress exerted by another person.

This patient's husband cannot consent on her behalf. Before accepting a patient's consent, you must consider whether they have been given the information they want or need, and how well they understand the details and implications of what is proposed. This is more important than how their consent is expressed or recorded. Although consent is often obtained on the day of the operation, in this situation, it could leave the woman (who may not want the operation) in a situation where she feels she cannot now avoid it. Verbal consent is inappropriate in the elective setting. If a patient is unable physically to sign the form, a witness must sign for them.

→ www.gmc-uk.org/guidance/ethical_guidance/consent_guidance_ ensuring_decisions_are_voluntary.asp

77. E ★★★

This is available in combination with magnesium oxide (in the commercially available Picolax®). Preoperative bowel preparation often differs between surgeons and local protocols. Those who use Picolax® believe that the bowel should be emptied before the operation, whilst others believe that use of this preparation, instead of a phosphate enema, increases the risk of an anastomotic leak due to the spill of bowel contents. The use of bowel preparation prior to surgery depends very much on the surgeon, so always check what each individual wants for their patients. The other laxatives on the list are all useful in the gradual softening of stool and are thus more often employed as laxatives, rather than in bowel preparation.

78. C ★★★   OHCM 10th ed. → p. 598

A fluctuant mass that rises on swallowing and protrusion of the tongue is a thyroglossal cyst. These grow in the midline between the isthmus of the thyroid and the hyoid bone. They are normally asymptomatic but can cause anxieties, as in this case, and so are resected surgically.

Cystic hygromas arise from the jugular lymph sac. A submandibular salivary stone would cause a lump inferior to the angle of the mandible. A branchial cyst arises from the upper third of the sternocleidomastoid. Carotid body tumours arise from superior to the carotid bifurcation.

79. C ★★★   OHCM 10th ed. → p. 636

This man presents with symptoms of acute pancreatitis. The modified Glasgow score used to be used to assess the severity of presentation and as a prognostic guide. However, increasingly, evidence demonstrates that the early warning score is a far more useful prognostic indicator than the Glasgow score.

Jones MJ, Neal CP, Ngu WS, Dennison AR, and Garcea G. Early warning score independently predicts adverse outcome and mortality in patients with acute pancreatitis. *Langenbecks Arch Surg.* 2017;**402**:811–19.

80. A ★★★   OHCM 10th ed. → pp. 374, 554

Anti-phospholipid syndrome significantly increases the risk of venous and arterial thrombosis. The other diagnostic tests are predictive of an increased risk of venous thrombosis.

→ emedicine.medscape.com/article/333221-overview

81. D ★★★

Placement or removal of an epidural catheter should be 10–12 hours after the last dose of low-molecular-weight heparin (LMWH) thromboprophylaxis. If the patient is receiving a treatment dose of LMWH, this time should be extended to 24 hours. Following removal, subsequent LMWH should be given no sooner than 4 hours. These precautions reduce the chances of developing epidural haematomas.

→ www.aagbi.org/sites/default/files/rapac_2013_web.pdf

82. E ★★★★   OHCM 10th ed. → p. 533

If the as-required morphine liquid is being used as regularly as this for as long as this, then the regime needs to be rethought. To do this, the amount of as-required liquid (10 mg/4 hours = 60 mg) taken daily should be added to the amount of modified-release (MR) (60 mg) to give a total daily dose (TDD = 120 mg). The new dose of MR can be calculated by dividing the new TDD by 2 (= 60 mg). The new as-required liquid dose can be calculated by dividing the new TDD by 6 (= 20 mg).

83. C ★★★★   OHCM 10th ed. → p. 742

Although post-endoscopic retrograde cholangiopancreatography (ERCP) pancreatitis is common, this man's amylase level is normal and the pain distribution is not typical. He has, in fact, perforated his duodenum following the sphincterotomy. A computed tomography (CT) scan would be the best modality, as it would show a collection and free air in the retroperitoneal space. He has guarding as a result of peritoneal inflammation caused by the retroperitoneal collection.

84. E ★★★★

The National Institute for Health and Care Excellence (NICE) recommendations are available for recommended preoperative tests. This man is an American Society of Anesthesiologists (ASA) grade 1 or a 'normal healthy patient'. The surgery he is awaiting is graded as grade 2 (intermediate). The recommendations suggest that no tests are required.

National Institute for Health and Care Excellence (2016). *Routine preoperative tests for elective surgery*. NICE guideline [NG45].

→ www.nice.org.uk/guidance/NG45

85. B ★★★★   OHCM 10th ed. → p. 571

The majority of surgical skin incisions are closed with an absorbable suture in a subcuticular plane. Monocryl®, which absorbs in approximately 3 weeks, is the most appropriate choice. As a monofilament, the risk of wound infection is lower than with braided sutures.

Ethilon® (nylon) is a non-absorbable monofilament, which is most commonly used to repair hernias which are too small to require mesh repair.

PDS® is an absorbable monofilament but absorbs more slowly, over approximately 9 weeks, and is therefore more appropriate for bowel anastomoses. Silk is non-absorbable and is used most commonly for securing drains. Vicryl® is a braided suture which is most commonly used for layered fascial closure. It is absorbed over approximately 4–5 weeks.

86. E ★★★★   OHCM 10th ed. → p. 756

The dose that is due should be omitted, and the level should be repeated 12 hours later, when, with normal renal function, it should be in range. At this point, a reduced dose can be give. Intravenous (IV) vancomycin therapy requires monitoring to ensure efficacy and minimize toxicity. Vancomycin has linear kinetics, so a proportional reduction in dose should yield similar results in the level. A dose of 750 mg twice daily will ensure an adequate trough level that will be for an effective bactericidal agent. Vancomycin activity is time-dependent, with anti-microbial activity depending on the length of time vancomycin is above the minimum inhibitory concentration of the organism.

Chapter 12

Clinical chemistry

Dan Furmedge

With so many tests available and increasingly fast laboratory processors, there is a growing temptation to request large numbers of blood tests on each and every patient. What we should remember is that they should be used as an adjunct to the history and clinical examination. Test results should reinforce the likely diagnosis and rule out our differentials, rather than be used to try and make the diagnosis per se.

What makes things easier is to know how serum biochemistry and homeostasis are regulated and then to consider a number of questions:

- Which hormones are involved in the control of this electrolyte?
- What happens when these are increased or decreased?
- Does the patient have any renal or hepatic impairment?
- Are they taking any drugs that might be affecting serum electrolyte levels?
- Have they taken an overdose?
- Is the patient dehydrated/hypovolaemic/hypoxic?

It can seem daunting at first when results come back unexpectedly out of range. They must be considered in combination with the patient's clinical status; if the numbers just do not fit, then repeat the test—they may not be right.

However, there are a few 'unmissable' electrolyte derangements that need to be dealt with immediately. Once detected, they should trigger the thoughts shown in Table 12.1.

Interpreting serum values is important, but to prevent iatrogenic derangement, careful use and prescription of intravenous fluids are also needed. Does a patient who looks hypovolaemic, has a low blood pressure, and is tachycardic need crystalloids or blood? Colloids, such as 'Gelofusine®' or 'Volplex®', are now largely out of date, with evidence

Table 12.1 Issues to consider when faced with abnormal biochemistry

Deranged serum level	Issues to consider	Check
Sodium	Patient dehydrated? Oedematous? Drugs?	Urine sodium Urine osmolality
Potassium	In keeping with clinical picture or repeat sample?	Urea and electrolytes (U&Es), 12-lead ECG
Calcium	Is the albumin normal?	U&Es, phosphate, and alkaline phosphatase

not supporting their use. Are they frail or do they have cardiac failure and therefore require cautious replacement? Do they have liver failure? Is their fluid balance so critical that close fluid monitoring in a level 2 critical care setting required? Gone are the days when central venous lines are used on the wards for fluid balance. This chapter will help consideration of the whole picture before putting pen to paper and (potentially) wrongly prescribing 4 L of fluids a day for a frail older man with left ventricular failure.

Another incredibly useful test are blood gases. There are occasions when an arterial sample is needed, but otherwise the majority of information can be gleaned from a venous sample. It is one of the most useful tools available and invaluable in an emergency, particularly when there is little history available or the patient is very unwell. Hydration status, oxygenation (arterial blood gases), acid–base balance, and response to the treatment being given can be easily followed using this test. This is another unmissable area that needs to be comprehensively understood for the examination room and emergency room alike.

QUESTIONS

1. A 28-year-old woman has been short of breath for 12 hours and feels generally unwell. An arterial blood gas is taken:

pH 7.50, PaCO$_2$ 3.2 kPa, PaO$_2$ 8.8 kPa, base excess −0.2 mmol/L, bicarbonate (HCO$_3$) 18.0 mmol/L.

Which is the *single* most likely diagnosis? ★

A Diabetic ketoacidosis

B Methanol overdose

C Panic attack

D Pulmonary embolus

E Vomiting

2. A 66-year-old woman has had pain in her left thigh for the past 6 months. She is slightly unsteady on her feet and has begun to limp.

Haemoglobin (Hb) 111 g/L, white cell count (WCC) 5.5 × 10^9/L, platelets 230 × 10^9/L.

Calcium 2.55 mmol/L, phosphate 1.0 mmol/L, alkaline phosphatase (ALP) 455 IU/L.

Which is the *single* most likely cause of this woman's symptoms? ★

A Chronic myeloid leukaemia

B Lymphoma

C Osteomalacia

D Osteoporosis

E Paget's disease

3. A 50-year-old man has vomited blood. He has had an urgent endoscopy and band ligation of oesophageal varices and is recovering in hospital. He is haemodynamically stable and is nil by mouth post-procedure. He is receiving intravenous (IV) fluid therapy:

Sodium chloride (saline) 0.9% 1 L/8 hours.

Glucose 5% 1 L/8 hours.

Sodium chloride (saline) 0.9% 1 L + 20 mmol potassium chloride/ 8 hours.

The medical registrar crosses out the above regimen and explains to the junior doctor he has made a mistake. Which is the *single* most likely explanation of the junior doctor's mistake? ★

A The patient already has raised total body sodium and needs dextrose instead

B The patient has suffered losses and needs more rapid replacement

C The patient is likely to be hypoglycaemic and needs more sugar infused

D The patient is likely to be hypokalaemic and needs more potassium

E The patient is likely to be oedematous and should be fluid-restricted

4. A 72-year-old woman is being treated for a urinary tract infection. The laboratory rings the ward with some urgent blood results: sodium 140 mmol/L, potassium 6.8 mmol/L, creatinine 95 micromol/L, urea 4.2 mmol/L.

Which is the *single* most appropriate next step? ★

A Calcium chloride 10% 10 mL intravenous (IV)

B Calcium resonium 15 g oral (PO) three times daily

C Electrocardiogram (ECG) and repeat sample

D Glucose/insulin infusion

E IV sodium chloride (saline) 1 L/4 hours

5. A 66-year-old man has noticed tingling around his mouth for the past few weeks. It was very subtle at first but has become increasingly apparent. He also feels tired, unmotivated, and low in mood. He has type 1 diabetes and uses regular non-steroidal anti-inflammatory drugs (NSAIDs) for osteoarthritis and gout. Which *single* examination finding is most likely to support the diagnosis? ★

A Carotid bruit

B Neck goitre

C Nystagmus

D Parotid gland swelling

E Twitching facial muscles

6. A 62-year-old man is recovering after an emergency hemicolectomy for a ruptured appendix abscess. On the second day after surgery, the registrar asks for potassium to be added to the man's intravenous (IV) fluid therapy.

Day 2 fluid balance:

- In: 3100 mL

    - Hartmann's IV 3000 mL
    - Water oral (PO) 100 mL

- Out: 3450 mL

    - Urine 1400 mL
    - Stoma 1800 mL
    - Abdominal drain 180 mL
    - Vomit 50 mL

Which is the *single* most likely reason the registrar has made this request? ★

A Due to excessive blood loss

B Due to high output from the stoma

C Prophylaxis against further vomiting

D Standard after every colectomy

E Standard if the fluid regimen is Hartmann's

7. A 64-year-old man has felt unwell for the past 5 days. He has been nauseated and has had sweats and shakes at night. He has hypertension and had a metallic mitral valve replacement 2 years ago.

T 37.9°C, HR 110 bpm, BP 85/60 mmHg.

He is clammy and cold peripherally. His abdomen is tender in the right upper quadrant.

Which is the *single* most appropriate next step? ★

A Give a STAT dose of intravenous (IV) gentamicin prior to any further action

B Only start broad-spectrum IV antibiotics if T >38°C

C Start empirical treatment with broad-spectrum IV antibiotics

D Start empirical treatment with broad-spectrum oral antibiotics

E Take multiple blood cultures prior to starting any antibiotics

8. A 72-year-old woman has had muscle cramps for the last hour. She feels dizzy and weak. She has been receiving furosemide 80 mg intravenous (IV) twice daily for an exacerbation of congestive cardiac failure.

T 35.6°C, HR 100 bpm, BP 100/75 mmHg.

She has decreased tone in all four limbs. Which *single* management option would be most likely to improve this woman's symptoms? ★

A Digoxin 500 micrograms IV

B Potassium chloride 10 mmol/hour IV

C Quinine sulfate 300 mg oral (PO) once every night

D Sotalol 80 mg PO twice a day

E Spironolactone 25 mg PO once a day

9. A 43-year-old man has severe epigastric pain with radiation to his back and three episodes of vomiting. He has recently returned from a stag party in Eastern Europe. He looks unwell.

T 36.9°C, HR 120 bpm, BP 107/74 mmHg, RR 18/min, SaO₂ 96% on air.

Which of the following blood tests is the *single* most likely test to confirm the diagnosis? ★

A Amylase

B B-type natriuretic peptide (BNP)

C CA19-9

D Gamma-glutamyl transpeptidase (GGT)

E Troponin

10. A 94-year-old woman fell and was found on the floor by her daughter. It is unclear how long she had been on the floor but was last seen well 4 days previously.

Urea 18 mmol/L, creatinine 257 micromol/L, potassium 6.1 mmol/L, sodium 127 mmol/L.

Which of the following blood tests is the *single* most likely test to explain the cause of this lady's acute kidney injury? ★

A Cortisol

B Creatinine kinase

C C-reactive protein (CRP)

D Lactate dehydrogenase

E Troponin

11. A 76-year-old man has become increasingly confused over a 24-hour period. In the 4 or 5 days prior to this, he has felt lethargic and weak but had a very powerful thirst. He is well known to the palliative care team at the hospital for the management of his multiple myeloma. Which would be the *single* most important step in management from the following options? ★ ★

A Bendroflumethiazide 2.5 mg oral (PO) once daily

B Calcium gluconate 10% 10 mL intravenous (IV) over 2 min

C Dexamethasone 8 mg PO twice daily

D Glucose 10% 200 mL IV STAT

E Pamidronate 30 mg IV over 3 hours

12. A 54-year-old woman with a history of rheumatoid arthritis and who is a current smoker is referred for a dual-energy X-ray absorptiometry (DEXA) scan by her general practitioner (GP) who feels she is at high risk for osteoporosis.

Which *single* cause from the following additional options is most likely to increase this lady's osteoporosis risk further? ★ ★

A Body mass index (BMI) 32

B Human immunodeficiency virus (HIV)

C Hypothyroidism

D Ischaemic heart disease

E Type 2 diabetes

13. A 72-year-old man has felt increasingly lethargic over the last week. He ran out of his prescription tablets around 10 days ago and comes to the emergency department with shortness of breath.

T 36.9°C, HR 85 bpm, BP 137/87 mmHg, SaO$_2$ 95% on air.

Capillary refill time (CRT): 2 s, jugular venous pressure (JVP) 4 cm, normal skin turgor, bilateral pedal oedema.

Serum sodium 124 mmol/L, urine sodium 18 mmol/L.

What is the *single* most likely cause of his hyponatraemia? ★ ★

A Addison's disease

B Diuretic therapy

C Heart failure

D Nephrotic syndrome

E Syndrome of inappropriate antidiuretic secretion (SIADH)

14. A 69-year-old man has a third episode of pain and swelling in his right first toe. Each time, the symptoms have improved with a short course of non-steroidal anti-inflammatory drugs (NSAIDs).

Urate: 624 mmol/L.

What is the *single* most likely contributing factor? ★★

A Allopurinol

B Bendroflumethiazide

C Febuxostat

D Lamotrigine

E Levetiracetam

15. A 60-year-old man attends a private health screening. He is asked to return to discuss some abnormalities in his blood results.

Haemoglobin (Hb) 131 g/L, white cell count (WCC) 6.4 × 10⁹/L, platelets 350 × 10⁹/L, mean corpuscular volume (MCV) 102 fL.

Urea 4.6 mmol/L, creatinine 100 micromol/L, sodium 134 mmol/L, potassium 4.1 mmol/L.

Bilirubin 15 micromol/L, alanine aminotransferase (ALT) 30 IU/L, alkaline phosphatase (ALP) 120 IU/L, gamma-glutamyl transpeptidase (GGT) 147 IU/L.

What is the *single* most likely explanation for these blood results? ★★

A Alcohol excess

B Gallstones

C Hepatitis B infection

D Primary biliary cholangitis

E Primary sclerosing cholangitis

16. A 19-year-old woman is being treated for severe pyelonephritis with co-amoxiclav and gentamicin.

She received her first dose of gentamicin 24 hours ago at 5 mg/kg.

T 38.9°C, HR 120 bpm, BP 96/67 mmHg, RR 18/min, SaO₂ 97% on air.

Urea 4.2 micromol/L, creatinine 72 micromol/L.

Gentamicin level: 1.7 mg/L.

What is the *single* most appropriate next course of action? ★★

A Give the next dose of gentamicin now at 3 mg/kg

B Give the next dose of gentamicin now at 5 mg/kg

C Hold the next dose and repeat gentamicin level in 12–24 hours

D Repeat gentamicin level immediately

E Stop gentamicin

17. An 84-year-old woman reports feeling muddled, generally unwell, and with yellow vision in the last 48 hours. She has recently been started on furosemide for leg swelling.

Her other medications include allopurinol, aspirin, calcium and colecalciferol, digoxin, phenytoin, rivaroxaban, and simvastatin.

Which blood test is the *single* most likely to reveal the cause for her symptoms? ★★

A Calcium

B Digoxin level

C Factor Xa level

D Phenytoin level

E Rivaroxaban level

18. A 32-year-old man is started on a course of chemotherapy for acute lymphoblastic leukaemia. Two days after his first dose of chemotherapy, he becomes unwell and is admitted to hospital following a seizure.

T 37.2°C, HR 85 bpm, BP 140/75 mmHg.

Which *single* biochemical finding is most consistent with the diagnosis? ★ ★ ★

A Hypercalcaemia

B Hyperuricaemia

C Hypokalaemia

D Hypomagnesaemia

E Hypophosphataemia

19. An 82-year old woman has a fall at home. A plain X-ray of her pelvis confirms a fracture of the left femoral neck. She has a left dynamic hip screw inserted and is discharged after 12 days of rehabilitation.

Sodium 137 mmol/L, potassium 4.0 mmol/L, creatinine 229 micromol/L, estimated glomerular filtration rate (eGFR) 20, vitamin D 89 nmol/L.

What is the *single* most appropriate bone protection agent for this woman? ★ ★ ★

A Alendronic acid

B Denosumab

C Strontium ranelate

D Teriparatide

E Zoledronic acid

20. A 56-year-old man is brought to the emergency department (ED) with a tonic–clonic seizure. This resolves with rectal diazepam, but he has a further 3-minute tonic–clonic seizure. His partner who attends with him reports confusion, dizziness, and unsteadiness over the last 48 hours. The biochemistry technician calls the ED resus with his sodium result: sodium 112 mmol/L.

What is the *single* most appropriate course of action? ★ ★ ★

A 0.45% sodium chloride

B 0.9% sodium chloride

C 1.8% sodium chloride

D 5% dextrose and 0.9% sodium chloride

E Hartmann's solution

ANSWERS

1. D ★   OHCM 10th ed. → p. 670

This woman has become acutely breathless. She is hypoxic and, as a reflex to this, is hyperventilating (as evidenced by the low $PaCO_2$—there is increased excretion of carbon dioxide via increased respiration). As a result, she has developed respiratory alkalosis.

Diabetic ketoacidosis and methanol overdose are both causes of metabolic acidosis (with a raised anion gap). Panic attacks can cause acute alkalosis via hyperventilation (and therefore low $PaCO_2$ and a high pH) but tends to happen in the absence of hypoxia, rather than as a response to it (as in pulmonary embolism). The symptoms of a panic attack would also be unlikely to persist for 12 hours. Vomiting causes metabolic alkalosis (i.e. a high pH with a high bicarbonate).

2. E ★   OHCM 10th ed. → p. 685

This is Paget's disease of the bone. An increase in bone turnover, followed by remodelling, bone enlargement, deformity, and weakness is typical—though often Paget's does not present in such a classical way. Calcium and phosphate are normal, with a markedly raised alkaline phosphatase (ALP), reflecting high bone turnover. An important differential not listed would be a sarcoma, and plain X-rays would be needed initially of the affected area. The other options would not cause the symptoms and an isolated ALP rise which has been described.

3. A ★   OHCM 10th ed. → p. 667

Given his diagnosis of oesophageal varices, this man most likely has liver failure, and therefore a total body sodium excess. Saline fluid therapies should therefore not be used in such patients, where possible (unless urgently required as an emergency), to reduce the risk of worsening ascites and oedema. He is haemodynamically stable so does not need urgent rapid replacement. There is nothing to suggest he is hypoglycaemic or hypokalaemic, and in fact, if he has ingested blood or been given intravenous (IV) blood products, his potassium may be high. He may be oedematous, but whilst nil by mouth, he should have some maintenance fluid—this should be carefully calculated in the context of a careful fluid balance examination.

4. C ★   OHCM 10th ed. → p. 674

Her potassium level is clearly raised, and if electrocardiogram (ECG) changes were present, this would merit emergency treatment with calcium chloride or calcium gluconate. The most worrying findings would be decreased or absent P waves, PR-interval prolongation, widened QRS, atrioventricular dissociation, or tall tented T waves. However, a high serum potassium level with a normal creatinine level raises the possibility that the sample has haemolysed, and therefore, the sample should be repeated. Other causes for pseudohyperkalaemia are prolonged tourniquet time, the sample taking a long time to get to the lab, a 'drip-arm' sample taken whilst potassium-containing fluids are being infused, or secondary to thrombocytosis (raised platelets).

Calcium gluconate/carbonate does not reduce the potassium level. It protects the cardiac membrane, and an improvement in ECG findings demonstrating temporary stabilization of the myocardium is often seen within a few minutes. It can be repeated multiple times, if needed. Calcium resonium is a polystyrene resin that binds potassium in the gut, although it does have a slow (2-hour) onset of action and can cause faecal impaction. Soluble insulin (10 U) and 50 mL of 50% glucose shift potassium into the cells and can be repeated, but blood glucose should be monitored. Simple sodium chloride is unlikely to have much effect on the overall potassium concentration.

5. E ★   OHCM 10th ed. → p. 678

This is a vague and rather uncommon presentation but is a useful reminder of some important physiology. Although the current complaints may seem disparate and benign, the clue lies in the past medical history—this man has insulin-dependent diabetes and gout and uses high-dose anti-inflammatory medications. He is almost certain to have a degree of chronic renal impairment and, as a result, some filtration imbalances. The tingling around his mouth is perioral paraesthesiae, which, in combination with depressive symptoms in someone with renal impairment, is suggestive of hypocalcaemia. The examination findings that illustrate this deficit are: Trousseau's sign and carpopedal spasm, in which the wrist flexes and the fingers are drawn together in response to occlusion of the brachial artery, and Chvostek's sign in which facial muscles twitch in response to tapping over the parotid, revealing neuromuscular excitability due to low calcium.

A carotid bruit is a non-specific finding, which can indicate an occlusive atheromatous plaque in the carotid arteries which can be a risk factor for stroke and transient ischaemic attack (TIA). A thyroid goitre may support a putative diagnosis of hypothyroidism, which could present with symptoms of lethargy and depression, as here, but would not cause the distinctive perioral tingling. Nystagmus alone is a non-specific finding, suggestive mainly of cerebellar disease, vestibular dysfunction, or thiamine deficiency in prolonged alcohol use. Parotitis can be found in sarcoidosis, chronic alcohol use, or anorexia nervosa; there is no suggestion of that here, the only link being the fact that it is the parotid that is tapped on to elicit Chvostek's sign in hypocalcaemia.

6. B ★   OHCM 10th ed. → p. 674

Just as for a patient who has diarrhoea, potassium depletion is common in the setting of a high output from the stoma and should be monitored closely and replaced. If this continues once oral fluids are introduced and increased, medication to slow down the bowel transit can be used, i.e.

codeine or loperamide. Fluid restriction (1–1.5 L/ day) and regular electrolyte solutions, as part of this restriction, may also be used. It is vitally important when prescribing fluids to remember which electrolytes may be lost. Vomiting, diarrhoea, or a high-output stoma can cause particularly high losses of potassium or magnesium.

7. E ★   OHCM 10th ed. → p. 792

The scenario suggests a patient in septic shock, with the source possibly from the gall bladder/biliary tree. This will need urgent treatment with intravenous (IV) fluids and antibiotics. However, given the history of the metallic valve, there is a chance that any circulating sepsis may have settled here. In order to be able to treat this appropriately, it is vital to take blood cultures before any antibiotics are on board. This is a rule that can be applied generally in the investigation and treatment of infection—culture and then treat. However, as per the Surviving Sepsis campaign, this should be done rapidly to ensure antibiotics have been given within an hour—any further delay is associated with an increase in mortality.

8. B ★   OHCM 10th ed. → p. 674

The symptoms and drug history are suggestive of hypokalaemia. Apart from blood tests, a useful measure in suspected derangement of electrolytes is an electrocardiogram (ECG). There may be no changes, but severe hypokalaemia can cause an 'apparent prolonged QT interval', in which T waves are replaced by U waves, which are bigger and occur later.

If potassium is >2.5 mmol/L and the patient is asymptomatic, it can be treated with oral supplements, but if—as in this case—there are symptoms, treatment should be intravenous (IV) at no more than 20 mmol/hour and not more concentrated than 40 mmol/L. This would always be diluted in sodium chloride, and it is no longer possible to find undilute concentrated potassium outside of a critical care environment due to the risk of causing a cardiac arrest if given too rapidly.

Digoxin may be used to treat atrial fibrillation, with a rapid response, if other agents are not appropriate; quinine sulfate is used as a treatment for chronic muscle cramps; sotalol is an antiarrhythmic drug occasionally used by specialist cardiologists, and spironolactone is a potassium-sparing diuretic—it is not useful in the acute setting of hypokalaemia but is an option in the longer term to try to avoid a repeat episode.

9. A ★   OHCM 10th ed. → p. 688

An amylase >5 times the upper limit of normal is diagnostic of acute pancreatitis, which this man has probably precipitated with an alcohol binge. It can also be raised in severe uraemia, diabetic ketoacidosis (DKA), gastroenteritis, and peptic ulcer disease, but the rise is usually more moderate.

10. B ★   OHCM 10th ed. → p. 688

This lady has fallen and has likely been on the floor for some time. This has caused muscle breakdown and obstruction of the glomeruli by myoglobin, and hence renal failure and acute kidney injury (AKI). A full screen for reasons for this lady's AKI will need to be considered (sepsis, drugs, dehydration, urinary retention, etc.), but a significantly raised creatinine kinase will suggest that rhabdomyolysis is likely to be a significant contributing factor.

11. E ★★   OHCM 10th ed. → pp. 528–9, 676

This man has a malignancy and some neurological (confusion and lethargy) and renal (polydipsia) symptoms of hypercalcaemia. Multiple myeloma is a malignancy typically associated with hypercalcaemia. The speed of onset and the extent of symptoms should prompt treatment with intravenous (IV) fluids, even without knowing the serum calcium level. In the first instance, patients need to be rehydrated before treatment with a bisphosphonate which works by inhibiting osteoclastic bone resorption and has its maximal effect around a week after administration.

Thiazide diuretics are contraindicated in hypercalcaemia, as they increase absorption at the renal tubules. Loop diuretics, on the other hand, inhibit absorption at the loop of Henle, thus increasing urinary excretion of calcium, but—given the need for hydration—they need to be used with caution.

Calcium gluconate is used in the acute management of hyperkalaemia. Dexamethasone is used, among other things, to control the symptoms of raised intracranial pressure caused by cerebral oedema. It may be used, in some cases, to treat hypercalcaemia of malignancy or granulomatous disease such as sarcoidosis but would not commonly be used first line. Whilst it is important to rehydrate, somewhere nearer 4 or 5 L is usually required in the first 24 hours and 0.9% sodium chloride would be the fluid of choice.

12. B ★★   OHCM 10th ed. → p. 683

There are many risk factors for osteoporosis, of which human immunodeficiency virus (HIV) is the only one on this list. Hyper-, not hypo-, thyroidism and a low, rather than high, body mass index (BMI) are risk factors. Type 1 diabetes is a risk factor, not type 2. Ischaemic heart disease is not a risk factor.

Patients with risk factors should undergo risk scoring stratification and should start appropriate treatment if osteoporosis is identified.

13. C ★★   OHCM 10th ed. → p. 672

The history here is one of a patient who usually takes oral diuretics for heart failure and whose fluid overload has worsened since stopping these, causing increased fluid retention and hypervolaemic hyponatraemia.

14. B ★★   OHCM 10th ed. → p. 680

Diuretics (loop and thiazide) are classic culprits for raising urate levels by reducing its excretion from the kidney and therefore contributing to episodes of gout.

Anticonvulsants like lamotrigine and levetiracetam do not affect urate levels. Allopurinol and febuxostat are both treatments for gout prophylaxis and work by lowering urate levels.

Hui M, Carr A, Cameron S, et al. (2017). The British Society for Rheumatology guideline for the management of gout.

→ academic.oup.com/rheumatology/article/56/7/e1/3855179

15. A ★★   OHCM 10th ed. → p. 664

All of the options, except hepatitis B, could cause a raised gamma-glutamyl transpeptidase (GGT) level, but usually in combination with a raised alkaline phosphatase (ALP) level or other non-specific abnormalities in the liver function tests. The additional clue is the raised mean corpuscular volume (MCV), which suggests that alcohol excess is the cause for this man.

16. C ★★   OHCM 10th ed. → p. 756

Gentamicin has high potential for oto- and nephrotoxicity, and levels must be monitored carefully in all patients, especially those with renal impairment. This lady had a correct dose given 24 hours ago and has had a trough level (taken immediately before the next dose is due). Despite her normal renal function, the level is high and it would be dangerous to give further gentamicin at this time. The correct action would be to repeat the gentamicin level in 12–24 hours and, if <1 mg/L, to give a proportionally reduced dose, again checking the level after 24 hours. It is always worth considering when antibiotics can be stopped, but this lady is still clearly septic and without organism sensitivities, it may be unwise to stop at this point without further clinical information and evidence of improvement.

17. B ★★   OHCM 10th ed. → p. 756

Yellow vision (xanthopsia) is characteristic of digoxin toxicity. This is likely to have been precipitated by the recent addition of diuretics to this lady's medication regime. An electrocardiogram (ECG) and a digoxin level would help to confirm the diagnosis. Calcium should be checked in anyone with confusion; phenytoin toxicity does not usually present in this way. Factor Xa and rivaroxaban levels are unlikely to be helpful in this scenario.

18. B ★★★   OHCM 10th ed. → p. 529

Tumour lysis syndrome is associated mostly with poorly differentiated lymphomas (e.g. Burkitt's lymphoma) and the leukaemias acute lymphoblastic leukaemia (ALL) and acute myeloid leukaemia (AML). Combination chemotherapy and steroids trigger the death of large numbers of cancer cells, leading to high potassium, high phosphate, and high uric acid levels, with low calcium levels (which can lead to seizures). This leads to uric acid nephropathy and acute renal failure. The risk of this is usually mitigated by the use of good hydration and drugs such as allopurinol or rasburicase. Occasionally, tumour lysis syndrome can be triggered in a patient who is given high-dose steroids, e.g. for asthma, where there is an underlying undiagnosed lymphoma.

19. B ★★★   OHCM 10th ed. → p. 682

This lady has osteoporosis, as defined by her age, sex, and her fractured neck of femur (classed as a fragility fracture). According to the National Institute for Health and Care Excellence (NICE) guidelines, there is no need to perform further tests to confirm osteoporosis in this group; the advice is to get on and treat. All of the options listed are treatments for osteoporosis. Alendronic acid, often used first line as a weekly oral tablet, is contraindicated due to the poor renal function, as is zoledronic acid which is an annual intravenous infusion. Strontium ranelate is used infrequently now due to a high risk of deep vein thrombosis (DVT). Teriparatide is reserved for severe osteoporosis affecting the spine. Denosumab is an effective monoclonal antibody and is usually the first choice for patients with severe renal impairment—it is given twice yearly as a subcutaneous injection. As with all agents, patients must have their vitamin D replaced if insufficient prior to therapy.

National Osteoporosis Guideline Group (2017). *NOGG 2017: Clinical guideline for the prevention and treatment of osteoporosis.*

→ www.sheffield.ac.uk/NOGG/NOGG%20Guideline%202017.pdf

20. C ★★★   OHCM 10th ed. → p. 672

Hyponatraemia is a very common problem and has a multitude of causes. In most cases, treatment is assessing the underlying cause and treating with fluid restriction, fluids, or other treatment, depending on the cause. In this case, the onset appears to have been rapid and the patient now has serious neurological complications of hyponatraemia—he is having seizures. This is an emergency and one of the few indications for 'hypertonic' saline (1.8% or 2.7% sodium chloride). Giving this is dangerous, due to the possibility of correcting the sodium too quickly and causing central pontine demyelination. Although this is the correct treatment in such an emergency, replacement should be done cautiously, by body weight and in a high dependency environment where response and sodium levels can be monitored frequently.

Eponymous syndromes

*Rudy Sinharay, Doug Fink, Shelly Griffiths, Maria
Phylactou, Ricky Sinharay, Will White, and
Dominik Vogel*

Medicine has long been riddled with diseases and tests named after
things, places, and people. Whilst this can be fun to learn and remember
for pub quiz answers, this can become increasingly difficult and does not
lend itself well to medical education assessment theory which would
class recall of these names as rote learning.

In this chapter, which looks at such syndromes, we have aimed to
cover some of these eponymous syndromes but using their generic features, rather than focusing on their specific historical names.

QUESTIONS

1. A 28-year-old male Russian is admitted to hospital after a drug overdose in prison. He acquired human immunodeficiency virus (HIV) through intravenous drug use 3 years ago and has poor adherence to his anti-retroviral therapy. He is underweight and has stigmata consistent with recent injections. He has multiple violaceous plaques on his face, oral mucosa, and legs. He has a detectable viral load, and his CD4 count is 396 cells/microlitre.

What is the *single* most likely cause of his skin lesions? ★

A Bacillary angiomatosis

B Basal cell carcinoma

C Idiosyncratic drug reaction

D Kaposi's sarcoma

E *Mycobacterium tuberculosis*

2. A 78-year-old man with a history of heavy smoking is seen in the ambulatory care clinic. He is concerned he is having a stroke. On examination, he has miosis of his right eye and a partial right-sided ptosis. His hands are nicotine-stained and he is clubbed.

What is the *single* most appropriate next investigation? ★

A Chest X-ray

B Computed tomography (CT) head

C Doppler ultrasound of carotid arteries

D Lumbar puncture

E Magnetic resonance imaging (MRI) of whole spine

3. A 54-year-old Chilean woman comes to the United Kingdom to visit her daughter. She was born in a small village outside Santiago. She develops severe breathlessness during her flight and presents to the hospital nearest the airport. Clinically, she is in heart failure. Her chest X-ray demonstrates an enlarged cardiac shadow. Her electrocardiogram shows type I second-degree atrioventricular block. She is moved to the cardiology ward for monitoring and consideration of a permanent pacemaker.

Which is the *single* most likely syndrome to be causing this patient's condition? ★★

A Chagas' disease

B Hansen's disease

C Lyme disease

D Machupo virus

E Weil's disease

4. A 23-year-old female presents with several months of intermittent right upper quadrant pain. Blood tests are unremarkable, and an abdominal ultrasound demonstrates multiple calculi within a thin-walled gall bladder. Laparoscopy is performed with a view to proceeding to cholecystectomy, when numerous liver capsule adhesions are identified.

What is the *single* most likely cause of her symptoms? ★ ★

A Budd–Chiari syndrome

B Crigler–Najjar syndrome

C Dubin–Johnson syndrome

D Fitz–Hugh-Curtis syndrome

E Gilbert's syndrome

5. A 27-year-old female presented to the emergency department after coughing up four tablespoons of fresh blood in the last 3 days. As well as feeling generally unwell, she has developed puffy legs in the last week and noted her urine to be dark and frothy. She does not have any other co-morbidities and she is a current smoker. A chest X-ray (CXR) shows bilateral lower zone infiltrates.

HR 98 bpm, BP 181/102 mmHg, RR 20/min, SaO$_2$ 98%.

Urine dipstick: protein +++ blood ++.

Haemoglobin 8.8 g/L, sodium 134 mmol/L, potassium 6.3 mmol/L, urea 29 mmol/L, creatinine 340 micromol/L, albumin 23 g/L.

What is the *single* most likely diagnosis? ★ ★

A Community-acquired pneumonia

B Congestive cardiac failure

C Goodpasture's disease

D Henoch–Schönlein purpura (HSP)

E Immunoglobulin A (IgA) nephropathy

6. A 19-year-old medical student was brought to the emergency department by his flatmate after he was found collapsed on the floor. He had been complaining of a headache, vomiting, and abdominal pain in the days prior to his admission. He had a fever of 39.9°C, a wide-spread non-blanching rash, and photophobia. Kernig's sign was positive.

HR 124 bpm, BP 83/52 mmHg.

White cell count (WCC) 17.8 × 10⁹/L, C-reactive protein (CRP) 269 mg/L, sodium 121 mmol/L, potassium 6.3 mmol/L, urea 13.6 mmol/L, creatinine 98 micromol/L.

A computed tomography (CT) scan of his head did not reveal any space-occupying lesions or acute bleed. He is started on intravenous (IV) ceftriaxone to cover for meningococcal septicaemia, and the medical registrar on call is going to do a lumbar puncture.

What *single* other intervention would prove to be lifesaving in this patient's case? ★ ★

A Aciclovir 10 mg/kg IV

B Dexamethasone 8 mg oral (PO)

C Dextrose 10% 1000 mL over 8 hours

D Hydrocortisone IV 100 mg

E Sodium chloride 0.9% 500 mL IV over 4 hours

7. A 19-year-old woman presents with a 2-week history where her mother noticed increasing unsteadiness on her feet, tremor, and her dropping her keys. In the last 2 days, she had become increasingly drowsy and jaundiced. ★ ★

Haemoglobin (Hb) 78 g/L, bilirubin 248, alkaline phosphatase (ALP) 160, prothrombin time 19.1 s.

Which *single* next investigation is most likely to support the diagnosis?

A Anti-mitochondrial antibodies

B Ferritin levels

C Serum ammonia levels

D Serum copper

E Serum ethanol levels

8. A 32-year-old woman presents to the emergency department with acute-onset wheeze and breathlessness. She says her symptoms have been worsening over the last 3 months and have not improved despite being prescribed a salbutamol inhaler by her general practitioner (GP). She does not smoke, works in a post office, and is originally from India. She has had a recent trip to Kolkata. On examination, she has widespread bilateral wheeze in her lungs. You notice a serpiginous maculopapular rash on her back.

Her chest radiograph shows bilateral infiltrates.

T 37.7°C, HR 96 bpm, RR 26/min, SaO$_2$ 97% on air.

Haemoglobin 12.9 g/L, neutrophils 6.9 × 10^9/L, eosinophils 1.4 × 10^9/L.

What is the *single* most likely diagnosis? ★★★

A Asthma

B Eosinophilic granulomatosis with polyangiitis (Churg–Strauss syndrome)

C Löffler syndrome

D Löfgren's syndrome

E Pulmonary Langerhans cell histiocytosis

9. A 56-year-old man attends the emergency department, complaining of central chest pain worsening on deep inspiration. He is haemodynamically stable and reports having felt unwell for the past 2 days with shivering and sweating. He was discharged a month ago after an ST-elevation myocardial infarction (STEMI), had undergone percutaneous revascularization of his left anterior descending artery (LAD) and has been started on dual antiplatelet therapy with aspirin and prasugrel, as well as bisoprolol, ramipril, and atorvastatin.

What is the *single* most likely mechanism accounting for his condition? ★★★

A Antibody-mediated

B Bacterial

C Drug-induced

D Ischaemic

E Viral

10. A 27-year-old man is referred to the nephrology clinic by his general practitioner (GP) with significant renal impairment (creatinine 240). He has been seen by many doctors in the past due to unexplained abdominal pains, fatigue, and high blood pressure. The nephrologist notes red, painless papules over his buttocks and thighs.

Which *single* investigation is likely to be diagnostic of his underlying condition? ★ ★ ★ ★

A Blood test for alpha-galactosidase activity

B Audiometry

C Echocardiography

D Kidney biopsy

E Ultrasound (US) kidneys, ureters, and bladder (KUB)

11. A 26-year-old man presented to the emergency department with chest pain and was found to have a large right-sided pneumothorax. His history revealed that he currently smokes 20 cigarettes a day. A 12-French chest drain was inserted, but despite applying wall suction at 2 kPa to the drain, the pneumothorax persisted. A computed tomography (CT) thorax was requested and showed small peribronchiolar nodules and multiple irregularly shaped, thin-walled cysts in the upper and mid zones.

What is the *single* most likely diagnosis? ★ ★ ★ ★

A Birt–Hogg–Dubé syndrome

B Desquamative interstitial pneumonia

C Lymphangioleiomyomatosis

D Lymphocytic interstitial pneumonitis

E Pulmonary Langerhans cell histiocytosis

ANSWERS

1. D ★   OHCM 10th ed. → p. 400

The Hungarian dermatologist Moritz Kaposi originally described Kaposi's sarcoma (KS) in Vienna in the late nineteenth century. It is an angioproliferative disorder associated with human herpesvirus 8 (HHV-8). Kaposi described 'classic' KS in older men of Mediterranean or Eastern European heritage which is usually indolent. Acquired immune deficiency syndrome (AIDS)-associated KS can actually occur at any level of immunosuppression, despite a well-preserved T-cell count. However, disseminated and visceral disease is more common with poor human immunodeficiency virus (HIV) control. Bacillary angiomatosis is the main differential diagnosis. It is a bacterial infection, but not typically diffuse or plaque-like. The distribution of lesions would be unusual for basal cell carcinoma. *Mycobacterium tuberculosis* can cause skin lesions, but these are relatively rare. Plaque lesions are not associated with anti-retroviral therapy (ART) drug reactions.

2. A ★   OHCM 10th ed.→ pp. 702, 708

This man has Horner's syndrome (triad of miosis, partial ptosis, and anhidrosis), with central causes (such as stroke, encephalitis, and brain tumours), preganglionic causes such as a Pancoast's tumour, and post-ganglionic causes such as carotid artery dissection. The most likely cause in this case is a Pancoast's tumour situated in the right apex of the lung, as this patient is a heavy smoker with clubbing. The tumour invades the sympathetic plexus in the neck, as well as occasionally the brachial plexus, causing arm pain and weakness. The recurrent laryngeal nerve can also be affected, causing a hoarse voice. A chest X-ray would there-fore be the first port of call to diagnose the patient, followed by further cross-sectional imaging.

3. A ★★   OHCM 10th ed. → p. 423

Chronic Chagas' disease (or American trypanosomiasis) is caused by the protozoa *Trypanosoma cruzi*. It is endemic to large parts of South America and associated with poverty where poor housing offers no pro-tection to the flying triatomine, or 'kissing bug', vectors. Around 25% of untreated individuals seropositive for *T. cruzi* will develop Chagas' car-diomyopathy. This is typically years after infection. Conduction abnor-malities are common in this cohort. Established cardiomyopathy is not thought to be sensitive to anti-trypanosomal therapy. Carlos Chagas was a Brazilian physician in the early twentieth century who originally ob-served the disease in railroad workers working in remote parts of the Amazon region. Hansen's disease is the eponym for leprosy, which is endemic in parts of South America. Lyme disease is a rickettsial infection of the eastern border of North America. Machupo virus is also known as Bolivian haemorrhagic fever. Weil's disease describes the most severe clinical manifestation of leptospirosis.

4. D ★★   OHCM 10th ed. → pp. 696–8

Transabdominal spread of chlamydial or gonococcal infection from pelvic inflammatory disease (PID) results in liver capsule inflammation and the development of numerous string-like adhesions between the liver and anterior abdominal wall. Liver function tests remain normal, and treatment is with antibiotics for PID.

Budd–Chiari syndrome occurs when the hepatic vein is obstructed by a clot or tumour, resulting in congestive ischaemia. As well as right upper quadrant (RUQ) pain, an alanine aminotransferase (ALT) rise is seen due to hepatocyte damage. Crigler–Najjar and Dubin–Johnson syndrome are inherited conditions presenting with jaundice in the first days of life (Crigler–Najjar) or in teenage years (Dubin–Johnson). Gilbert's syndrome is a benign condition presenting with unconjugated hyperbilirubinaemia normally during an unassociated illness.

5. C ★★   OHCM 10th ed. → p. 700

This patient is suffering from a pulmonary–renal syndrome. She has significant haemoptysis and evidence of an acute glomerular nephritis caused, in this case, by anti-glomerular basement membrane antibodies (binding the kidney's basement membrane and alveolar membrane). This is classic of Goodpasture's syndrome.

A. Respiratory infections can cause haemoptysis and an acute kidney injury (AKI) when the patient becomes septic, but they do not usually cause acute glomerulonephritis (note that atypical infections such as *Legionella* occasionally can).

B. Acute pulmonary oedema can cause pink frothy sputum that can appear to be like haemoptysis, and can be associated with an AKI. The patient would, however, be in respiratory failure.

D and E. Both are associated with deposition of immunoglobulin A (IgA) immune complexes and occasionally can cause a pulmonary–renal syndrome. Henoch–Schönlein purpura (HSP) is a small-vessel vasculitis associated with purpuric rashes.

6. D ★★   OHCM 10th ed. → p. 714

This patient has evidence of bacterial meningitis and meningococcal septicaemia. He is also hypotensive, tachycardic, hyponatraemic, and hyperkalaemic. Therefore, the possibility of Waterhouse–Friderichsen syndrome should be considered. This is characterized by adrenal failure following bleeding into the adrenal glands. It is caused by severe bacterial infection. Waterhouse and Friderichsen first described this syndrome in 1911 in a patient who had *Neisseria meningitidis*. However, haemorrhagic adrenalitis due to severe infection has since been associated with a plethora of other pathogens such as *Pseudomonas aeruginosa, Enterococcus coli, Staphylococcus aureus,* and *Streptococcus pneumoniae*. Intravenous (IV) hydrocortisone will, in this case, be a lifesaving intervention.

B. There is evidence that dexamethasone can improve mortality in patients with *S. pneumoniae* meningitis. However, the most pressing step here would be to recognize that the patient is having an adrenal crisis and to proceed to give IV hydrocortisone.

D and E. This patient is shocked and will need fluid resuscitation. This should be given in the form of fluid challenges, as acute boluses, instead of over a few hours.

7. D ★★   OHCM 10th ed. → p. 285

In young patients with abrupt-onset Coombs'-negative haemolytic anaemia, neurological symptoms, and a high bilirubin-to-alkaline phosphatase ratio, think of Wilson's disease. An autosomal recessive disorder that affects the *ATP7A* gene on chromosome 13, it causes retention of copper in the liver and central nervous system (CNS). Investigations show low serum copper, low serum caeruloplasmin, and elevated urinary copper levels, although liver biopsy is often required due to diagnostic uncertainty. Kayser–Fleischer rings are present on slit-lamp examination in around 50%. Treatment acutely is with albumin dialysis, haemofiltration plasmapheresis, plasma exchange, or liver transplantation. Penicillamine acutely has a risk of hypersensitivity.

8. C ★★★   OHCM 10th ed. → p. 704

A cause of pulmonary eosinophilia, named after Wilhelm Löffler, Swiss physician (1887–1972) who first described case histories in 1932. Eosinophils infiltrate the lungs following exposures to allergens that include parasites (*Ascaris lumbricoides, Trichinella spiralis, Fasciola hepatica, Strongyloides, Ankylostoma, Toxocara*) and drugs (sulfonamides, hydralazine, nitrofurantoin). In this case, the likely cause is *Strongyloides*, as the patient has the pathognomonic rash of larva currens. The diagnosis would be confirmed with *Strongyloides* serology/polymerase chain reaction (PCR), and treatment in this case would be with either mebendazole or ivermectin.

B. A rare small- to medium-vessel vasculitis that can present in a similar manner. The presentation is usually that of asthma and paranasal infiltrates. Around 30–40% of patients are antineutrophil cytoplasmic antibodies (ANCA)-positive, particularly perinuclear staining (p-ANCA) positive (anti-myeloperoxidase antibodies).

D. Löfgren's syndrome is an acute form of sarcoidosis that is benign and usually self-limiting. It is characterized by erythema nodosum, bilateral hilar lymphadenopathy (BHL), and polyarthralgia or polyarthritis.

9. A ★★★   OHCM 10th ed. → pp. 154, 698

The combination of pleuritic/pericardial chest pain and recurring fever occurring a few weeks after an acute myocardial infarction is suggestive of Dressler's syndrome—also known as post-myocardial infarction syndrome. It is thought that the underlying mechanism is the formation of autoantibodies against the myocardium after the primary cardiac event.

The presentation is not typical of an acute coronary syndrome (D), but in-stent thrombosis may occur and this needs to be excluded. Apart from the clinical picture, the electrocardiogram (ECG) will provide useful information with more localized signs in left anterior descending artery (LAD) occlusion. Also, pulmonary embolism should be included into the list of differential diagnosis.

Any kind of infection may cause these symptoms, but viral pericarditis (E) or tuberculosis (B) would rather be a coincidence with this history. None of the above drugs are known to cause drug-induced pericarditis (C).

10. A ★★★★   OHCM 10th ed. → p. 698

This gentleman may have Fabry disease, an X-linked lysosomal storage disorder caused by abnormalities in the *GLA* gene, leading to a deficiency in alpha-galactosidase A. This leads to accumulation of glycosphingolipids in the skin (angiokeratomas in the classic 'swimming trunk' distribution), eyes, heart, kidneys, and nerves. Treatment is with enzyme replacement with alpha or beta human galactosidase.

11. E ★★★★   OHCM 10th ed. → p. 704

Pulmonary Langerhans cell histiocytosis usually occurs in young adults (20–40 years of age), and in up to 95% of cases, a history of current or previous smoking is present. Langerhans cells proliferate and form granulomas in the bronchiolar and bronchial epithelium. The resultant fibrosis causes traction on the central bronchiole that becomes cyst-like. Computed tomography (CT) imaging reveals multiple nodules, which may be cavitating, and thin-walled cysts which predominate in the upper and mid zones.

A. This is a genetic multi-system disorder characterized by multiple lung cysts, renal tumours, and cutaneous manifestations such as angiofibromas and perifollicular fibromas. The cysts tend to be multiple and have a predilection for the lower zones.

B. A rare idiopathic interstitial pneumonia that also occurs in those who are heavy smokers. It is associated with diffuse ground-glass changes on CT, with small cystic changes that represent lung fibrosis.

C. This is a rare multi-system disorder that almost exclusively affects women of childbearing age. It can be associated with tuberous sclerosis. CT imaging shows thin-walled cysts of variable sizes, surrounded by normal lung parenchyma, that occur throughout the lungs.

D. This is a benign lymphoproliferative disorder associated with infiltration of lymphocytes into the lungs. It can be indicative of the presence of human immunodeficiency virus (HIV) infection and autoimmune diseases such as Sjögren's. Computed tomography (CT) features include thickening of bronchovascular bundles, interstitial thickening, small pulmonary nodules, and scattered thin-walled cysts with a predilection for mid to lower zones.

Radiology

Rudy Sinharay

You have teased out the history, elicited the signs, and generated a list of differential diagnoses—now to confirm your suspicions, by selecting an appropriate radiological investigation. From the ubiquitous chest X-ray for diagnosing community-acquired pneumonia or congestive cardiac failure to an urgent computed tomography (CT) scan of the brain to confirm a suspected subarachnoid haemorrhage, radiological investigations are an essential (if sometimes overused) resource for diagnosing disease. When working in the acute hospital setting, some knowledge and experience in interpreting X-rays and some types of CT imaging are important in order to ensure your patient is managed correctly and quickly. Going back to basic principles and using your hard-learnt anatomy will set you in good stead when looking at both X-rays and cross-sectional imaging.

This chapter has been written to expose you to clinical situations where imaging is required to make a diagnosis or to make a decision on patient management. As well as this, I hope the questions in this chapter will help you think about what the correct modality of imaging to request would be to investigate pathology in the various body systems. For instance, an ultrasound of the liver may be more useful to assess liver cirrhosis than a CT scan (as well as preventing exposures to high-dose radiation). And again, in practice, if there is any doubt about the result of a radiological investigation, or indeed which type of investigation to request, your local radiologist would be more than happy to help.

QUESTIONS

1. A 26-year-old man has been suffering with a stiff back for the past year. The pain is very low down and especially bad first thing in the morning. He is a keen sportsman and has noticed that the pain eases the more activity he does. Which *single* arrow in the image in Figure 14.1 is most likely to indicate the anatomical origin of symptoms? ★

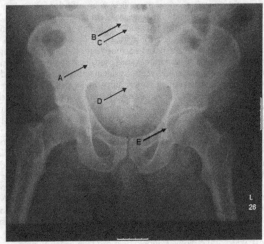

Figure 14.1

A Arrow A
B Arrow B
C Arrow C
D Arrow D
E Arrow E

2. A 62-year-old man has pain in his left knee. It is particularly bad after long days on his feet but is not especially stiff in the morning. He has otherwise been fit and well. An X-ray is arranged (Figure 14.2).

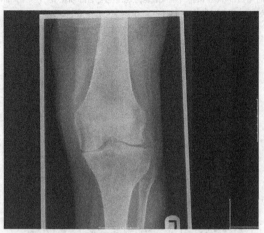

Figure 14.2

Which is the *single* most appropriate initial treatment for his pain? ★

A Celecoxib 100 mg oral (PO) twice daily

B Diclofenac 50 mg PO three times daily

C Glucosamine 1.5 g PO once daily

D Paracetamol 1 g PO four times daily

E Tramadol 50 mg PO four times daily

3. A 37-year-old man has had 12 hours of severe abdominal pain. It comes in waves and is associated with nausea.

He has had this pain once before, but it passed without him having to resort to medical help. His kidneys, ureters, and bladder (KUB) film is shown in Figure 14.3.

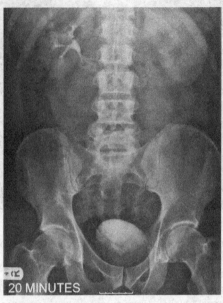

Figure 14.3

Which *single* finding on the image is most supportive of the likely diagnosis? ★

A Calculus at the left vesico-ureteric junction

B Calculus at the right vesico-ureteric junction

C Dilated right pelvic calyces

D Distended bladder

E Right delayed nephrogram

4. A 28-year-old man has had 3 days of abdominal pain. He is vomiting and does not want to eat. He feels the need to belch regularly and has not had his bowels open in 5 days. He suffers with acid reflux and had a laparotomy following a stab wound 3 years previously. He has a distended abdomen that is diffusely tender, with high-pitched bowel sounds. An abdominal X-ray is performed (Figure 14.4).

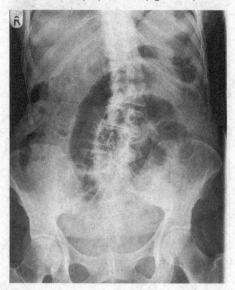

Figure 14.4

T 36.9°C, HR 100 bpm, BP 115/80 mmHg.

Which would be the *single* most appropriate next step in management? ★

A Computed tomography (CT) scan of the abdomen

B Insert a nasogastric tube

C Regular high-dose laxatives

D Urgent colonoscopy

E Urgent laparotomy

5. A 55-year-old woman has had abdominal pain for a week. She has had a total abdominal hysterectomy and an appendicectomy 5 years ago. An abdominal X-ray is performed (Figure 14.5).

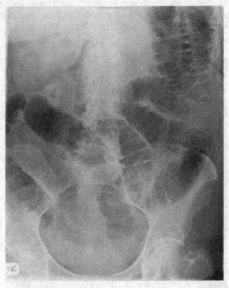

Figure 14.5

T 37.1°C, HR 115 bpm, BP 140/90 mmHg.

Which *single* pair of details from the history would be most likely to support the diagnosis? ★

A Diarrhoea + recent foreign travel

B Dizziness + melaena

C Fluctuating bowel habit + weight loss

D Intermittent constipation + rectal bleeding

E Vomiting + bowels not open for several days

6. A 77-year-old man has had a headache for the past 24 hours. He has vomited and is increasingly drowsy and confused. An urgent computed tomography (CT) scan of his head is performed (Figure 14.6).

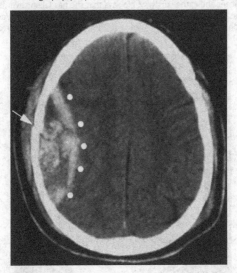

Figure 14.6
Courtesy of Dr James Holt.

Which *single* further detail from the history would be most supportive of the likely diagnosis? ★

A He has had a high fever for several days

B He sustained a head injury 3 days previously

C His level of consciousness has fluctuated for many weeks

D Onset of headache was sudden and devastating

E Reported personality change over the past few months

7. A 75-year-old woman has had a headache for a number of days. She cannot remember when it started but feels that it is getting worse. Her husband reports that she has had intermittent episodes of being vacant and rather drowsy. He says that she has fallen several times in the past few months, and he feels she is unsafe in their current accommodation. A computed tomography (CT) scan of her head is performed (Figure 14.7).

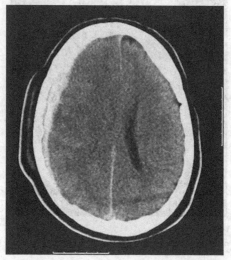

Figure 14.7

Which is the *single* most appropriate next step? ★

A Ceftriaxone 2 g intravenous (IV) STAT

B Contact the neurosurgeons

C Dexamethasone 8 mg oral (PO) STAT

D Lumbar puncture

E Magnetic resonance imaging (MRI) of the brain

8. A 31-year-old man has been increasingly short of breath for the past 3 weeks. He sweats at night, had a non-productive cough, and has lost 5 kg in weight.

T 37.6°C, HR 95 bpm, BP 100/60 mmHg, SaO$_2$ 92% on air (desaturation to 86% on exertion).

He is cachectic and has thick, white patches on his tongue. His chest X-ray is shown in Figure 14.8.

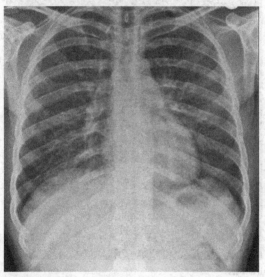

Figure 14.8

Which is the *single* most likely diagnosis? ★★

A Bronchial carcinoma

B Lymphoma

C Pulmonary tuberculosis

D *Pneumocystis jiroveci* pneumonia

E Sarcoidosis

9. A 56-year-old woman has had painful fingertips in her left hand for the past 3 months. She is now finding it difficult to fulfil her duties as a practice nurse. She had a similar episode with the fingers of her right hand 3 years previously (Figure 14.9). There is swelling and tenderness of the distal interphalangeal joints of the first two fingers of her left hand. On the right hand, there are deformities and swellings at the distal interphalangeal joints of the first three fingers.

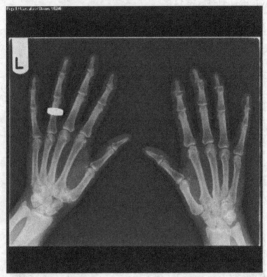

Figure 14.9

Which is the *single* most appropriate treatment? ★★

A Azathioprine 150 mg oral (PO) once daily

B Colchicine 250 mg PO twice daily

C Methylprednisolone 40 mg STAT intra-articular

D Naproxen 500 mg PO twice daily

E Prednisolone 50 mg PO once daily

10. An 80-year-old woman has had intermittent headaches for 6 months. Aside from various aches and pain in her hips, she has hearing loss which has gradually developed after months of tinnitus. Figure 14.10 shows the results of her plain skull X-ray.

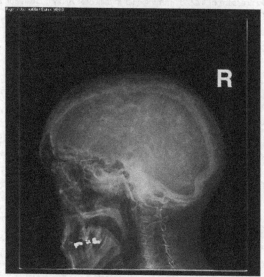

Figure 14.10

Which is the *single* best explanation for the pathological process behind her symptoms? ★★

A Defective osteoclast function leading to increased bone density

B High proportion of uncalcified osteoid and cartilage

C Increased bone turnover with disorganized formation of new bone

D Reduced density of cortical bone

E Reduced density of trabecular bone

11. A 25-year-old woman becomes acutely short of breath 1 week postpartum. On examination, she has mild pitting oedema in both legs, and the left leg is 3 cm larger than the right in circumference. She has a heart rate of 115 bpm, oxygen saturations of 95% on air, and a blood pressure of 122/85 mmHg. Her initial chest X-ray is clear. She has a ventilation/perfusion (V/Q) scan (Figure 14.11).

(a)

(b)

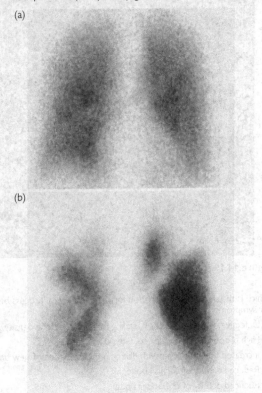

Figure 14.11 (a) Ventilation; (b) Perfusion. Courtesy of Norwich Radiology Department.

What is the *single* most appropriate next step in the patient's management? ★★

A Request an echocardiogram

B Request an ultrasound Doppler of her left leg

C Start antibiotic therapy

D Start diuretic therapy

E Start treatment-dose low-molecular-weight heparin

12. A 65-year-old woman has fallen at home. She has had increasingly regular headaches for several weeks. She has hypertension, type 2 diabetes, and Crohn's disease and takes amlodipine, azathioprine, bendroflumethiazide, metformin, gliclazide, and prednisolone. A computed tomography (CT) head scan is carried out (Figure 14.12).

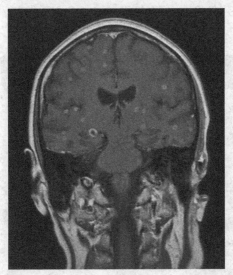

Figure 14.12
Courtesy of Dr James Holt.

Which is the *single* most likely pathological process at the root of this woman's condition? ★★

A Atherosclerosis

B Immunosuppression

C Inflammation

D Malignancy

E Seroconversion

13. A 48-year-old man has developed a non-productive cough. Previously, he felt as if he had 'flu' with aching muscles and general malaise. He is normally fit and well and returned from a trip overseas a week ago. He visited no rural areas and does not remember being bitten by anything.

T 37.7°C, HR 100 bpm, BP 110/75 mmHg, SaO₂ 94% on air.

His chest X-ray is shown in Figure 14.13.

Which is the *single* most likely causative organism? ★★★

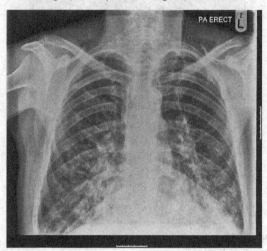

Figure 14.13

A *Chlamydia pneumoniae*

B *Legionella pneumophila*

C *Pneumocystis jiroveci*

D *Staphylococcus aureus*

E *Streptococcus pneumoniae*

14. A 55-year-old woman has been increasingly short of breath for 2 weeks. She has felt feverish and has been coughing up green-coloured sputum for the past 5 days. She smokes ten cigarettes a day and drinks 20 units of alcohol a week.

T 38.8°C, HR 115 bpm, BP 110/65 mmHg, RR 22/min, SaO₂ 91% on air.

Percussion of the chest reveals stony dullness up to the mid zone on the right. Her chest X-ray is shown in Figure 14.14.

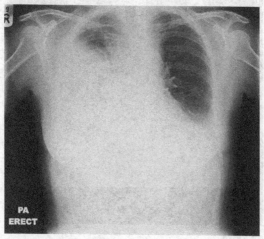

Figure 14.14

Which *single* pathological process is the most likely cause? ★ ★ ★

A Decreased colloid osmotic pressure

B Elevated hydrostatic pressure

C Impaired lymphatic drainage of the pleural space

D Increased capillary permeability

E Passage of peritoneal fluid through spaces in the diaphragm

15. An 82-year-old man has had a productive cough for 3 days and has been even more short of breath than usual. His exercise tolerance is reduced, such that he is breathless, even standing from his chair. His chest X-ray is shown in Figure 14.15.

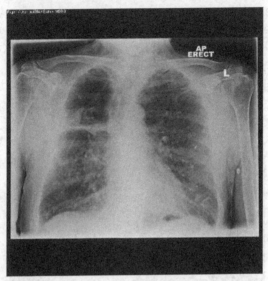

Figure 14.15

Which is the *single* most likely diagnosis? ★★★

A Cor pulmonale

B Exacerbation of chronic obstructive pulmonary disease (COPD)

C Lobar pneumonia

D Pneumothorax

E Reactivation of tuberculosis

16. An 82-year-old woman has been found on the floor of her residential home. She recently has had a painful right knee (Figure 14.16). The knee is warm and tender, with a palpable effusion.

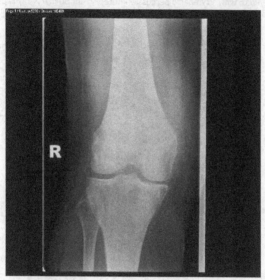

Figure 14.16

T 37.2°C, HR 90 bpm, BP 125/70 mmHg.

Which is the *single* most likely explanation for the effusion? ★ ★ ★

A Degeneration of the articular cartilage and subchondral bone

B Immune reaction to an infectious organism infiltrating the joint

C Inflammatory destruction of the articular cartilage

D Precipitation of calcium pyrophosphate crystals in the joint

E Precipitation of monosodium urate crystals in the joint

17. An 81-year-old woman has had central abdominal pain over the last 24 hours. She usually has difficulty opening her bowels and has been passing minimal flatus for the past 3 days. Her abdomen is distended, with a tympanic percussion note. An abdominal X-ray is performed (Figure 14.17).

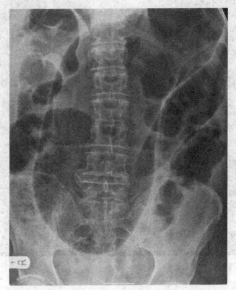

Figure 14.17

T 36.7°C, HR 88 bpm, BP 155/86 mmHg.

Haemoglobin (Hb) 126 g/L, white cell count (WCC) 8.5 × 10⁹/L.

Venous blood gas: pH 7.44, base excess –0.7.

Which is the *single* most appropriate initial management? ★★★

A Barium enema

B Computed tomography (CT) scan of the abdomen

C Flexible sigmoidoscopy

D Laparotomy

E Laxative therapy

18. A 74-year-old woman has had lower abdominal pain and vomiting for 5 days. Her bowels have not opened in this time and she feels extremely bloated. She is in a considerable amount of pain. She takes levothyroxine 100 micrograms oral (PO) once daily. She smokes 20 cigarettes a day and drinks 15 units of alcohol a week. An abdominal X-ray is performed (Figure 14.18).

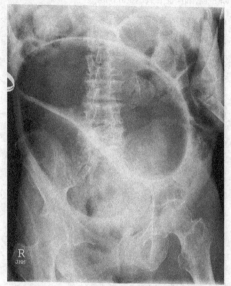

Figure 14.18

T 36.4°C, HR 90 bpm, BP 128/80 mmHg.

Which is the *single* most likely diagnosis? ★★★

A Incarcerated umbilical hernia

B Gallstone ileus

C Perforated duodenal ulcer

D Severe constipation

E Sigmoid volvulus

19. A 68-year-old woman has had central abdominal pain for 3 days. Over the last 12 hours, the pain has become more intense and she has vomited four times. She has not opened her bowels for 2 days.

T 36.4°C, HR 90 bpm, BP 128/80 mmHg.

An abdominal X-ray is performed (Figure 14.19). Her abdomen is distended, with a tympanic percussion note.

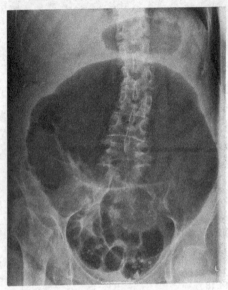

Figure 14.19

Which is the *single* most likely diagnosis? ★★★

A Absolute constipation

B Caecal volvulus

C Incarcerated epigastric hernia

D Perforated gastric ulcer

E Small bowel obstruction

20. A 67-year-old man has had a 15-year history of intermittent chest pain associated with dysphagia. His symptoms are distressing and can be associated with the regurgitation of food. He had an outpatient barium swallow which is shown in Figure 14.20.

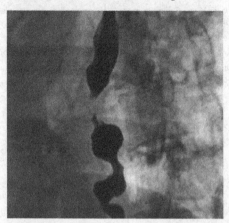

Figure 14.20
Courtesy of Norwich Radiology Department.

What is the *single* most likely diagnosis? ★ ★ ★

A Achalasia

B Benign oesophageal stricture

C Diffuse oesophageal spasm

D Hiatus hernia

E Oesophageal cancer

21. A central venous catheter (CVC) is inserted for central potassium replacement and amiodarone infusion in a patient with severe left ventricular systolic dysfunction, fluid overload requiring intravenous (IV) diuretics, and atrial fibrillation.

Which *single* X-ray finding is most likely to confirm correct placement of the line? ★ ★ ★

A Both ends of the line can be seen

B The line is lying laterally to the upper thoracic transverse processes

C The line tip is between the first and third sternocostal joints

D The line tip is in the midline above the level of the clavicles

E There is no obvious intrapleural air

ANSWERS

1. A ★   OHCM 10th ed. → p. 550

Arrow A is pointing to the sacroiliac joints. Although a plain X-ray may be normal in early ankylosing spondylitis, it is the sacroiliac joints that are first affected—usually the lower half of the joints on the iliac side. For a better image of sacroiliitis, magnetic resonance imaging (MRI) is preferable.

B. This is the lumbar vertebral body.

C. This is the lumbar spinous process.

D. This is the sacral spinous process.

E. This is the sacroischial joint.

2. D ★   OHCM 10th ed. → p. 544

The X-ray shows the classical findings of osteoarthritis: loss of joint space, subchondral bone cysts, and osteophytes. The first-line treatment is regular paracetamol with topical non-steroidal anti-inflammatory drugs (NSAIDs) for the knees and hands. Should this provide insufficient pain relief, oral NSAIDs, opioids, and, if severely affecting function, then joint replacement could then be considered. As shown in Figure 14.21, these 'relatively safe pharmaceutical options' are the next stage after the core treatments (in the central circle) have been considered.

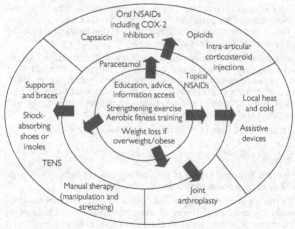

Figure 14.21

National Institute for Health and Care Excellence (2014). *Osteoarthritis: care and management.* Clinical guideline [CG177].

→ www.nice.org.uk/guidance/cg177

3. E ★   OHCM 10th ed. → p. 728

Although all options fit with the history, only **E** is present on the film. It is an intravenous (IV) urogram taken 20 minutes after injection of the contrast dye. Immediately following this infusion, the contrast should be promptly taken up by a normal kidney and would create a distinct outline (or 'nephrogram') on the initial 1-minute film. A well-demarcated kidney on a 20-minute film, as in this case—a 'delayed nephrogram'—is a sensitive indicator of ureteral obstruction and renal function derangement. If the obstruction is acute, the delay is usually only for a few minutes, whilst in long-standing obstruction, the uptake of contrast by the kidney can be 1 hour or longer, leading to a persistently dense nephrogram.

Schwartz DT and Residorff EF (eds) (2000). *Emergency Radiology.* McGraw-Hill: New York, NY.

4. B ★   OHCM 10th ed. → p. 610

This man has a bowel obstruction. His history is very suggestive and is confirmed by an X-ray showing dilated loops of the small bowel. Given his surgical history, the most likely cause is adhesions. The aim in managing the condition is to relieve pressure on the bowel—conservative management will be instigated by passing a nasogastric tube and rehydrating with intravenous (IV) fluids. In most cases, surgery will not be necessary; indeed, the goal is to avoid surgery for fear of producing more adhesions and a cycle of recurrent pain and obstruction.

There is often no need for further imaging in simple adhesional small bowel obstruction, particularly in patients who have had previous episodes. However, computed tomography (CT) may be useful in excluding other more sinister causes of obstruction.

Laxatives would not be helpful in this situation. A colonoscopy will not aid a diagnosis of small bowel obstruction. Surgery is indicated when there is evidence of compromise of the bowel's viability, e.g. in closed-loop obstructions. It is often possible to manage small bowel obstruction through a laparoscopic approach, rather than a laparotomy, with resulting benefits from a minimally invasive approach.

Griffiths S and Glancy D. Intestinal obstruction. *Surgery.* 2017;**35**:157–64.

5. E ★   OHCM 10th ed. → p. 581

From the X-ray and history of previous abdominal surgery, this woman is likely to have bowel obstruction due to adhesions.

Diarrhoea and recent foreign travel would indicate gastroenteritis, which would not cause small bowel obstruction. Melaena is a feature of an upper gastrointestinal bleed. A change in bowel habit and weight loss are suggestive of a colorectal malignancy. Intermittent constipation and rectal bleeding are not specific and can be features of a number of different pathologies.

6. B ★   OHCM 10th ed. → p. 482

The man is showing symptoms of raised intracranial pressure (ICP). The computed tomography (CT) scan shows blood in the extradural space. Typical of this type of bleed is the 'lucid interval', in which consciousness holds steady for several days after the initial insult before the rising ICP takes its toll. Unlike a subdural bleed, extradural bleeds cannot take weeks or months to declare themselves.

A. This could be due to any infective cause.

C. This could occur in a subdural bleed.

D. This indicates a subarachnoid haemorrhage.

E. This may be more suggestive of a space-occupying lesion.

7. B ★   OHCM 10th ed. → p. 482

The history suggests, and the image confirms, the diagnosis of a subdural haematoma. The only immediate course of action for the junior doctor is to ask for a neurosurgical opinion, with a view to carry out a burr-hole procedure to evacuate the clot, if appropriate; many subdurals are managed conservatively. A lumbar puncture (D) would be dangerous in this setting (probable raised intracranial pressure). Steroids (C) would not reduce the raised intracranial pressure (they just reduce oedema around tumours). There is no suggestion of meningo-encephalitis (A), and there is no need for further imaging (E).

8. D ★★   OHCM 10th ed. → pp. 168, 400

The history of a dry cough with exertional dyspnoea and hypoxia is typical, as is the X-ray showing bilateral pulmonary infiltrates. Another clue are the patches on the tongue, which may be *Candida*, an opportunistic infection in immunosuppression. In a man of this age with these two unusual infections, a human immunodeficiency virus (HIV) test is essential.

A. This is unlikely in someone of this age and with no obvious mass lesion on X-ray.

B. Weight loss and night sweats in a young adult should raise the suspicion of a haematological malignancy, but with such an obvious respiratory source, it is unlikely in this case. A more common presentation would be weight loss and night sweats and the finding of a non-tender superficial lymph node.

C. This is probably the best differential, as the weight loss, cough, and night sweats fit, but the exertional dyspnoea does not and the chest X-ray is not typical.

E. Like tuberculosis, this is a granulomatous disease that affects the lungs, but it does not present in this way—breathlessness is not normally the main feature; indeed, it is often discovered incidentally.

9. **D** ★★   OHCM 10th ed. → p. 544

Although osteoarthritis is often thought of as a gradual, benign process, it can be more dramatic and consequently more debilitating. Whilst 'wear and tear' is certainly at the heart of the problem, during the acute phase, there is active synovitis that can be very painful and—as here—cause functional upset.

The X-ray findings are supportive in this case, showing marked degenerative changes in the right hand, with less advanced—but more active—changes in the left. This woman has asymmetrical distal interphalangeal joint deformity, with Heberden's nodes in her right hand. These nodes are no longer painful but will restrict joint mobility. The active inflammation is in her left hand, and for this, she will need a short course of strong non-steroidal anti-inflammatory drugs (NSAIDs), as well as some targeted physiotherapy.

A, C, and E. These are all treatments for inflammatory arthropathies and would not be appropriate in this case.

B. This is most commonly used for the symptomatic relief of gout.

10. **C** ★★   OHCM 10th ed. → p. 685

A history of bone pain, together with hearing deficit, in someone over 65 should prompt you to think of Paget's disease. In essence, Paget's disease is a metabolic bone disorder characterized by cycling osteoclastic and then osteoblastic activity, mainly affecting the axial skeleton, but also the proximal long bones and the skull.

The cycle starts with a lytic phase driven by osteoclasts, resulting in the presence of lucent regions on plain X-rays. This is followed by uncontrolled new bone formation—driven by osteoblasts—that leads to cortical thickening. In the skull—as shown on this woman's X-ray—this results in the classical 'cotton-wool' appearance: demineralized areas on the outside surrounding sclerotic areas on the inside.

Although Paget's disease is often detected incidentally—on blood tests [normal calcium and phosphate, with raised alkaline phosphatase (ALP) levels] or plain X-rays—it can present with musculoskeletal pain and/or neurological or cardiovascular complications. The most common neurological complication is deafness—in fact, hearing loss affects up to 50% of those with Paget's disease of the skull, due to an overgrown petrous temporal bone compressing the auditory nerve.

A. This refers to the pathological process behind osteopetrosis (a very rare inherited disorder), in which the fine balance behind osteoblast and osteoclast activity is lost—osteoclasts are unable to resorb as normal, but osteoblasts continue to make new bone, resulting in hyperdense, but brittle, bone.

B. This refers to the fundamental problem in osteomalacia—that there is a normal amount of bone but that its density is low.

D and E. These refer to osteoporosis. It can affect both cortical and trabecular bone, leading to differing presentations—if cortical bone is more affected, then crush fractures of the vertebrae will be a problem, whilst if trabecular bone is affected, then long bones are more likely to be damaged, particularly the neck of femur.

11. E ★★ OHCM 10th ed. → p. 738

Figure 14.11 is a ventilation/perfusion (V/Q) scan that demonstrates multiple perfusion mismatches in the perfusion scintigram, compared to the ventilation scintigram, which is consistent with an acute pulmonary embolism (PE). This is a nuclear medicine scan that usually uses inhaled technetium (Tc) plus injected 99mTc macro-aggregates which circulate into the lung capillaries. Normal perfusion excludes PEs, but a normal ventilatory component is required to increase the sensitivity of this investigation. Owing to the number of indeterminate scans, computed tomography pulmonary angiogram (CTPA) imaging is more commonly used. A V/Q scan was chosen in this case, as the patient is postpartum and is likely to have developed increased breast tissue volume, which makes her more susceptible to the effects of higher-dose radiation.

As this patient has had a PE, she should be immediately anticoagulated with low-molecular-weight heparin and subsequently started on either a direct-acting oral anticoagulant (DOAC) or warfarin for up to 6 months.

A. This may be required if pulmonary hypertension were suspected (there were possible signs of right heart failure, with leg oedema), but it is not immediately the next step.

B. This is likely to find a deep vein thrombosis (DVT), given the clinical findings, but will not change the management of this patient.

C and D. These are not currently indicated.

12. B ★★ OHCM 10th ed. → p. 498

The brief history is suggestive of cerebral space-occupying masses. The magnetic resonance imaging (MRI) scan (coronal view) shows multiple discrete ring-enhancing lesions. Differentials for these appearances include metastases (most commonly from the lung, kidney, breast, melanoma, and colon), demyelination, multiple infarcts, and, in patients who are human immunodeficiency virus (HIV)-positive, lymphoma. However, in those who have been on long-term immunosuppression, like this woman, the most likely cause are abscesses. The most common infections that can cause multiple small lesions are toxoplasmosis, cryptococcosis, and cysticercosis.

Chapman S and Nakielny R (eds) (2003). *Aids to Radiological Differential Diagnosis*, 4th edn. Saunders: London.

13. B ★ ★ ★   OHCM 10th ed. → p. 168

An atypical pneumonia, *Legionella* colonizes water tanks—classically in hotels—causing a 'flu-like' illness, followed by a dry cough and breathlessness. X-ray findings vary and often lag behind symptoms but may show bilateral consolidation of the lower zones (as in this case). It should be considered in previously fit patients who present with a cough and hypoxia (particularly if they have had recent trips overseas).

A. *Chlamydia* typically begins with a combination of pharyngitis and otitis before progressing to a pneumonia.

C. *Pneumocystis jiroveci* causes pneumonia symptoms in the immunosuppressed [classically those with human immunodeficiency virus (HIV)].

D. *Staphylococcus* causes a cavitating pneumonia in those at either end of the age spectrum or those with an underlying lung disease.

E. Although *Streptococcus pneumoniae* is the most common causative organism, it tends to affect the elderly or those with some kind of compromise such as alcohol users and those with heart failure or an underlying lung disease.

14. D ★ ★ ★   OHCM 10th ed. → p. 192

The history is suggestive of an infective process, whilst the clinical findings are those of a pleural effusion. Fluid accumulation in the pleural space in the setting of an infection is known as a 'parapneumonic effusion'. The fluid is an exudate and seeps into the pleural space, following inflammation of the lung and resulting increased capillary permeability. Following Light's criteria, effusions are either transudates or exudates (based on ratios of fluid:serum protein and lactate dehydrogenase). Those that occur due to systemic disturbances are usually transudates, whilst those that are a response to local factors are usually exudates.

A. This occurs due to hypoproteinaemia, as seen in liver cirrhosis and the nephrotic syndrome (transudate).

B. This is a consequence of an increased venous pressure, as in heart failure or constrictive pericarditis (transudate).

C. This follows an obstruction of the superior vena cava and results in a decreased absorption of pleural fluid, and hence leaking into pleural spaces (exudate).

E. This occurs in liver disease with ascites (transudate).

15. B ★ ★ ★   OHCM 10th ed. → p. 184

The key here is not to get distracted by the X-ray, but to focus instead on the history. Whilst this X-ray is quite difficult to interpret, the short history is very suggestive of an exacerbation of chronic obstructive pulmonary disease (COPD). With this in mind, the X-ray can be tackled—chest films of those with COPD are often very striking, particularly in those patients who are towards the emphysema end of the spectrum. This disease is characterized by widespread air-trapping within the lungs.

This may be hard to visualize radiographically unless—as in this case—the trapped air forms 'bullae' as large as those seen here.

A. Whilst a productive cough can feature in heart failure (here right-sided failure secondary to lung disease), the speed of the deterioration and the appearance of the X-ray are not typical.

C. Although the history is suggestive, there is not enough organized consolidation on the X-ray to classify this as a pneumonia.

D. This is the best differential and indeed needs to be carefully considered in such a situation. For a start, pneumothorax can commonly happen in those who have apical bullous disease. Secondly, it can be very difficult to tell large bullae apart from pneumothoraces. Whilst the edge of a pneumothorax normally runs parallel with the chest wall, the edge of a bulla will often curve away from the chest wall. In difficult images—like this one—computed tomography (CT) will often be required to further differentiate.

E. Although tuberculosis does affect the apices, a reactivation would not present in this acute way.

16. D ★★★   OHCM 10th ed. → p. 549

The most common cause of an acute monoarthropathy in a woman over 65 years of age is pseudogout. The history is typically that of the rapid onset of severe pain—often in the knee—with a reduced range of movement and mobility, leading to falls. Clinical examination reveals a warm, swollen knee that is tender to touch. Both diagnosis and treatment rely on aspiration of the joint—the fluid is sent for microscopy and culture, as well as for examination for crystals. Under a polarized filter, their behaviour can be examined—in pseudogout, the crystals are rhomboid-shaped and exhibit positive birefringence (Positive = Pseudogout). Plain X-ray findings are also supportive—the joint space is narrowed and full of debris, such as in this case where there is a clear wedge of calcification at the medial aspect.

A. This refers to osteoarthritis. Although it can flare and indeed cause joint effusions, it is unlikely to present in such an acute fashion. Plain X-ray findings would be different, instead showing the classical features of narrowed joint space, subchondral bone cysts, osteophytes, and peri-articular sclerosis.

B. This refers to the process behind septic arthritis. Always a vital differential to exclude in acute monoarthropathy, it would usually cause more systemic upset, as well as more dramatic local signs. The plain film findings may include: an effusion, swelling of the surrounding soft tissues, periarticular osteoporosis, loss of joint space, and marginal and central erosions.

C. This refers to rheumatoid arthritis (RA). Flares of RA can lead to acute presentations, such as this, with grossly elevated inflammatory markers [C-reactive protein (CRP) >250 mg/L] and occasionally accompanying delirium. However, it would be unlikely to present for the first time in someone of this age. On the X-ray, there may be few changes in early disease, but as it progresses, there may be osteopenia around the joint, as well as narrowing of the joint space and soft tissue swelling.

E. This refers to the pathological process behind gout. It is another good differential and probably the next best answer here, as clinically, the crystal arthropathies (gout and pseudogout) can be indistinguishable. However, gout is nine times more common in men than in women and crucially does not show many changes on a plain X-ray. Certainly, in the first presentation of gout, the X-ray may be completely normal. Only after repeated attacks would radiographic signs develop, and these are normally in the form of sclerotic regions on the joint surfaces.

17. C ★★ OHCM 10th ed. → p. 611

This is a sigmoid volvulus, and the treatment of choice, if there is no evidence of ischaemic bowel, is the placement of a rectal flatus tube under sigmoidoscopic guidance (either rigid or flexible). This is effective in 60–95% of cases.

The presence of blood-stained effluent and devitalized mucosa on sigmoidoscopy suggests ischaemia. Sigmoid resection is indicated in such cases and those where endoscopic decompression is not possible or successful. Barium enema and laxatives are not indicated whilst the volvulus is ongoing, but may be appropriate for subsequent bowel preparation should a resection be considered.

→ www.fascrs.org/sites/default/files/downloads/publication/clinical_practice_guidelines_for_colon_volvulus.pdf

18. E ★★★ OHCM 10th ed. → p. 611

The history of progressive distension is suggestive of some form of bowel obstruction. The cause of the obstruction in this case is a sigmoid volvulus—chronic constipation (often in institutionalized patients) results in the faecally and gas-loaded segment of bowel twisting on its mesenteric pedicle, creating a closed loop. The result is a single grossly dilated loop of bowel, seen on X-ray as showing the 'coffee bean' sign. It reaches up towards the xiphisternum and has oedematous walls, seen as thick, white boundaries replacing the usual haustra.

An incarcerated umbilical hernia or gallstone ileus may cause intestinal obstruction but would be unlikely to create the closed loop seen here. A perforated duodenal ulcer will present with sudden-onset epigastric pain, likely on a background of dyspeptic symptoms.

19. B ★★★ OHCM 10th ed. → p. 613

Caecal volvulus commonly presents with large bowel obstruction and a classical 'comma-shaped' shadow in the mid abdomen. Treatment involves colonoscopic decompression or a right hemicolectomy if the colon is ischaemic.

Absolute constipation is a description of symptoms, rather than a diagnosis. An incarcerated epigastric hernia may present with bowel obstruction (though rarely, as they normally contain just pre-peritoneal fat), but a tender irreducible lump would be present on examination. A perforated gastric ulcer would be more likely to present with sudden-onset epigastric pain; a delay of 3 days before presenting for medical attention would be most unlikely. The appearance of small bowel obstruction on an abdominal X-ray is characteristic and very different to that seen with a caecal volvulus.

→ www.fascrs.org/sites/default/files/downloads/publication/clinical_practice_guidelines_for_colon_volvulus.pdf

20. C ★★★   OHCM 10th ed. → p. 743

Figure 14.20 shows a 'corkscrew appearance' of the oesophagus, a rare, but classical, finding associated with diffuse oesophageal spasm.

A. This would be associated with a dilated tapering oesophagus.

B and E. These would both be associated with luminal narrowing.

D. This would be associated with the stomach protruding through the hiatus. If it is a sliding hernia, this may be observed as a dynamic process.

21. C ★★★   OHCM 10th ed. → p. 774

This is a decreasingly common task for the on-call junior doctor outside of the critical care environment. A post-insertion X-ray should always be requested to check for two main things: (1) that there are no complications from the procedure; and (2) that the line is lying in the correct place for use. The most common immediate complication that can be screened for on an chest X-ray is a pneumothorax. If the junior doctor is happy that there are no intrapleural slivers of air and he or she can confirm that the line tip lies between the first and third sternocostal joints—i.e. in the superior vena cava—then he or she can say that there have been no immediate complications from the procedure and that the line is lying in the correct place, ready for use.

Emergencies

Tom Coryndon, Chris Parnell, James Harnett, and
Dan Furmedge

All doctors have to deal with emergencies—this can be a daunting prospect, particularly when first on the scene. The fear may be that one
wrong decision could be crucial and that the recovery of the patient depends entirely on what is done at this moment. The truth is that doctors
are rarely—if ever—alone for long and that senior help is, for the most
part, just a few seconds away. It should also serve as some consolation
that the approach to any clinical emergency should be much the same
and depends heavily on the basic and advanced life support algorithms
(Figures 15.1 and 15.2).

This chapter is written in the spirit that any clinical encounter should
be approached as if it is an emergency—this means resorting to the
ABCDE (airway, breathing, circulation, disability, exposure) approach.
Clearly, if the patient to whom we are called is sitting up in bed talking
and drinking a cup of tea, then expectations can be tailored accordingly.

As it is so hard to categorize what constitutes a clinical emergency, it
is better that we go into every encounter expecting one. It is easier
to taper down one's level of urgency than it is to suddenly escalate
treatment in the light of sudden surprising findings. In this way, the
idiosyncratic situations—such as the call regarding the post-op thyroid
patient—should be considered just as urgent as the seemingly clear cardiac arrest calls.

Having performed the systematic ABCDE assessment of each situation, the next stage is to develop the knowledge and confidence to go on
and diagnose which specific emergency is unfolding and to apply appropriate management plans. Questions in this chapter aim to reinforce the
ability to perform this assessment, as well as outlining some of the specific therapies that are required to manage individual emergencies.

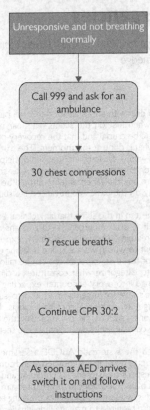

Figure 15.1
Reproduced with the kind permission of the Resuscitation Council (UK).

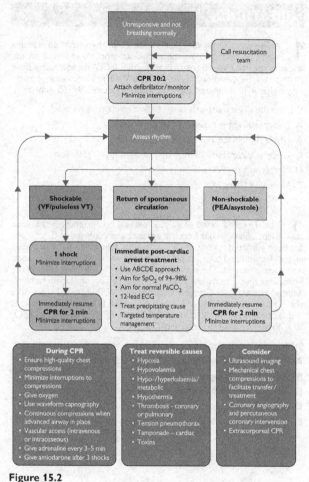

Figure 15.2
Reproduced with the kind permission of the Resuscitation Council (UK).

QUESTIONS

1. A 64-year-old man with type 2 diabetes and hypertension presents with 3 hours of ongoing epigastric discomfort, shortness of breath, and ongoing vomiting. His electrocardiogram (ECG) demonstrates sinus rhythm with ST elevation in II, III, aVF, and V1. The ST elevation is markedly higher in III compared to II. His blood pressure is 98/65 mmHg.

What is the *single* most appropriate agent to improve his pain? ★

A Aspirin 300 mg + ticagrelor 180 mg oral (PO)

B Glyceryl trinitrate 2–4 sprays sublingual (SL)

C Glyceryl trinitrate 1–10 mcg/min intravenous (IV) infusion

D Morphine 5 mg IV

E Morphine 10 mg PO

2. You are called to see an 82-year-old lady on the emergency assessment unit who has become agitated and confused at 3 a.m. She has been admitted for observation overnight, following a fall with a head injury. A computed tomography (CT) head and C-spine 6 hours post-injury were normal. The nurses do not report any further falls on the ward. Her medications are amlodipine, atorvastatin, apixaban, ramipril, and temazepam. Her Glasgow Coma Scale (GCS) score is E4, V4, M6; she is not orientated to time, place, or person but follows commands and is compliant. Her vitals are: HR 52 bpm, BP 173/87 mmHg, SpO_2 97% on room air, RR 18/min, and T 37.2°C.

Which is the most appropriate *single* first step from the options below? ★

A Immobilize her C-spine and commence vitamin K intravenous (IV)

B Perform a neurological exam

C Prescribe her regular temazepam

D Review her chart for any missed/new medications

E Send bloods for thyroid function, bone profile, vitamin B12, and folate to complete a delirium screen

3. A 70-year-old lady with cervical spondylosis and no other history has collapsed after struggling to eat a steak sandwich on the ward. You attend a cardiac arrest call. The nurse reports ineffective coughing, stridor, and see-saw respiration before the collapse. She has lost her central pulse, with bradycardia on the monitor. Cardiopulmonary resuscitation (CPR) has been commenced, with the anaesthetist unable to intubate the patient and unable to ventilate with a bag–valve mask.

Which procedure should the team be preparing for? ★

A External (transcutaneous) pacing

B Fibreoptic intubation

C Heimlich manoeuvre

D Needle cricothyroidotomy

E Surgical cricothyroidotomy

4. A 32-year-old woman with type 1 diabetes and hypothyroidism presents to the emergency department with confusion and lethargy.

T 37.8°C, HR 110 bpm, BP 75/40 mmHg, SpO_2 97% on room air.

Glasgow Coma Scale (GCS) score 12/15 (E3, V4, M5), BM 4.0 mmol/L.

A venous blood gas is unremarkable, except for sodium 128 mmol/L and potassium 5.6 mmol/L. You note her thyroid-stimulating hormone (TSH) was within normal range at a routine endocrinology follow-up last week. What is the most appropriate first-line drug treatment? ★

A Glucose oral gel 75 g

B Hydrocortisone 100 mg intravenous (IV)

C Insulin Actrapid® 20 units + dextrose 50% 50 mL IV

D Metaraminol 0.5 mg IV

E Salbutamol 5 mg nebule

5. A 45-year-old man with previous unspecified mental health problems is brought to hospital by his family, having become progressively jaundiced over the last 2 days. On questioning, he discloses a paracetamol overdose 4 days ago but is unsure of the quantity. You arrange laboratory blood tests.

Which of the following of his results is an indication for referral to a specialist liver unit for consideration for liver transplantation? ★

A Activated partial thromboplastin time (aPTT) 104 s

B Alanine aminotransferase (ALT) 1079 U/L

C Bilirubin 247 micromol/L

D pH 7.28

E Urea 36 mmol/L

6. A 48-year-old man is brought to the emergency department with profound light-headedness. He describes feeling as if he is about to faint.

T 36.4°C, HR 26 bpm, BP 76/51 mmHg, RR 20/min, SpO₂ 98% on air.

What is the *single* most appropriate initial treatment? ★

A Adenosine 6 mg intravenous (IV)

B Adenosine 12 mg IV

C Atropine 500 micrograms IV

D Atropine 3 mg IV

E Transcutaneous pacing

7. A 24-year-old man arrives confused and agitated and holding his head as if in pain. He threatens to stab the matron with a syringe from the sharps bin, claiming she is the devil. He has no psychiatric or medical history. No collateral history is available. He has violently refused all observations and investigations. What is the most appropriate medication for the patient? ★

A Aciclovir intravenous (IV)

B Lorazepam intramuscular (IM)

C Olanzapine oral (PO)

D Pabrinex® IM

E Phenytoin IV

8. You are working in the emergency department of a large teaching hospital with a hyperacute stroke unit. You are talking to a paramedic colleague who is at the end of a busy and stressful night shift. Whilst speaking, she suddenly begins to slur her words and drops the paperwork from her left hand. She is unable to pick it up, as her hand is very clumsy. She has a history of type 2 diabetes and hypertension.

What is the *single* most appropriate course of action? ★

A Ask the triage nurse to book her in for review in majors

B Bleep the on-call neurology specialty registrar (SpR) and ask for an urgent review

C Phone switchboard and activate a thrombolysis call

D Request an urgent computed tomography (CT) brain

E Request an urgent electrocardigram (ECG)

9. An on-call junior doctor responds to a crash call from an acute medical ward. She is the first to arrive at the bedside. The patient, a 56-year-old man, does not respond to voice or pain. His breathing is not audible from the end of the bed. On inspiration, his chest is drawn in, whilst his abdomen expands, the opposite occurring on expiration. Which is the *single* most appropriate next step? ★

A Auscultate the chest

B Check the position of the trachea

C Ensure the airway is open and clear

D Give high-flow oxygen

E Percuss the chest

10. A 78-year-old man is found unresponsive, and a doctor on the ward is called to the patient's bedside. The nurse has not been able to detect a blood pressure during routine observations. The patient is displaying no signs of life. He is not breathing and has no detectable pulse. Which is the *single* most appropriate next step? ★

A Get the resuscitation trolley from the nurses' station

B Give two rescue breaths immediately

C Go and check the notes for a Do Not Attempt Resuscitation (DNAR) order

D Insert two wide-bore cannulae into each antecubital fossa

E Start chest compressions at a rate of 30:2

11. A 46-year-old man is brought into the emergency department by paramedics and, whilst being assessed, becomes unresponsive. He has no signs of life and no pulse. The team start cardiopulmonary resuscitation (CPR) and begin the advanced life support algorithm. After 3 minutes, no peripheral intravenous access has been obtained despite multiple attempts.

What is the next *single* most appropriate course of action? ★

A Administer drugs via an endotracheal tube

B Central venous access via a femoral line

C Intraosseous access via the humeral head

D Intravenous access via the external jugular vein

E Repeat attempts at peripheral venous access

12. A 55-year-old man has collapsed. He has had abdominal pain and vomited several times in the last 3 days. He takes sodium valproate for generalized epilepsy. He is drowsy and clammy, with cool peripheries.

T 37.2°C, HR 140 bpm, BP 95/65 mmHg.

Abdomen: epigastric tenderness.

Haemoglobin (Hb) 91 g/L, white cell count (WCC) 12.5 × 10⁹/L.

Sodium 132 mmol/L, potassium 4.9 mmol/L, urea 15.8 mmol/L, creatinine 89 micromol/L.

Which *single* supplementary clinical examination would be the most informative at this stage? ★ ★

A Chest

B Digital rectal

C Gait, arms, legs, and spine (GALS)

D Inguinal and testicular

E Neurological including cranial nerves

13. A 15-year-old girl has taken an overdose of 30 paracetamol tablets 3 hours ago. She is extremely anxious, but otherwise asymptomatic. She has no past medical history. She weighs 45 kg.

BP 125/65 mmHg, HR 95 bpm, SaO₂ 98% on air.

Which is the *single* most appropriate next step? ★

A Activated charcoal

B N-acetylcysteine infusion

C Paracetamol plasma level at 4 hours

D Refer to psychiatry

E Urgent liver function tests + clotting screen

14. A 21-year-old woman has been found unconscious by her partner. There are several packets of paracetamol and an empty bottle of vodka alongside her. When she comes to in the emergency department, she is confused and unable to estimate when she took the tablets.

Glasgow Coma Scale (GCS) score: 14/15.

Which is the *single* most appropriate next step? ★ ★

A Observe the woman's GCS score in the emergency department

B Refer her to the renal unit for haemodialysis

C Start *N*-acetylcysteine immediately

D Start *N*-acetylcysteine 4 hours after presentation

E Take paracetamol levels and treat if raised

15. A 66-year-old woman has suddenly become short of breath. She suffered no chest pain at the time but is now in discomfort with every deep breath in. Six days previously, she underwent the resection of a caecal carcinoma. Which is the *single* additional feature that should prompt the most urgent attention? ★

A Blood pressure (BP) 80/60 mmHg

B Erythematous, swollen right calf

C Heart rate (HR) 120 bpm

D Raised jugular venous pressure (JVP)

E Oxygen saturations (SaO$_2$) 95% on 5 L oxygen

16. A 61-year-old man has suddenly become very short of breath. In the last hour, he has had a computed tomography (CT)-guided biopsy of a mass in the right lung.

T 36.4°C, HR 120 bpm, BP 100/60 mmHg, SaO$_2$ 75% on 15L O$_2$.

He looks cyanosed; his trachea is deviated towards the left, and his breath sounds are much louder over the left hemithorax. Which is the *single* most appropriate course of action? ★

A Arterial blood gas

B Insertion of a cannula into the right second intercostal space

C Insertion of a chest drain

D Insertion of an airway adjunct

E Chest X-ray

17. A 64-year-old woman is in theatre recovery post-operatively, following a left hemicolectomy for colorectal cancer. She reports feeling very unwell (Figure 15.3).

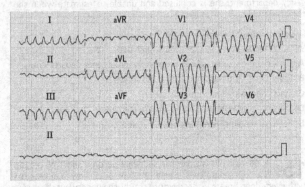

Figure 15.3
Reproduced with permission from Wilkinson I.B, Raine T., Wiles K. *et al*, *Oxford Handbook of Clinical Medicine*, Tenth edition, figure 3.12, p. 106. Copyright (2017) with permission from Oxford University Press.

T 35.9°C, HR 180 bpm, BP 65/40 mmHg, RR 20/min, SaO₂ 98% on 2 L O₂ via nasal specs.

What is the next *single* most appropriate treatment? ★

A Adenosine 6 mg intravenous (IV)

B Amiodarone 300 mg IV

C Commence chest compressions [cardiopulmonary resuscitation (CPR)]

D Magnesium 2 g IV

E Synchronized direct current (DC) cardioversion

18. A 32-year-old woman has a 2-day history of severe headache, malaise, myalgia, and nausea. The headache was gradual in onset and is described as 'all over'. Her two young children have similar symptoms and are being seen in the children's area of the department. Her sister who visited today found her asleep and difficult to rouse. An ambulance was called. On examination, she is now awake and co-operative, but very tired. Observations are within normal limits, other than tachycardia of 110 bpm. There is no fever. Neurological examination is normal. What is the most appropriate investigation? ★★

A Arterial blood gas

B Blood cultures

C Computed tomography (CT) head

D Lumbar puncture

E Upper respiratory viral swab

19. A 22-year-old woman with no past medical history is brought in by ambulance, following a witnessed generalized tonic–clonic seizure. Her seizure terminates on arrival to the emergency department after 15 minutes, with no medications given. She remains drowsy and disorientated. Whilst transferring her from the ambulance trolley with the nurse, she begins to seize again. What is your most appropriate initial action? ★★

A Check and open her airway

B Check glucose

C Levetiracetam 500 mg intravenous (IV)

D Lorazepam 4 mg IV

E Midazolam 10 mg buccal

20. You are performing the first round of chest compressions on a patient in confirmed cardiac arrest with the crash team. The 2-minute rhythm check reveals tachycardia with a wide sinusoidal QRS complex and no palpable pulse. They are on high-flow oxygen, and you are still waiting for the first arterial blood gas (ABG) result. What is the next step? ★★

A Continue cardiopulmonary resuscitation (CPR) whilst charging the defibrillator to the manufacturer's instructions, shock the patient, and immediately resume CPR

B Continue CPR whilst charging the defibrillator to the manufacturer's instructions, shock the patient, and immediately perform a rhythm check and pulse check

C Give adrenaline 1 mg intravenous (IV) (1 in 10 000) and continue CPR

D Give amiodarone 300 mg IV and continue CPR

E Resume chest compressions for a further 2 minutes in a 30:2 ratio to rescue breaths

21. An 18-year-old man has an acute episode of wheeze and chest tightness. He is unable to talk and is brought to the emergency department on high-flow oxygen. After back-to-back salbutamol 5 mg nebules and one ipratropium bromide 500 micrograms nebule, he remains very breathless. Arterial blood gases are taken on arrival and 20 minutes into treatment (Table 15.1).

Table 15.1 Arterial blood gas results taken on 15 L oxygen delivered via a non-rebreathe mask

	Arrival	20 minutes later
pH	7.37	7.32
PaO₂ (kPa)	9.22	8.85
PaCO₂ (kPa)	4.49	5.89
HCO₃⁻ (mmol/L)	23	21

Which is the *single* most appropriate immediate management? ★ ★

A Aminophylline 5 mg/kg intravenous (IV) infusion

B Hydrocortisone 200 mg IV

C Magnesium sulfate 2 g IV infusion

D Refer to the intensive therapy unit (ITU)

E Salbutamol 5 mg nebulized (NEB)

22. A 78-year-old woman has a collapse witnessed by her son. He calls the paramedics when she is unable to stand and seems weak down her right side. On arrival in the emergency department, her Glasgow Coma Scale (GCS) score is 13/15, with a right hemiparesis. She is increasingly agitated and within an hour, her GCS score is 8/15. Which is the *single* most appropriate next course of action? ★ ★

A Ask for an urgent anaesthetic review

B Arrange to start thrombolysis treatment for a probable stroke

C Give aspirin 300 mg per rectum (PR)

D Give lorazepam 2 mg intravenous (IV)

E Request an urgent computed tomography (CT) scan of the head

23. A 24-year-old man has a painful right testis, lower abdominal pain, and nausea. The testis is swollen, hot, and extremely tender. The emergency department triage nurse contacts the junior doctor to discuss the patient over the telephone. Which is the *single* most appropriate question in the immediate assessment of this patient? ★★★★

A Are there associated rigors?

B Has there been vomiting?

C Has this happened before?

D How quickly did the pain come on?

E Is there pain on passing urine?

24. An 18-year-old man is bought to the emergency department from a nightclub by his friends, acting strangely following snorting half a gram of an unknown white powder. He is agitated and combative when examined, but you note he is diaphoretic, with dilated pupils. An electrocardiogram (ECG) shows sinus tachycardia at 145 bpm.

T 37.8°C, BP 185/95 mmHg.

What is the *single* most appropriate initial treatment? ★★★

A Dantrolene 1 mg/kg intravenous (IV)

B Glyceryl trinitrate (GTN) infusion 1–2 mg/hour IV

C Lorazepam 1–2 mg IV

D Metoprolol 5 mg IV

E Paracetamol 1 g IV

25. A 32-year-old woman is found collapsed in a train station.

Glasgow Coma Scale (GCS) score 10/15.

T 35.3°C, HR 115 bpm, BP 108/68 mmHg, RR 8/min, SpO$_2$ 88% on room air.

Pinpoint pupils.

An arterial blood gas (ABG) on air reveals: pH 7.25, PCO$_2$ 7.99, PO$_2$ 7.68, HCO$_3^-$ 26, base excess 1, lactate 2.3, glucose 5.4.

What is the *single* most appropriate next step? ★★★

A High-flow oxygen, 400 micrograms naloxone intravenous (IV)

B High-flow oxygen, 500 mL Hartmann's solution IV

C High-flow oxygen, sodium bicarbonate 1.26% IV

D Oxygen via Venturi mask, 500 mL Hartmann's solution IV

E Start non-invasive ventilation

26. A 15-year-old boy has dropped a pan of boiling water on himself, whilst cooking for his family on mother's day. He has a very painful, red, and blistered rash covering the whole front of his left thigh and some blistering to the dorsum of his left (non-dominant) hand. There is no hand joint involvement; none of the burns are circumferential, and sensation is preserved. He is very stoic and denies severe pain post-analgesia and burns dressing. His observations are normal.

What is the *single* most appropriate follow-up for this patient? ★ ★ ★

A Admit for intravenous (IV) fluids and therapeutic wound cooling

B Discharge with follow-up in 48 hours with the general practitioner (GP)

C Discharge with follow-up in 48 hours in the paediatric emergency department

D Discharge with open follow-up in the emergency department if ongoing concerns

E Refer to the regional burns unit

27. A 39-year-old breastfeeding mother presents 2 days post-delivery of her third child with a 3-day crescendo severe headache, flashing lights in her vision, and epigastric pain. Her pregnancies were uncomplicated, and she has no other medical problems.

T 37.1°C, HR 45 bpm, BP 185/95 mmHg, RR 22/min, SpO₂ 98% on room air.

Glucose: 6.3.

Her full blood count (FBC) and C-reactive protein (CRP) are normal. Her liver function tests (LFTs) are mildly raised, but unchanged from the time of delivery. Before you manage a neurological exam, she begins to have a generalized tonic–clonic seizure. Her plantars are upgoing.

Which medication(s) is most likely to benefit here? ★ ★ ★

A Ceftriaxone 2 g intravenous (IV)

B Diazepam 10 mg per rectum (PR)

C Lorazepam 4 mg IV

D Magnesium sulfate 4 g IV

E Phenytoin 18 mg/kg infusion

28. The emergency department charge nurse calls you to urgently review a 29-year-old woman who has taken a paracetamol overdose of 50 tablets 7 hours ago. Your registrar has prescribed N-acetylcysteine (NAC), and the first bag was commenced 10 minutes ago. The patient complains of itching, and on examination, you find widespread urticaria to the torso and limbs. Observations are within normal limits. What is the most appropriate action? ★★★

A Adrenaline 500 micrograms intramuscular (IM)

B Chlorphenamine 4 mg intravenous (IV)

C Document NAC allergy on the drug chart

D Slow the infusion

E Stop the infusion

29. A 40-year-old man is bought in by the ambulance service in cardiac arrest, having fallen into a lake whilst fishing. His temperature is 28°C. Which of the following is an appropriate modification to the advanced life support (ALS) algorithm in hypothermic cardiac arrest? ★★★

A Defibrillation energy should be halved

B Defibrillation should be withheld until temperature >30°C

C Drug doses should be doubled

D Drug intervals should be halved

E Drugs should be withheld until temperature >30°C

30. A frail 94-year-old lady is in hospital for pneumonia. She has dementia and lives in a nursing care home where she requires prompting and assistance with all activities of daily living. She is transferred, using a hoist, and does not mobilize. She has a grade 3 pressure sore and is doubly incontinent, with fixed limb contractures in the lower limbs.

She is found unresponsive and pulseless by the nursing staff who begin cardiopulmonary resuscitation (CPR) and call the cardiac arrest team. The cardiac arrest team arrive.

Which is the *single* most appropriate course of action? ★★★★

A Adrenaline 1 mg intravenous (IV)

B Cease cardiopulmonary resuscitation (CPR)

C Contact the next of kin to discuss a 'Do Not Attempt Resuscitation' order

D Continue uninterrupted chest compressions

E Intubate

ANSWERS

1. D ★   OHCM 10th ed. → p. 796

Morphine intravenous (IV) is the recommended first-line analgesic route in the management of ST-elevation myocardial infarction (STEMI)— always remember to give an antiemetic to counter the commonly experienced nausea. The oral route is less appropriate here, as the patient is vomiting and is not first line in acute coronary syndrome (ACS). This patient has an inferior STEMI with right ventricular involvement, as evidenced by ST elevation in V1 and a higher degree of ST elevation in III, compared to II. These patients are highly preload-dependent. Nitrates should be avoided in such patients, as they can precipitate a catastrophic drop in blood pressure—this is already low. Aspirin, in combination with another antiplatelet agents, are certainly indicated in the immediate management of this patient but will not improve his pain.

2. B ★   OHCM 10th ed. → p. 828

All agitated patients do require a chart review; however, this is not the first step for this lady. Although rare after an initially normal computed tomography (CT) brain, this lady has a delayed intracranial bleed until proven otherwise. A brief, but thorough, neurological exam should be performed emergently to identify any new deficit. This lady is on a novel oral anticoagulant (NOAC), and a repeat CT head may be indicated. All sedating medications should be avoided in the context of recent head injury, as they may mask changes in the mental state. Avoid using benzodiazepines as much as possible in the elderly, but be aware of withdrawal symptoms if patients have been taking regular doses. In the absence of new trauma, a new C-spine injury since her previous clear CT C-spine is exceptionally unlikely. Vitamin K has no significant reversal effect for patients receiving a NOAC. This could well be a presentation of delirium from another cause, and a full delirium screen should be considered once a delayed intracranial bleed has been excluded.

3. E ★   OHCM 10th ed. → p. 772

This patient has a history consistent with a partial, and now complete, airway obstruction. After cough becomes ineffective, back slaps and abdominal thrusts would be appropriate first aid. This is now impossible with an arrested patient. Vigorous cardiopulmonary resuscitation (CPR) may help dislodge the fatal food bolus, but the anaesthetist is likely unable to remove it due to her rigid neck deformity. In a 'can't intubate, can't ventilate' situation, hypoxic brain damage is inevitable and will occur in minutes. The most senior anaesthetist available must attend immediately. Fibreoptic intubation will take too long. Needle cricothyrotomy may buy some time but is frequently ineffective. Surgical cricothyrotomy is indicated and will allow ventilation if the obstruction is at the level of the vocal cords and above.

4. B ★   OHCM 10th ed. → p. 836

This is adrenal insufficiency until proven otherwise. Addison's disease is often associated with other autoimmune conditions. It would also be prudent to administer fluid resuscitation for hypotension. Vasopressors should only be considered if hypotension persists despite adequate fluid resuscitation. Addisonian crises can be associated with fever, although careful investigation for an infective source should also be undertaken. The hyperkalaemia is mild and should not need urgent correction at this level, unless associated with ECG changes; however, it should be monitored.

5. D ★   OHCM 10th ed. → pp. 275, 844

The Kings College criteria for referral for liver transplantation in paracetamol toxicity is either:

- pH <7.30
- Or all three of:
  - Prothrombin time (PT) >100 s
  - Grade III or IV encephalopathy
  - Serum creatinine >300 micromol/L.

6. C ★   OHCM 10th ed. → p. 808

This man has profound bradycardia with adverse features. Adenosine is used for supraventricular tachycardia and is not appropriate here. Atropine is used for bradycardia in increments of 500 micrograms at a time, to a maximum of 3 mg in total. Hence, C is the correct response here. If after 3 mg atropine, there has been little or no effect, other options may need to be considered. Transcutaneous pacing is one option which may need to be used until a more definitive method of pacing can be achieved.

7. B ★

This type of severe agitated delirium or encephalopathy may be secondary to drugs, head injury, hypoglycaemia, or infection, or it could be a psychiatric disorder. However, this man presents an immediate risk to himself, your colleagues, and other patients. He requires rapid tranquilization to allow essential observations, investigations, and management to start. Intramuscular (IM) benzodiazepine is the safest method of achieving this, but always ensure the patient can be moved to an appropriate area for monitoring and airway management, with senior support. Antivirals and antibiotics may be indicated if fever or signs of meningitis/encephalitis are present. Temporal lobe epileptic seizure may respond to benzodiazepines or require further treatment. Only after organic causes have been excluded, then treatment of primary psychosis may be necessary.

8. C ★ OHCM 10th ed. → p. 470

This lady has signs of an acute stroke. Activating the thrombolysis team as early as possible is essential, as she remains within the thrombolysis window (<4.5 hours). Her hospital check-in can be sorted at the bedside in tandem. She is lucky to be in a stroke centre—were you to be in a smaller centre, calling 999 and asking for an emergency transfer to the nearest stroke centre could be an appropriate option. Other investigations are important, but given the time window—activating the local stroke pathway will lead to all other interventions being undertaken, and rapidly.

9. C ★ OHCM 10th ed. → p. 779

The signs elicited by the junior doctor—silent breathing and 'see-saw' breathing—are those of complete airway obstruction. However, the key learning point here is that, even if the junior doctor failed to recognize these signs, the patient could be treated by sticking to the ABCDE mantra of resuscitation. Rather than second-guessing what is going on ('Maybe he's got a pneumothorax ... '), by working systematically from the airway onwards, the problem may be treated without having to diagnose it. In this case, positioning, basic airway manoeuvres, airway suction, insertion of an oropharyngeal airway, and then high-flow oxygen may be enough to alleviate the patient's breathing problems.

→ www.resus.org.uk/pages/guide.htm

10. E ★ OHCM 10th ed. → p. 894

This man has had a cardiac arrest. Chest compressions should be started as soon as possible.

The ratio of compressions to breaths should be 30:2, and these should be started whilst waiting for the resuscitation trolley and other help to arrive. Rescue breaths were part of the old guidelines. Chest compressions are more important and have thus superseded previous guidelines. If there is ambiguity over a patient's resuscitation status, then cardiopulmonary resuscitation (CPR) should always be started and can be stopped once this is clarified. Clearly, if CPR is futile, it may be appropriate to stop the resuscitation attempt early, but until more information is available, CPR should begin. The man has no cardiac output and, although intravenous (IV) access is indicated, as part of the advanced life Support algorithm, this should not be the first thing to do.

→ www.resus.org.uk

11. C ★ OHCM 10th ed. → p. 894

Obtaining intravenous access during cardiac arrest is a common challenging problem. Whilst external jugular and central femoral access and further attempts at peripheral access may all be appropriate, the Resuscitation Council guidelines are now very clear that if no venous access has been obtained by 2 minutes, then intraosseous access should be gained at the humeral head or the anterior tibia. This is fast and is obtained via an intraosseous gun. This has superseded previous recommendations about giving drugs down an endotracheal tube, which is no longer recommended. Once intraosseous access is obtained, drugs can be given via this route and this allows more time for other access to be sought.

12. B ★   OHCM 10th ed. → p. 790

The initial clinical findings are that of shock. The blood results suggest acute blood loss. Against the background history—disregarding the distracting concurrent epilepsy—the likely source is the upper gastrointestinal tract. A digital rectal examination (DRE), looking for fresh blood or melaena, provides vital information in this instance but remains underperformed in the acute setting.

13. C ★   OHCM 10th ed. → p. 844

Blood taken before 4 hours is unreliable because the drug is still being absorbed and distributed. The N-acetylcysteine infusion does not need to be started, unless the time of the overdose is unknown or has been staggered over a few hours. Initial symptoms are often limited to nausea and vomiting, but liver damage is possible in adults who have taken 10 g or more (20 tablets) or as little as 5 g in those with risk factors. These include those on liver enzyme-inducing drugs, chronic alcohol abusers, and those who are likely to be deficient in glutathione such as people who have cystic fibrosis, human immunodeficiency virus (HIV) infection, or an eating disorder or those who are cachexic or starved.

A. This should be considered if the overdose has been taken within 1 hour.

B. This should not be started until the blood test has been taken at 4 hours and as long as the results are returned by 8 hours. If the level is below the treatment line and the patient is asymptomatic, no further medical treatment is required.

D. A referral to psychiatry would be important for all patients who have taken an overdose. However, assessing and treating the effects of the overdose takes immediate priority, unless there is severe active ongoing suicidal intent.

E. There is often no change in these values acutely.

14. C ★   OHCM 10th ed. → p. 844

In cases like this, where a serious overdose is suspected and where the time and amount of ingestion are unknown, it is advisable to give the paracetamol antidote N-acetylcysteine immediately. The 4-hour figure refers to the time after ingestion at which plasma levels can be interpreted. If levels turn out to be below the treatment line or if after 24 hours of treatment, there are no adverse features to suggest treatment should be continued, N-acetylcysteine can be stopped without harm.

→ www.rcem.ac.uk/docs/Paracetamol%2Overdose/Paracetamol_
Poisoning%2Proforma_ED%2Management%2of%2Oral%2inges-
tions%2in%2adults.pdf

15. A ★   OHCM 10th ed. → pp. 790, 819

This woman has likely suffered a pulmonary embolus (PE). However,
the key for the doctor on call attempting to prioritize referrals is the
patient's cardiovascular status—here, the systolic blood pressure (BP)
of <90 mmHg suggests haemodynamic instability secondary to a massive
PE, and therefore, one that needs urgent assessment with consideration
of thrombolysis. The other features may be useful in confirming the diagnosis (apart from D which cues pulmonary oedema, rather than PE).

16. B ★   OHCM 10th ed. → pp. 54, 814

This man has rapidly developed the signs of a pneumothorax. Having
just had a needle inserted into his chest, this is almost certainly an iatrogenic pneumothorax (the incidence of which outnumbers spontaneous
pneumothoraces in several large studies). The deviation of the trachea
suggests that it is under tension (i.e. the intrapleural pressure exceeds
the atmospheric pressure through both inspiration and expiration) and
so needs urgent reversal or he may rapidly proceed to a cardiac arrest.
This is done by introducing a cannula into the pleural space, usually in
the second anterior intercostal space mid-clavicular line. Air should be
removed until the patient is no longer compromised, and then a chest
drain can be inserted into the pleural space for definitive management.

A and E. The tension under which the right chest is means the mediastinum is shifted to the left, causing compression of the great veins and
an impaired venous return. This is a serious situation that would lead to
cardiorespiratory arrest, unless addressed, leaving no time for any further investigations.

C. A chest drain will be needed ultimately, but a more urgent relief of
the tension is needed prior to this.

D. Whilst it is right to begin the management of this emergency situation by addressing the airway, there is no suggestion that this man is
unconscious enough to tolerate either a Guedel or a nasopharyngeal
airway. He should be put on high-flow oxygen, whilst attention is directed towards the air in his pleural space.

17. E ★   OHCM 10th edn → p. 804

This lady has a post-operative broad complex tachycardia (ventricular
tachycardia). She has profound hypotension and presyncope, which
are both adverse features requiring immediate correction. The most
appropriate option here, according to the Resuscitation Council guidance, would be for an immediate synchronized direct current (DC)
cardioversion. Adenosine might be appropriate if there were no adverse
features and if this were a narrow complex tachycardia. Amiodarone
may be required, in addition to direct current (DC) cardioversion, but

this would not be the immediate lifesaving step. Intravenous (IV) magnesium can help in polymorphic ventricular tachycardia (torsades de pointes). Cardiopulmonary resuscitation (CPR) would be inappropriate, as this lady is still alert and clearly has signs of life and a recordable blood pressure—therefore, she has a pulse.

18. A ★★   OHCM 10th ed. → p. 842

Whilst an infective cause seems most likely in a household collectively experiencing viral-like symptoms, carbon monoxide poisoning must be considered, especially in view of the improved drowsiness. This can rapidly be established with blood gas analysis. A patient with a carboxy-haemoglobin (COHb) level above 3% (10–15% in smokers) should be placed on high-flow oxygen. The half-life of COHb in room air is around 300 minutes; high-flow oxygen reduces this to 90 minutes. The history of difficulty rousing must be probed further, as loss of consciousness may be an indication for hyperbaric oxygen therapy. The case should be discussed with the local hyperbaric medicine unit for advice.

19. A ★★   OHCM 10th ed. → p. 826

This patient is in status epilepticus, and her airway is at risk. Protecting and supporting the patient's airway is critical and must be achieved before other interventions are commenced. You will need help in this situation. Suction may also be required. Intravenous (IV) lorazepam is the first IV agent of choice. Intraosseous access may be required if IV access cannot be rapidly established, and buccal midazolam may be an appropriate first-line agent where IV access is unavailable. Levetiracetam is not a first-line emergent anticonvulsant, though it may be started later down the line. A glucose check is vital in all seizing patients once the airway is supported.

20. A ★★   OHCM 10th ed. → p. 894

This question asks about the details of the Resuscitation Council UK advanced life support (ALS) algorithm for the management of cardiac arrest. A pulseless wide complex tachycardia, as mentioned here, should always be considered to be pulseless ventricular tachycardia (VT). This is a shockable rhythm, and the most immediate management therefore is to deliver cardioversion. Cardiopulmonary resuscitation (CPR) should be immediately continued for 2 minutes before the next rhythm check. Amiodarone is not a first-line drug in ALS but can be given after three unsuccessful shocks in a patient who remains in a shockable rhythm. Adrenaline should be given every 3–5 minutes in CPR but is not the most important option in this scenario.

21. D ★★   OHCM 10th ed. → p. 810

This man presents with severe asthma and does not respond to initial treatment (as evidenced by hypercapnia on the arterial blood gases). According to British Thoracic Society guidelines, this meets the criteria for intensive therapy unit (ITU) referral. The rising PaCO$_2$ suggests tiredness, and thus the need for airway support to maximize ventilation—he may well need intubation. (Note: it would not be wrong to give this man another nebulizer, intravenous steroids, magnesium, or a theophylline, but the most pressing step at this time is to contact an anaesthetist with a view to securing the airway, as it is unlikely that these measures would be sufficient.)

→ www.brit-thoracic.org.uk/document-library/clinical-information/asthma/btssign-asthma-guideline-2016/

22. **A** ★★   OHCM 10th ed. → pp. 470, 786

The history and examination are convincing for a stroke, and a computed tomography (CT) scan will certainly be needed. However, the patient has rapidly dropped her consciousness level, and before any investigations and treatment can happen, this needs to be addressed. An anaesthetist would rather know at this stage, rather than when a peri-arrest call is put out as her Glasgow Coma Scale (GCS) score reaches 4 or 5. The airway can be stabilized, so that a CT scan can be performed safely and further care of the patient can then be co-ordinated.

Agitation is common in intracranial events, especially haemorrhages, but should not be treated with sedation, unless administered and monitored by an anaesthetist. Thrombolysis or aspirin are the treatment options for ischaemic strokes but cannot be started until a CT scan excludes a haemorrhage.

23. **D** ★★   OHCM 10th ed. → p. 652

The key here is to explore the possibility of testicular torsion. The main differential is usually epididymo-orchitis, in which the onset of pain is much more gradual. In a patient in whom the onset is dramatic and sudden, then torsion becomes the most likely cause. Whilst urinary symptoms (**E**) are also more common in epididymo-orchitis, they may overlap as part of the general extreme lower abdominal pain seen in torsion. Once torsion tops the list, the junior doctor's priority is getting a urological or surgical opinion; definitive treatment is surgery (for detorsion and bilateral orchidopexy)—the sooner this happens, the greater the chance of the testis being saved. Rigors cue an infective cause. Vomiting is rather too non-specific to be immediately useful. A previous similar episode may be suggestive of a hydrocele.

24. **C** ★★★   OHCM 10th ed. → p. 843

This patient is displaying a sympathomimetic toxidrome and should be treated supportively. Identification of the exact drug may not be possible but could be one or a combination of 3,4-methylenedioxymethamphetamine (MDMA), cocaine, or synthetic cathinones ('legal highs'). Control of agitation with benzodiazepines is often sufficient to also settle associated tachycardia and hypertension. This patient has mild hyperthermia, and cooling methods should be considered. Calming agitation may also reduce heat production from muscular hyperactivity, although the temperature should be closely monitored and dantrolene considered in worsening hyperpyrexia. Paracetamol is unlikely to be effective in drug-related hyperthermia. Beta-blockers should be avoided in sympathomimetic toxicity, as unopposed alpha-adrenergic activity may worsen hypertension.

25. A ★★★   OHCM 10th ed. → p. 842

This patient has hypoventilation secondary to opiate overdose. High-flow oxygen with an appropriate initial dose of intravenous (IV) naloxone (to look for reversibility) would be the most appropriate course of action. This can be repeated up to every 2 minutes until ventilation and arterial blood gases (ABGs) improve (maximum of 10 mg). A high initial dose may lead to frank withdrawal features. Remember the half-life of naloxone is short, and some patients may require an infusion (seek senior advice for this). Oxygen and fluids would be reasonable but would not reverse the likely problem. The patient's age and pinpoint pupils make type 2 respiratory failure secondary to chronic lung disease unlikely, and we do not have to worry about loss of hypoxic drive. Altered consciousness level is a relative contraindication to non-invasive ventilation (NIV), and NIV is not a treatment for opiate overdose. Bicarbonate is used in the management of severe tricyclic poisoning, which classically produces a different toxidrome to that seen here.

26. E ★★★   OHCM 10th ed. → p. 846

A specialist burns centre referral is indicated for all partial-thickness burns of >10% of the body surface area in adults and >5% in paediatrics. This patient is technically paediatric, and by using a Lund and Browder chart (essential for all burns patients), we can see that his burn area is over 5%. Other body map charts are available for use in infants and young children. Local follow-up could be used for an otherwise well adult with <10% uncomplicated partial-thickness burns. Admission for fluid resuscitation is indicated for >10% partial-thickness burns in a child and >15% for adults. Use the Parkland formula to calculate fluid requirements (but check the local protocol, as these can vary).

27. D ★★★

This lady is eclamptic. Remember that pre-eclampsia/eclampsia can occur up to 6 weeks post-delivery, although rare. This lady also potentially has HELLP (haemolysis, elevated liver enzymes, and low platelet count) syndrome, with her elevated liver function tests (LFTs). Magnesium sulfate 4 g intravenous (IV) over 5 minutes is the first-line treatment of choice, followed by an infusion. An absence of infective signs/symptoms makes meningitis unlikely here but should be considered. Current guidelines (as above) recommend avoiding diazepam in eclampsia, though in an emergency, this or lorazepam IV may have already been given. Phenytoin is not a first-line anticonvulsant and will not address the primary process here.

28. D ★★★   OHCM 10th ed. → p. 844

Hypersensitivity-like reactions to N-acetylcysteine (NAC) are common and involve direct release of mediators from inflammatory cells, without involving antibodies. Adrenaline is not appropriate in this situation, as there is no clinical evidence of anaphylaxis. Stopping the infusion can be undertaken in a severe reaction, but it should be restarted as soon as possible; NAC is essential to protect against hepatotoxicity, and this patient has taken a significant overdose. Slowing the infusion is often sufficient to control the reaction. Additionally, antihistamines are useful for treatment of associated rashes. However, 4 mg is the oral dose of chlorphenamine; 10 mg would be an appropriate intravenous dose in this situation.

29. E ★★★   OHCM 10th ed. → p. 848

Drugs will undergo reduced metabolism in hypothermic arrest and so are withheld below 30°C. Above this, intervals should be doubled until normothermic, i.e. adrenaline would be given every 8–10 minutes. Defibrillation is also less effective and should only be tried three times below 30°C, then not again until the temperature reaches 30°C.

30. B ★★★★   OHCM 10th ed. → p. 894

A, D, and E are all part of the advanced life support algorithm and may be appropriate in a patient in whom continued cardiopulmonary resuscitation (CPR) is felt to have a chance of success. In this lady who has an advanced age, with clear evidence of marked background physical (cachexia, dependence on others, limited mobility) and cognitive (dementia) frailty, CPR should never have been started and a valid 'Do Not Attempt Resuscitation' order should have been in place prior to her deterioration. In the event that it is not and resuscitation is commenced, a sensible senior decision-maker should identify immediately that this attempt at resuscitating this patient will not be successful, discuss this with the arrest team to ensure agreement, and stop the attempt at an early stage, whilst attempting to preserve some dignity in such a patient whose death is not at all sudden or unexpected. Option C, discussion with the next of kin about a Do Not Attempt Cardiopulmonary Resuscitation (DNACPR) order should have happened on admission to hospital (or even better, it should have been done in the community prior to admission). In an emergency situation such as this, the decision must be taken in the patient's best interests. Contrary to widely held belief, it is perfectly reasonable to stop a resuscitation attempt immediately if it is clear that the patient will not have a good outcome (frail patients or those with severe medical disease).

Chapter 16

Geriatric medicine

Dan Furmedge

Geriatric medicine is the largest 'medical' specialty in the United Kingdom, with the number of geriatricians expanding at a huge rate with significant demand. Pragmatic specialists in frailty and complex co-morbidity, the work of geriatricians reaches across geriatric medicine wards, the acute medical unit, emergency departments and acute frailty units, surgical wards, and tertiary medical wards and in the community from inner city London to rural Scotland. They can be found in residential and nursing care homes, rehabilitation teams, and hospital at home teams.

Frailty, falls, delirium, dementia, continence, immobility, rehabilitation, polypharmacy, nutrition, end-of-life care, advanced care planning, community medicine, and legal and ethical medicine are all core features of a geriatrician's day. In this chapter, the questions give a taste of some of these concepts and will also demonstrate how geriatric medicine crosses almost every specialty.

QUESTIONS

1. A 94-year-old woman is reviewed in the falls clinic, having fallen eight times in the last year. Her regular medications are colecalciferol, digoxin, oxybutynin, simvastatin, and warfarin.

Which of her medications is the *single* most likely to be contributing to her falls risk? ★

A Colecalciferol

B Digoxin

C Oxybutinin

D Simvastatin

E Warfarin

2. A 93-year-old man has had several episodes of acute confusion recently associated with other illnesses. His daughter understands that these are episodes of delirium but is concerned that, after each episode, he never fully regains his previous cognitive level.

Which feature is not characteristic of delirium? ★

A Acute onset

B Attentional deficit

C Change in alertness

D Fluctuant

E Progressive

3. A 76-year-old man is admitted to hospital, having been found on the floor at home. He was last seen by his neighbour 2 weeks before. He is frail and cachexic. He has large necrotic pressure sores affecting his right side.

A nasogastric tube is inserted, as his swallowing is not safe and it is not felt he can meet his high nutritional needs orally. A feeding regime is started.

His blood tests are checked after 48 hours.

Sodium 132 mmol/L, potassium 2.9 mmol/L, phosphate 0.16 mmol/L, magnesium 0.23 mmol/L, corrected calcium 2.01 mmol/L, albumin 22 g/L.

What is the cause of the blood abnormalities above? ★

A Malabsorption

B Refeeding syndrome

C Thiamine deficiency

D Tissue necrosis

E Underlying malignancy

4. A 94-year-old woman is reviewed in the falls clinic, having fallen eight times in the last year. She describes a loss of balance, from which she is unable to correct herself and falls over. Her blood tests, including full blood count and renal and bone profiles, are in the normal range. Her electrocardiogram (ECG) shows a normal sinus rhythm.

Which assessment is most likely to leave to an intervention most likely to reduce her falls risk? ★ ★

A Dietician assessment

B Optician assessment

C Pharmacist assessment

D Physiotherapist assessment

E Social work assessment

5. An 86-year-old woman presented after a collapse. She was standing in the queue for the checkout at the supermarket. She told her husband she felt nauseated and unwell. She was then observed to become unresponsive and fell to the ground. She was unresponsive for around a minute, after which there was some twitching and jerking of her arms. She then made a full recovery after around 2 minutes.

Her electrocardiogram (ECG) revealed a normal sinus rhythm.

Which investigation is most likely to reveal the underlying diagnosis? ★ ★

A A 7-day ambulatory cardiac monitor

B Echocardiogram

C Electroencephalogram (EEG)

D Magnetic resonance imaging (MRI) of the brain

E Tilt test

6. An 81-year-old woman is admitted to the medical assessment unit with dehydration and pneumonia. The nursing staff are required to assess her risk of pressure sores and create an individualized care plan for managing this risk.

Which is the *single* most appropriate tool for this assessment? ★ ★

A 4AT

B Bartel index

C MUST score

D Tinetti score

E Waterlow score

7. A 91-year-old woman suffers from severe constipation. Over the years, she has tried many different laxatives, with varying effect. She is now stable on a regime of senna 15 mg at night, macrogol sachets twice daily, and a glycerin suppository given once weekly by the district nurse.

Which of the following options best describes the method of action of macrogol? ★★

A 5HT$_4$ agonist

B Bulking

C Osmotic

D Softening

E Stimulant

8. An 89-year-old woman has been in hospital for 3 weeks and has been treated for biliary sepsis with broad-spectrum antibiotics for 10 days. These have now stopped, but she has developed profuse diarrhoea and abdominal tenderness.

Her other medications are amlodipine 5 mg daily, aspirin 75 mg daily, omeprazole 20 mg daily, rivaroxaban 20 mg daily, and simvastatin 40 mg at night.

Stool microscopy, culture, and sensitivity (MC&S): negative

Stool *Clostridium difficile* antigen: positive

Stool *C. difficile* toxin: positive

Which is the *single* most appropriate medication to stop? ★★

A Amlodipine

B Aspirin

C Omeprazole

D Rivaroxaban

E Simvastatin

9. A 76-year-old woman is admitted following a fall. She sustained a left fractured neck of femur and underwent surgery with a left dynamic hip screw.

Her past medical history includes hypertension and severe gastro-oesophageal reflux disease with Barrett's oesophagus.

Regarding her bone health, what is the next appropriate step? ★★

A Alendronate 70 mg oral weekly

B Calcium and colecalciferol supplementation

C Dual-energy X-ray absorptiometry (DEXA) scan

D Measure serum calcium and vitamin D

E Zoledronic acid 5 mg intravenously yearly

10. A 78-year-old man with dementia is admitted from a residential care home overnight and is seen by you at 3.30 a.m. He has metastatic prostate cancer and looks very frail, but he is alert but confused and unable to engage in a conversation. He is clinically stable.

He does not seem to have a community 'Do Not Attempt Cardiopulmonary Resuscitation' order, but it seems entirely clinically appropriate for him to have one.

With regard to completing a 'Do Not Attempt Cardiopulmonary Resuscitation' (DNACPR) form in this situation, which of the following options is the *single* most appropriate? ★★

A The form should be completed immediately and a telephone call should be made to the next of kin at this time to inform them of the decision

B The form should be completed immediately and this should be discussed with his next of kin at the earliest opportunity tomorrow to inform them of the decision

C The form should be completed immediately and the patient should be informed of the decision

D The form should be completed immediately, with a second senior doctor's signature endorsing your decision

E The form should be completed tomorrow after a discussion has taken place with the next of kin to inform them of the decision

11. An 84-year-old man complained of tiredness and lethargy.

White cell count (WCC) 6.1 × 10⁹/L, haemoglobin (Hb) 87 g/L, platelets 201 × 10⁹/L.

Ferritin 206 micrograms/L, folate 0.6 micrograms/L, vitamin B12 0.12 mmol/L, thyroid-stimulating hormone (TSH) 3.2 mU/L.

What is the next *single* most appropriate course of action? ★★★

A Replace folate

B Replace iron

C Replace levothyroxine

D Replace niacin

E Replace vitamin B12

12. An 86-year-old man has become acutely confused. He is screaming, trying to climb out of bed, hitting and biting any member of staff who approaches him. He seems to be having visual hallucinations. Despite the efforts of nursing staff and a 1:1 nursing assistant trained in the management of delirium, he remains extremely distressed and at high risk of causing physical harm to himself. He clearly does not have capacity to make decisions about his own healthcare.

He has hypertension, Lewy body dementia, and osteoporosis.

What is the *single* most appropriate next course of action? ★ ★ ★

A Complete an application for a Deprivation of Liberty Safeguard (DOLS)

B Haloperidol 0.5 mg

C Lorazepam 0.5 mg

D Haloperidol 5 mg

E Lorazepam 5 mg

13. A 92-year-old woman has had very poor oral intake over the last 6 months. Her daughter reports that she eats only with direct feeding and manages only one or two small spoonfuls at a time. She is upset that her mother spends most of her time asleep and is very concerned that she is not getting enough in to sustain her nutritional requirements. She says her mother now never leaves the bed because she has lost strength due to not eating and drinking enough.

She has Alzheimer's dementia and osteoporosis.

Her daughter has been reading up on options for nutrition and would like her mother to have a percutaneous endoscopic gastrostomy (PEG) tube for feeding.

With regard to PEG tubes in patients with advanced dementia, which of the following is the most appropriate to tell her daughter? ★ ★ ★

A PEG feeding is associated with a higher mortality rate than oral feeding

B PEG feeding is associated with increased constipation

C PEG feeding will significantly reduce the risk of aspiration

D PEG tubes need to be changed every 12 weeks

E PEG tubes will allow the administration of usual oral medications

14. A 90-year-old man has been admitted to hospital for the fourth time in 6 weeks after being found at home on the floor, despite previously being discharged with carers four times daily. The ambulance staff report that his council-owned flat is in squalor and not habitable.

He is diagnosed with dementia, and a capacity assessment is undertaken whereby he is deemed not to have capacity to make a decision about a safe discharge destination. Despite this, his wishes remain clear that he wants to return to his flat. The multidisciplinary ward team feel he is not safe to return to his flat. He has no next of kin.

What is the next appropriate step in discharge planning? ★ ★ ★

A Apply for Court of Protection

B Apply for a Deprivation of Liberty Safeguard (DOLS)

C Apply for an Independent Mental Capacity Advocate (IMCA)

D Discharge home with carers four times daily

E Discharge to a care home in the patient's best interests

15. A 78-year-old man has moderate Alzheimer's dementia. Despite using an anticholinesterase inhibitor, his partner reports that there has been no change and that his cognition and behaviour appear to have worsened. His Montreal Cognitive Assessment (MoCA) score was 18/30 12 months ago and is now 14/30.

She has read about N-methyl-D-aspartate (NMDA) antagonists in dementia and wonders if these might help.

Which of these drugs is an NMDA antagonist? ★ ★ ★

A Donepezil

B Galantamine

C Memantine

D Rivastigmine

E Ropinirole

16. There are a number of physiological changes associated with normal ageing.

Which single option below is not associated with normal ageing? ★ ★ ★

A Impaired thermoregulation

B Increased gastric acid secretion

C Increased pulse pressure

D Reduced serum albumin concentration

E Reduced vital capacity

ANSWERS

1. C ★ OHCM 10th ed. → pp. 16, 28

Many medications are associated with an increased risk of falls. These include obvious culprits such as antihypertensives, but less widely appreciated are drugs with a high anticholinergic burden. These increase the risk of falls and cognitive impairment. In this case, both digoxin and oxybutynin have some anticholinergic activity, but oxybutynin has a much stronger (class 3) anticholinergic effect than digoxin (class 1). This has led to the recommendation from the National Institute for Health and Care Excellence (NICE) that oxybutynin for the use of urge urinary incontinence in frail older women should be avoided altogether.

2. E ★ OHCM 10th ed. → p. 484

Delirium is a set of symptoms which have been previously described as an 'acute confusional state', although this term is now avoided to ensure there is better awareness of the syndrome of delirium. The hallmark features of delirium are acute or subacute onset, disturbance of conscious level or alertness, reduced attention, and disorganized behaviour. Other features may include a reversal of the sleep–wake cycle and apparent psychotic features such as hallucinations or delusions. Delirium may completely resolve, but sometimes recovery is incomplete, particularly in frail older people after a severe or prolonged episode of delirium. However, treating the cause can usually halt or reverse the delirium. A progressive cognitive decline is a requirement for a diagnosis of dementia, not delirium.

3. B ★ OHCM 10th ed. → p. 587

Refeeding syndrome is a common and life-threatening side effect of enteral nutrition, following a period of malnutrition or minimal oral intake. Through an unknown mechanism, electrolytes are moved intracellularly and can fall to life-threatening levels, causing symptoms and arrhythmias. Phosphate is usually the most severely affected, but potassium, magnesium, and calcium levels can all fall. These electrolytes must be carefully monitored following the start of a feeding regime and replaced carefully, alongside intravenous thiamine. Thiamine deficiency in itself does not cause electrolyte abnormalities. Malabsorption and underlying malignancy may cause electrolyte disturbance, but this would be unlikely to be so acute. Tissue necrosis often causes raised electrolyte levels due to cellular breakdown and release of electrolytes into the bloodstream.

4. D ★★ OHCM 10th ed. → p. 16

Assessments by all of the listed professionals, as part of a multifactorial falls risk assessment, may contribute to an overall falls reduction in this lady. However, strength and balance training delivered by a physiotherapy-led service is the only stand-alone intervention which has evidence in falls prevention and should be offered to all frail older patients who are falling or are at high risk of falls.

5. E ★★ OHCM 10th ed. → p. 460

The history of this collapse is most consistent with a vasovagal syncope— a warning with nausea, a brief loss of consciousness with a rapid recovery, after a period of standing. Although there was some twitching and jerking, this can be a normal feature of a syncopal event and there were no other features to suggest this could have been a seizure, and an electroencephalogram (EEG) or magnetic resonance imaging (MRI) brain are therefore unlikely to be helpful in this context. With a normal electrocardiogram (ECG), cardiac conduction abnormalities are extremely unlikely, and therefore a cardiac monitor or an echocardiogram are likely to have a very low yield. Vasovagal syncope can often be demonstrated or induced using a tilt test, although this would only be indicated if these episodes were frequent or unexplained and after all causative agents, such as antihypertensive medications, have been stopped.

6. E ★★

Many tools and risk stratification scores are used in healthcare today, with many of these performed by nursing staff, to help create detailed individualized care plans for patients across a range of areas such as nutrition, falls risk, cognition, and pressure areas. The Waterlow score is a detailed assessment score which outputs a level of risk for acquiring pressure sores and tissue damage—this can then be used to, for example, highlight the need for a pressure-relieving mattress or instigate a regular turning regime to prevent such sores. The 4AT is a delirium screening tool; the Bartel index is a measure of dependence and looks at activities of daily living; the MUST score is a malnutrition screening tool also completed for many patients admitted to hospital, and the Tinetti test is a test which looks at gait and balance and is usually done by physiotherapists.

7. C ★★ OHCM 10th ed. → p. 260

Macrogol, like lactulose, is an osmotic laxative which retains fluid within the lumen of the bowel. These agents should not be used together. Bulking agents include ispaghula husk and methylcellulose; stimulant laxatives include senna and bisacodyl, and stool softeners include sodium docusate. Prucalopride is a less well-known, newer agent which is a $5HT_4$ agonist with prokinetic properties and has approval from the National Institute for Health and Care Excellence (NICE) for use in severe constipation.

8. C ★★ OHCM 10th ed. → p. 259

Proton pump inhibitors (PPIs) reduce gastric acid secretion, and it is thought that, in doing this, *Clostridium difficile* spores are more likely to survive. PPIs should therefore be stopped as soon as a case of *C. difficile* is suspected, alongside any laxatives and, where possible, any outstanding antibiotics which may have precipitated the infection. It may be appropriate to hold amlodipine in this case if she is hypotensive, but there is no definite reason to discontinue any of the other medications at this point.

9. D ★★ OHCM 10th ed. → p. 682

This woman has osteoporosis, as defined by her age (>75 years) and having sustained what is classed as a fragility fracture (neck of femur or wrist, some also class humerus). She therefore does not need a dual-energy X-ray absorptiometry (DEXA) scan for this but needs treatment for her osteoporosis. Alendronate would not be appropriate, given her recent history of severe reflux and Barrett's oesophagus. Zoledronic acid or denosumab are both possible appropriate treatment options, depending on local policies, but before embarking on these, calcium and vitamin D levels must be checked—and if low, vitamin D levels should be replaced before embarking on further osteoporosis therapy.

10. E ★★

This is a very frail man with multiple medical co-morbidities and a limited life expectancy, in whom a Do Not Attempt Cardiopulmonary Resuscitation (DNACPR) order is completely appropriate and would be a correct medical decision. In previous years, a DNACPR order would have been completed in a patient like this and the next of kin told at a later time, or never at all. Following a number of high-profile legal cases, the law has become quite clear on this. This man does not have capacity, and therefore informing him of the decision is not an option. If a DNACPR decision has been made in a patient without capacity, then their next of kin or an advocate must be informed about this decision or it is a breach of their human rights. In this man who is clinically stable and not at high risk of death overnight, best practice would be to document the medical decision and rationale for making it, but not completing the DNACPR officially until the discussion has taken place—which should happen first thing in the morning, accompanied by collateral history taking and a general update, so as not to call just to discuss CPR decisions. If the patient were unwell and there was a chance of deterioration and death, then it would be appropriate to contact the next of kin overnight in this context (and if the patient were this unwell, then it would be appropriate to do this anyway, regardless of CPR discussions). If the decision cannot wait and attempts have been made to contact the next of kin, but these have been unsuccessful, the DNACPR order can be placed, as long as this is carefully documented and a second doctor is in agreement with the DNACPR decision.

11. E ★★★ OHCM 10th ed. → p. 332

Although, in this case, both folate and vitamin B12 are low and likely to be the cause of this man's anaemia, it is important to ensure that vitamin

B12 replacement is started before folate. If folate is replaced without B12 and there is a concomitant vitamin B12 deficiency, then the neurological manifestations of vitamin B12 deficiency can be unmasked or exacerbated, leading to a subacute combined degeneration of the spinal cord and these changes may not be reversible.

12. C ★★★   OHCM 10th ed. → p. 484

This man is profoundly delirious, and despite excellent efforts to ensure his delirium is managed non-pharmacologically, he remains at risk to himself and others. This is one of the few indications for pharmacological treatment of delirium. Although haloperidol is often first line in most delirium guidance, in his case, using lorazepam is the only option. He has Lewy body dementia, which is a contraindication to the use of haloperidol and some antipsychotics—using them risks precipitating an acute parkinsonian rigidity neuroleptic malignant syndrome. Previously, it was common to use high doses of sedation in agitated patients. However, this is an older man and 5 mg of either would be inappropriate and risk respiratory depression or severe sedation for days. Therefore, the starting dose of either drug would be 0.5 mg. In some, this is adequate; in some, it allows the delirium to be managed using 1:1 nursing assistants. Very rarely, some patients may need a higher dose, and this can therefore be titrated in increments of 0.5 mg to allow a much more cautious and safe approach. A Deprivation of Liberty Safeguard (DOLS) is likely to be required for this man but is not the priority at this moment in time.

13. A ★★★

Patients with dementia who have percutaneous endocospic gastrostomy (PEG) tube insertion and feeding have a higher mortality rate at 6 months than those who do not, although the mortality rate in both groups is high. This is vital to communicate to worried relatives, as these patients are frail and are eating less, as part of the natural course of their dementia, which includes a change in anabolic cytokines. PEG feeding is associated with a high rate of diarrhoea, which may be uncomfortable and undignified; this often, but not always, settles after some time. PEG feeding does not reduce the risk of aspiration, contrary to common belief. PEG tubes do not need to be changed so regularly. Some oral medications can be given via a PEG, but some cannot if they cannot be crushed. Some cause blockage of PEG tubes. Overall, PEG tube feeding in patients with advanced dementia is inappropriate and oral feeding, despite a poor intake, is the preferred choice, in combination with good palliative care, carer education, and communication.

14. C ★★★

This is a difficult, but common, scenario on geriatric and medical wards throughout the UK. Despite several attempts at a safe discharge at home, this man is still clearly at very high risk to himself, leading to a recommendation by the multidisciplinary team that he moves to a 24-hour care environment. The one step which is required for this man who has no next of kin would be to instruct an Independent Mental Capacity Advocate (IMCA) to act as an independent advocate for him. They will carry out an independent assessment of all the facts and will help the team come to a reasonable best interests decision. An application for Court of Protection for this matter would be extremely unusual for a hospital. A Deprivation of Liberty Safeguard would be absolutely required for this man as, if he were to attempt to leave hospital, he would be stopped, but it is less likely to aid the discharge process than an IMCA. Discharge home with a restart of his previous care package would leave him open to a number of risks and needs careful further thought. Likewise, it would be inappropriate to discharge him to a care home against his wishes without the independent advocate being involved.

15. C ★★★   OHCM 10th ed. → p. 489

Traditional drugs for Alzheimer's dementia include anticholinesterase inhibitors (donepezil, galantamine, and rivastigmine). These are variably effective, with some patients having a noticeable response and others clearly with none. Memantine, an *N*-methyl-*D*-aspartate (NMDA) antagonist is a new drug which has approval from the National Institute for Health and Care Excellence (NICE) for moderate Alzheimer's dementia where anticholinergic drugs have been ineffective or not tolerated or for severe Alzheimer's disease. Ropinirole is a dopamine receptor agonist and has no role in the treatment of dementia.

16. B ★★★

There are a wide number of physiological changes associated with normal ageing—many of these leading to impaired function, reduced adaptability, and importantly altered pharmacokinetics and pharmacodynamics, e.g. due to changes in renal function. Normal changes include reduced vital capacity (lungs), increased pulse pressure (blood pressure), reduced serum albumin concentration, and impaired thermoregulation. Gastric acid secretion actually decreases, which leads to an overall slight increase in gastric pH with age.

Index

Note: Page numbers in *italics* denote answers to questions. Tables and figures are indicated by an italic t and f following the page number.